LASCIVIOUS BODIES

Lascivious Bodies

A sexual history of the eighteenth century

JULIE PEAKMAN

Atlantic Books
London

First published in Great Britain in hardback in 2004 by Atlantic Books, an imprint of Grove Atlantic Ltd

9 8 7 6 5 4 3 2 1

A CIP catalogue record for this book is available from the British Library.

ISBN
1 84354 156 4

Typeset by Avon DataSet Ltd, Bidford on Avon, Warwickshire
Printed in Great Britain by MPG Books Ltd, Bodmin, Cornwall

Atlantic Books
An imprint of Grove Atlantic Ltd
Ormond House
26–27 Boswell Street
London WC1N 3JZ

For Jad

Contents

Illustrations

Acknowledgements

My first thanks must go to Toby Mundy at Atlantic Books for having confidence in me and encouraging me to pursue the project. I am grateful to Bonnie Chiang for her careful editing, as well as for her jolly suggestions for the book. Also thanks to the various librarians who have helped me: at the British Library, London; the Wellcome Library, London; and the Library and the Artefact Museum of St Andrews University.

Specific thanks go to Lesley Hall who introduced me to colleagues at Oxford Brookes University, Steven King and Jonathan Andrews, who, in turn, helped in providing me with the opportunity of setting up a course called 'Sex In History 1650–1850'. Thanks are also due to my students for their enthusiastic questioning and avid interest in the subject, which made me realize there was a need for such a book.

I am grateful to Rictor Norton and Natsu Hattori for reading chapters of this book, and to Sean Brady and Deirdre Palk for struggling through the complete manuscript. Whole-hearted gratitude goes to Jad Adams for his suggestions and many re-reads, but most of all for his unending support. Finally, Roy Porter's many words of wisdom still echoed through my mind as I struggled towards the finish – his teaching is remembered.

The author and publishers are grateful to the following for permission to reproduce images:
15, Scottish National Portrait Gallery, Edinburgh/Bridgeman Art Library; 26, 27, 28, 29, University of St Andrews; 13, 18, 19, 20, 21, 25, 32, 34, 35, 36, 37, 38, 39, 49, 50 British Library

Introduction

Lascivious Bodies is a book about sex in England during the long eighteenth century stretching approximately from 1680 to 1830. It explores so-called 'normal' behaviour in courtship, marriage, adultery, divorce and prostitution and investigates heterosexual activities which were considered curious, such as flagellation, auto-asphyxiation and foot fetishism. It also delves into activities considered abnormal, such as bestiality and necrophilia, homosexuality (both male and female), and male and female cross-dressing. *Lascivious Bodies* is an investigation of sexual activities and people's reactions to them, looking at practices as well as ideas – not just what was considered acceptable or 'normal', but all sorts of sex, in all sorts of places, with all sorts of people.

The eighteenth century in England was an exuberant time with many variations of sexual experimentation. It was a time of social and economic flux, of confusion, when sexual boundaries were fluid and mutating. The world was expanding through exploration, leading to an increase in trade and luxury goods, and new freedoms were developing. With this new-found liberty came the perceived 'spread of vice', the idea that abominations were being introduced from France, Spain, Italy and Holland. In addition, this period saw the arrival of a new class system, which brought with it new methods and meanings to sex and, in reaction, new taboos and excitements.

This book mainly concentrates on England but it also touches on Scotland and Ireland. In certain chapters, where comparisons with other countries are helpful in understanding the progress of an activity, or where unusual cases have been found, I have looked to the Continent, as with the French male cross-dressers and cattle buggers, the Florentine lesbian nuns and the Prussian female husband.

The first half of the book, Chapters One to Six, concentrates on male and female heterosexuality, in terms of behaviour and opinion. Chapter One gives an overall picture of sex in London and the sexual activities available 'on the town'; prostitutes, their clients and moral reformers all figure in the battle to draw up sexual boundaries, as they pushed and pulled in a tug of war over a moveable sexual moral line. Chapter Two investigates sex inside and outside the marital relationship, concentrating on the heterosexual aspects of life; courtship, marriage, adultery and divorce. Chapters Three and Four explore the memoirs of British libertines and courtesans in an attempt to understand the difference in men's and women's attitudes to sex; Sexual Man is investigated through the dissipated lives described in the diaries of William Hickey, the well-travelled rake and lawyer, James Boswell, the Scottish biographer of Samuel Johnson, and Casanova, the Venetian memoirist, all of them out-and-out philanderers. The autobiographies of three famous courtesans, Mrs Margaret Leeson, Harriette Wilson and Julia Johnstone, shed light on the sometimes contradictory views of women who conducted their lives outside the realm of the 'respectable' household. Chapters Five and Six provide an inside view of the 'secret' societies of Sir Francis Dashwood and the Beggar's Benison to reveal how sex among the aristocracy and gentry was often connected with politics and financial machinations.

The second half of the book, Chapters Seven to Twelve, examines the sexual activities considered curious or 'abnormal' – men-with-men, women-with-women, cross-dressing, flagellation, bestiality, auto-asphyxiation, bestiality, oral activities, masturbation and group sex. It looks at those who chose to live their lives under the veil of secrecy because of the threat of capital punishment, harassment or persecution; and those who suffered social and economic stress because of their sexual preferences. For readers interested in the historiographical background, the appendix sums up some of the main theoretical arguments in the history of sexuality.

This book runs the gamut of sexualities and sexual activities available to men and women in the long eighteenth century – this period was one of multifarious sexual pleasures, experimentation and exploration of the lascivious body. An examination of newspapers, pamphlets, magazines, journals, diaries, memoirs, letters and trial reports has uncovered not only what these liberated men and women thought about themselves and their activities but also sheds light on the morals of a sometimes not-so-liberal society. Despite the image of the libertine Georgian era, there were, in fact, many who decried those who were more sexually unrestrained. But then there were also those who were brave enough to follow the sexual inclination of their choice in the pursuit of pleasure ...

CHAPTER ONE

The Streets of London

> The lewdest people upon earth, ourselves excepted, are not guilty of such open violations of the laws of decency. Go all the world over, and you'll see no such impudence as in the streets of London, which makes many foreigners give our women in general a bad character, from the vile specimens they meet with from one end of the town to the other.
>
> Daniel Defoe, *Augusta Triumphans* (1728)

As he walked through London, the writer and journalist Daniel Defoe collected all the information he needed on lewdness for *Augusta Triumphans* (1728). He subtitled the pamphlet 'the way to make London the most flourishing city in the universe' yet London was already the sex capital of Europe, with a reputation for insidious vice, both at home and abroad. As he patrolled the narrow streets, Defoe would have noticed the drunken rakes reeling from tavern to tavern, trawling Covent Garden for prostitutes. He no doubt saw the young harlots hanging out of street windows showing off their assets in low-cut blouses, and heard the moans of couples fornicating up back alleys in the darkened streets of the City or around the fields of St Martin's Church. Little would have changed when, half a decade later, portly Scottish lawyer James Boswell wandered up the Strand, eyeing the whores (**FIG. 1**) as he made his way towards St James's Park to meet his witty yet libidinous friend, the politician John Wilkes. En route, Boswell would have been accosted by young women plying their trade. Most likely, he would have passed the old woman who carried a basket of dildos disguised as dolls. Instead of legs, these dolls, had a cloth-covered cylinder about six inches long and one inch wide. One female customer had returned hers with the complaint that it was too big and

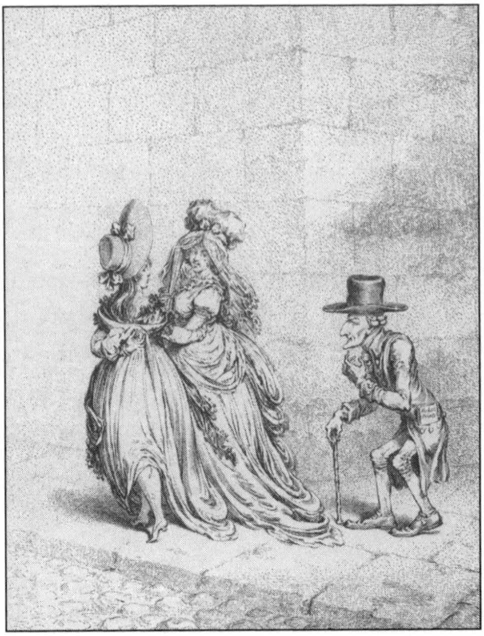

FIG. 1 James Gillray, *A Corner, Near the Bank*, 1797

ordered a smaller one. The saleswoman insisted that she pay in advance, explaining that if the lady changed her mind again she would not be able to sell a used doll.[1]

The metropolis bustled with life, with an estimated 675,000 people vying for space by the mid-century. This figure would grow to a million by the 1800s. Immigrants swelled the city, with migrants from the countryside filling it still further. Young people from all over came to London in search of employment: by 1700 about eight thousand of them were arriving every year looking for work and fun – and plenty could be had of both. Labourers found work as street-sellers of fruit, milk, coal, pasties, pickles, powder and gingerbread, or as knife-grinders, tinkers, watermen, sedan chairmen, coal heavers and chimney-sweeps. Lower down the scale, people eked out a living as rag-pickers, rat-catchers and scavengers. Women would sing ballads, take to sewing stockings or any amount of needlework; or they might fall into domestic service, the biggest employer of females. Many of these servants would, at some time, fall into prostitution as did Elizabeth Lancaster. Interviewed by the Overseers of the Poor in 1815, she told of how she had worked in domestic service in two different establishments for nine months before turning to prostitution, where she made a living for four and half years.[2] Domestic servants were particularly vulnerable to seduction by a male member of the household in which they worked. In more menacing incidents, threats of violence might induce a girl into sex, some of these from the master of the household.

Bawds like Mother Needham, depicted so adroitly by Hogarth (**FIG. 2**), kept an eye open for fresh-faced country girls in a bid to lure them back to their brothels with promises of food and lodgings. Indeed, London was the epicentre for hustlers, bawds, pimps and whores alike and a gentleman was just as likely to have his pocket picked as to have his lusts gratified. 'London is a really dangerous place,' rued the poet William Shenstone in mid-century; 'the pickpockets, formerly contented with mere filching, make no scruple to knock people down with bludgeons in Fleet Street and

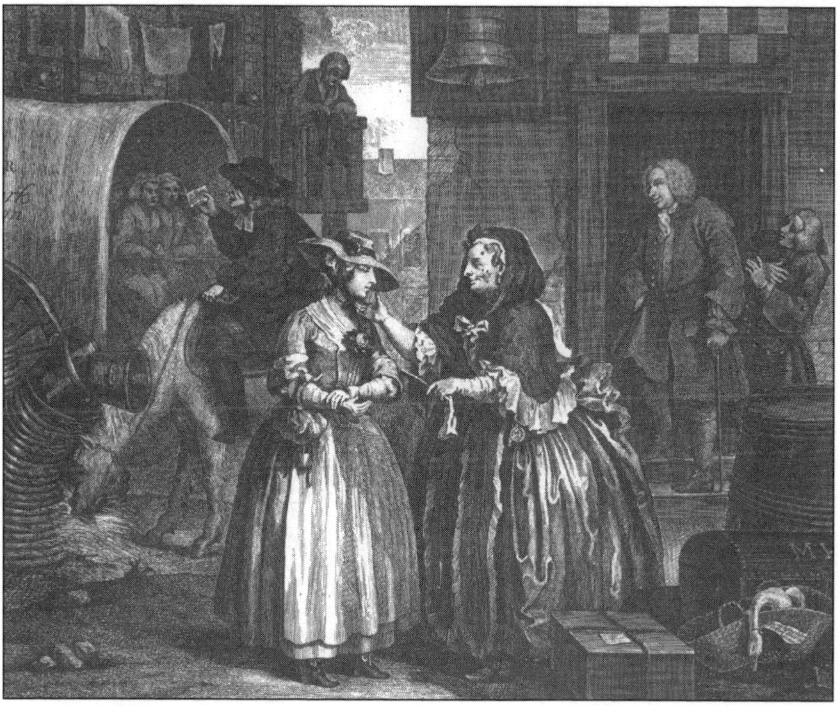

FIG. 2 William Hogarth, *A Harlot's Progress, Plate I*, 1732

the Strand, and that at no later hour than eight o'clock.'[3] Yet the policing system consisted of only a hodge-podge of amateurs and professionals made up of three thousand beadles, constables and the parish watch. 'London is guarded at night by old men', complained one French visitor, 'chosen from the dregs of the people who have no arms but a lantern and a pole, crying the hour every time the clock strikes . . . and whom it is the custom of young rakes to beat and use ill when they come reeling out of the taverns where they have passed the night.'[4]

Entertainment and sex went hand in hand. Covent Garden was a place where people met up, attracted by its colourful array of stalls offering all kinds of spectacles, from tumbling, juggling and dancers to waxworks and puppetry. Gaiety and dance could be found at any amount of balls and society gatherings. Conversation was sought in the burgeoning coffee-houses such as that run by Moll* and Tom King in Covent Garden (**FIG. 3**), which attracted hell-raisers, rakes and beaux as well as market traders.[5] By 1710, there were said to be two thousand all-male coffee-houses in London alone.[6] Customers would make their way to their favourite place then move on to meet up with other friends. 'About Twelve the *Beau-Monde* assembles in several Chocolate and Coffee Houses: The best of which are the *Cocoa-Tree* and *White's* Chocolate-Houses, *St James*, the *Smyrna*, and the *British Coffee-Houses*,' advised the traveller John Macky, 'and all are so near one another, that in less than an Hour you see the Company of them all.' Clubs were founded in coffee-shops where men went to share interests. James Boswell and Benjamin Franklin** belonged to a club at St Paul's coffee-house which met on alternate Thursdays. 'Wine and punch upon the table, some of us smoke a pipe . . . at nine there is a side-board with Welsh rabbits *[sic]* and apple puffs, porter and beer. Our reckoning is about eighteen pence a head,' calculated Boswell.[7]

Gentlemen took refreshments and read one of the newspapers left lying around for the benefit of customers. 'All Englishmen are great

* Moll King was a sparky businesswoman whose coffee-house was so popular during the 1720s and '30s that she bought two properties next door to expand the business, but even then it was full to capacity most nights.

** Franklin was a diplomat and a scientist most famed for his invention of the lightning rod. His experiments with electricity were renowned throughout Britain.

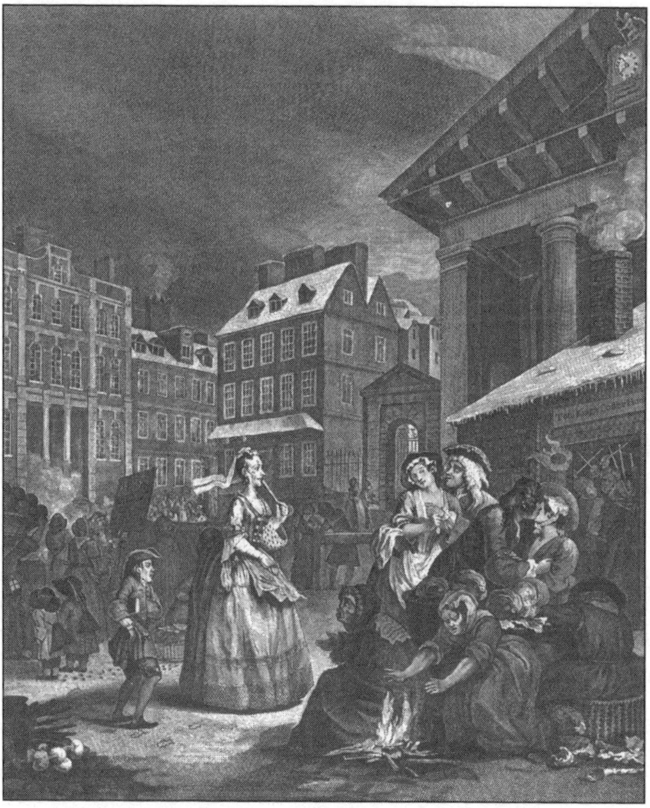

FIG. 3 William Hogarth, *Morning*, 1738

newsmongers,' reported the Swiss traveller César Saussure in 1730, 'workmen habitually begin the day by going to coffee-rooms in order to read the latest news.'[8] But even here, places rarely frequented by the opposite sex, men had a hard time keeping their eyes away from a pretty woman. Coffee-house owners were blamed for providing attractive barmaids:

> such tempting, deluging, ogling, pretty, young Hussies to be our Bar-keepers, as steal away our Hearts, and insensibly betray us to Extravagance. This has been a growing Evil for some Years, but it has now got to its full Height; and the sly young Dogs the Coffee-boys, when you call to pay, desire you

> please to pay at the Bar. This has often cost me a Compliment, which I invented for my Mistress, and very frequently a Glass or two of Ratifee or Dr *Stephen's* Water . . . These young Gipsies steal our Hearts with such sly alluring Looks, that a man must be a *Stoick* whose Blood is not put into a Fermentation at the Sight of them.[9]

Away from the smoky rooms of the coffee-houses, the *demi-monde* (those of doubtful reputation and social standing on the outskirts of society) were found in their own popular haunts, such as the Fountain Tavern with its walls resplendent with lascivious paintings depicting scenes from Ovid and Tibullus. Here, food was served in an elegantly furnished drawing-room, 'consisting of every delicacy in and out of season', an occurrence common to similar stylish establishments.[10] Meanwhile, pleasure gardens, parks and theatres were natural places for merrymaking to which people gravitated, including celebrated women of the day. Vauxhall and Ranelagh gardens (**FIGS.** 4 & 5), St James's Park and the Drury Lane Theatre were all in vogue as popular places of entertainment. Vauxhall, on the south side of the Thames, had been reorganized and reopened in 1732. For a shilling,

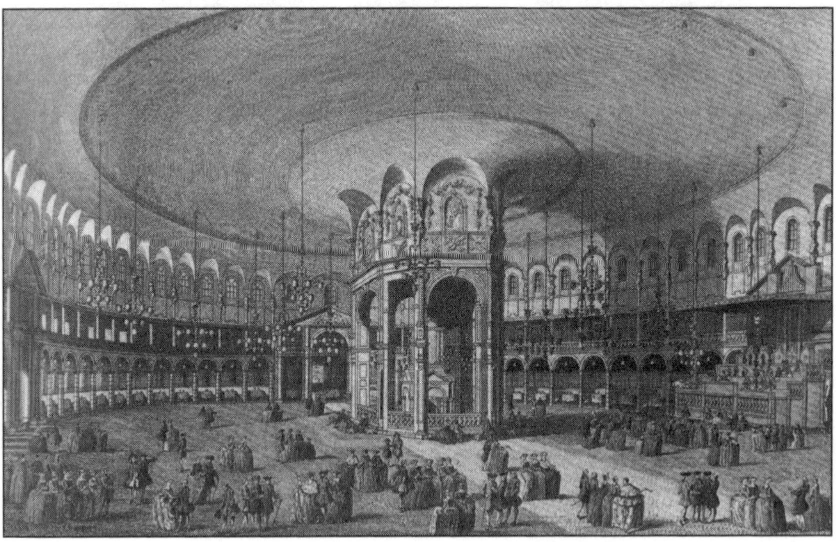

FIG. 4 Antonio Canaletto, *An Inside View of the Rotunda in Ranelagh*, 1751

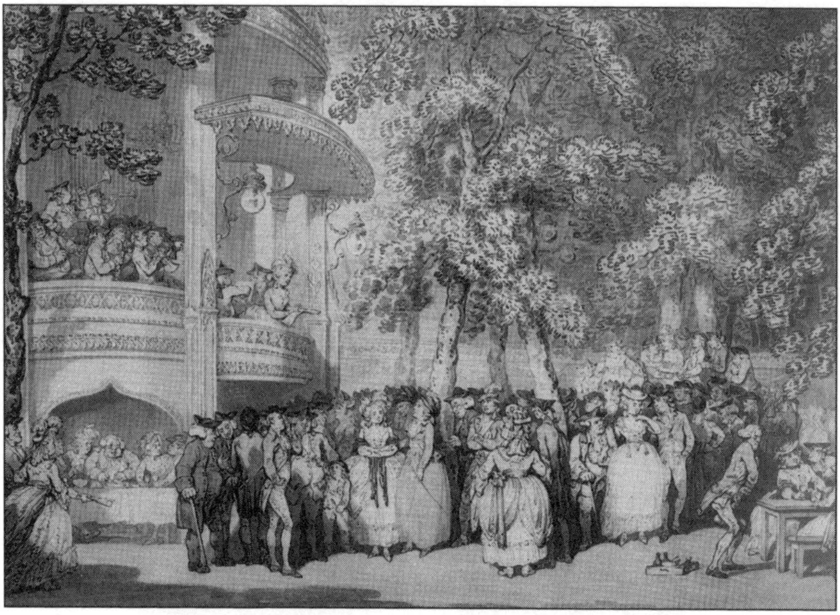

FIG. 5 Thomas Rowlandson, *Vauxhall Gardens*

anyone could stroll around the grottoes, statues, temples and waterfalls, listen to music and watch the firework displays.

In 1742, the more up-market Ranelagh Gardens opened on the north side of the Thames near Chelsea Hospital. In a letter to the *British Magazine* in 1748, one woman declared, 'I shall not scruple to spend an evening six times a week at Ranelagh, and that with no other company than my companion, when my female acquaintance happen'd to be engaged.'[11] The high price of 2s 6d aimed to keep out the riff-raff but allowed entrance to wealthier courtesans. The cost of admission did not, however, seem to have deterred two women who appeared content to make a spectacle of themselves. According to one observer at Ranelagh the previous evening, the women, dressed in the highest fashions, had broken into a fight. Ripping at each other's outrageously elaborate hairdos, they pulled unusual vegetable matter from within:

> her head, most unfortunately, became entangled in that of the wrathful antagonist, and she had one of her smartest feathers

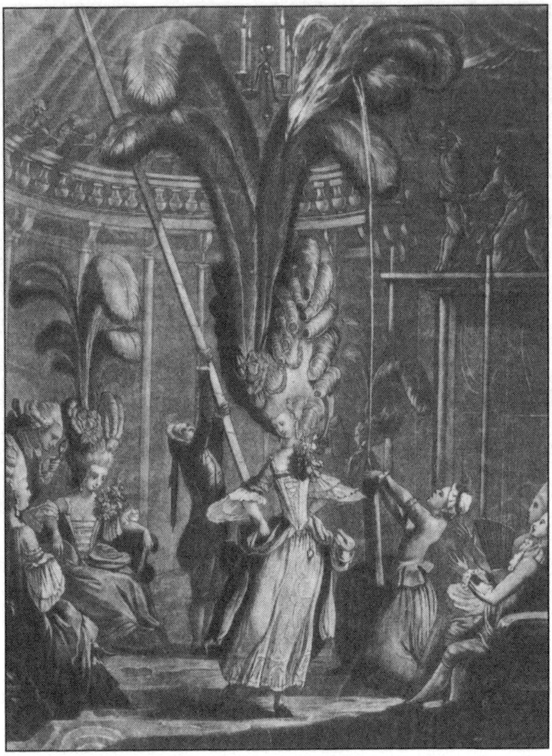

FIG. 6 Sayer, *A Hint to the Ladies to take Care of their Heads*, 1776

> instantly dislodged by a *raddish* which grew – a formidable excrescence – out of her neighbour's curls, . . . the latter caught hold of a huge *leek* staring in the front of the former's head-dress, and dragged it off . . .[12]

The fashion of wearing highly elaborate designs in the hair was a trend set by Georgiana, Duchess of Devonshire, who was particularly noted for her ridiculously outlandish head adornments (**FIG. 6**). Women built their wigs extremely high and ornamented them with fruit, feathers and even miniature ships.

Gossip in the daily newspapers related exciting occurrences of the previous day. In 1773, the *Covent Garden Magazine* boasted that they were issued 'solely for the entertaining of the polite world'. When the courtesan Kitty Fisher fell off her horse riding in Green Park, the story became worthy of nearly every newspaper in town. One snippet, *Horse and Away to St James's Park Or, a Trip for the Noontide Air. Who Rides Fastest, Miss Kitty Fisher or her Gay Gallant?*, regaled readers with the event:

> Upon our coming up, we found it to be the celebrated Miss Kitty Fisher: her military attendant had raised her from the Ground. – The Nymph was in tears, but rather from Apprehension of her Danger than the sense of Pain; for whether it was owing to any thing her Heroe said, or from finding the danger over, she, with a childishness, stopped the torrent of tears, and burst into a fit of Laughing.[13]

The *Universal Magazine* even produced a poem for her:

> *Dear Kitty had thy only fall*
> *Been that thou met'st with in the Mall*
> *Thou had'st deserved our pity.*
> *But long before that luckless day,*
> *With equal Justice might we say,*
> *Alas, poor fallen Kitty!*[14]

Kitty was well worthy of such reports, having made her reputation through her affairs with royalty and the gentry and was admired enough to have her portrait painted by Joshua Reynolds.

Men might use magazines and newspapers to solicit the attention of one of the many courtesans by publishing advertisements similar to our current 'lonely-hearts' columns. If a gentleman had admired a lady at a ball or a masquerade the previous evening, he might request to meet her. One London newspaper, dated 1 March 1754, contained such an appeal:

> If the Lady that was at the last Masquerade, dress'd in a white Domino, trimm'd with Purple, a Hat of the same, tall, and genteel in Person, will be so obliging as to favour the Gentleman who ask'd her to dance, but was refused, with a Line when and where he may have the Pleasure of seeing her, by directing for C.G. at the Cocoa-Tree in Pall-Mall, he intends to propose

> something greatly to her Advantage, and hopes it will meet with her Approbation. Note, A Coach and Six, and 7000 l. per Annum, at her Service if she don't think the Gentleman too old.[15]

This was a means for a man to obtain a mistress, to attract an admired courtesan by advertising his wealth. Courtesans were notoriously choosy about their clientele. Frequently they would refuse to meet a man at all unless he had been properly introduced. Nor was money the sole object of their attentions – a courtesan would consort with a man and become his companion only if she was attracted to him. If a man was merely after sex, better that he should look to the brothels and bagnios in town.

On the Town

All sorts of sexual practices were on offer in early-eighteenth-century London. Specialised brothels offered flagellation services where clients were whipped until blood ran down their backs. Alternatively, some men requested the assistance of prostitutes to help bring them to climax through strangulation. Yet others would prefer to seek their pleasure with another man, though they had to be more discreet than their heterosexual counterparts as buggery was still a crime punishable by death. Male youths could be picked up on the streets and their sexual services bought for a couple of pints of wine. Otherwise the comforts of the molly-houses, or male brothels, could be sought out where a larger choice was on offer. Meanwhile, for women, female-only houses could be found, such as Mother Courage's in Suffolk Street and Francis Bradshaw's house in Bow Street, where women of quality could go and relax. Women might also join the all-female flagellants' group which met in a house in Jermyn Street. Unfortunately, although this establishment is mentioned in one of the gentlemen's magazine's, little else is known about it.

A certain 'German Gentleman' believed there were 107 brothels in 1725 in the vicinity of Drury Lane alone.[16] In his *A Proposal To Render Effectual A Plan To Remove The Nuisance Of Common Prostitutes From The Streets Of This Metropolis* (1758), Saunders Welch estimated that there were approximately three thousand prostitutes active in London.[17]

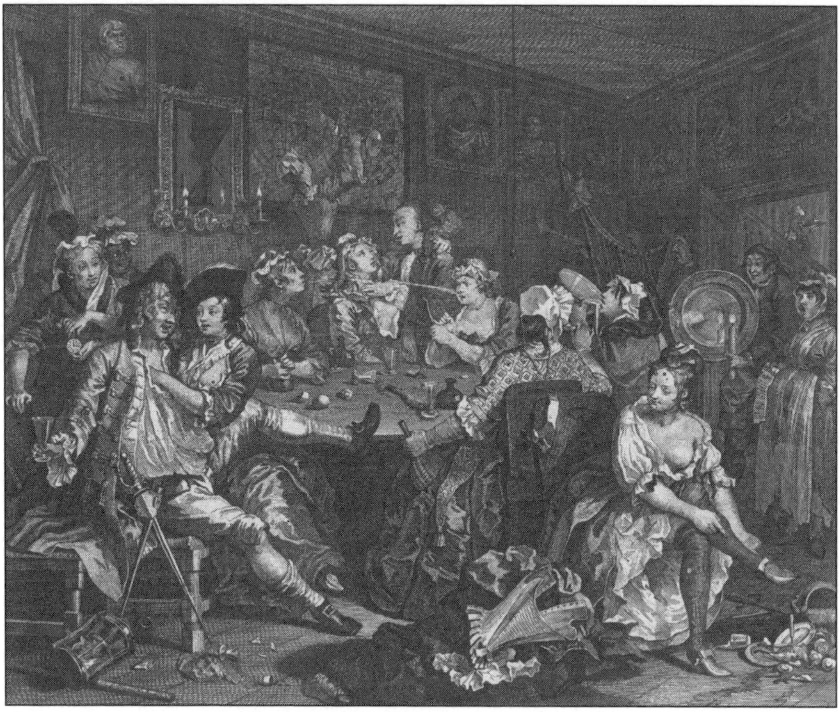

FIG. 7 William Hogarth, *A Rake's Progress*, 1735

According to Old Bailey records, a great many prostitutes were unmarried, with over half of them born outside London. Once in the city, whores mingled with the rest of the population, walking the same streets and frequenting the same parks, ale-houses and gin-shops as most other Londoners.[18]

Many taverns doubled as brothels where a man could buy a pint of ale in the front room, pick up a young woman and take her into the back room for sex. A French lawyer, Monsieur Pierre Jean Grosley, visiting London in 1765 duly noted how 'the low taverns serves them [the whores] as a retreat to receive their gallants in; there is always a room set aside for this purpose' (**FIG. 7**).[19] This was the case for James Boswell, who had sex with two young streetwalkers in the back room of Shakespear's Head Tavern, Covent Garden. He paid as little as between sixpence and a shilling for his outdoor activities, most notably with 'a strong, jolly damsel' under

Westminster Bridge and even less for 'a little profligate wretch'.[20] Whores could be bought for anything from a few pence to a few guineas. In 1762, Boswell noted the wide range of women available, 'from the splendid Madam at fifty guineas a night, down to the civil nymph with white-thread stockings who tramps along the Strand and will resign her engaging person to your honour for a pint of wine and a shilling'.[21]

High-class courtesans could earn a great deal of money, either kept in luxury by a wealthy protector or sharing their affections among a few rich clients. They traded from their sumptuous establishments in St James's Square, Pall Mall and Soho. As one visitor remarked of English courtesans, their 'apartments are elegantly, and sometimes magnificently furnished; they keep several servants, and some have their own carriages'.[22] Generally, women were in charge of their own élite establishments. Marylebone was a favoured neighbourhood for the richer sort of courtesan; here, one writer estimated, 'thirty thousand ladies of pleasure reside, of which seventeen hundred are reckoned to be house-keepers. They live very well, and without ever being disturbed by the magistrates. They are indeed so much their own mistress, that if a justice of the peace attempted to trouble them in their apartments, they might turn him out of doors.'[23] Or a gentleman could visit the public baths, or bagnois as they were then called. 'I visited the bagnios,' Jacques Casanova recalled in his *Memoirs*, 'where a rich man can sup, bathe and sleep with a fashionable courtesan, of which there are many in London. It makes a magnificent debauch and only costs six guineas . . .'

Lower down the economic scale, whores operated from the less salubrious bawdy-houses in Covent Garden and Holborn, with even seedier brothels alongside the Thames in Southwark and in the East End. Men tended not to be in charge of the running of female brothels, although male 'bullies' were sometimes employed to protect women in lower-class brothels and to throw out marauding customers. For those strapped for cash, down-and-out streetwalkers could be picked up in the Strand and purchased for a couple of pence. As Boswell pointed out, it was impossible to meander from Fleet Street to the Strand or around St James's Park without being accosted by streetwalkers. Grosley said much the same: 'About nightfall [the whores] range themselves in a file in the footpaths of all the great streets in companies of five or six, most of them dressed very genteely [*sic*]. Whole rows of them accost passengers in broad daylight . . .'[24] Unlike the courtesans, who entertained in high style, the poorer women were merely staying alive by prostitution, living hand-to-mouth, often breadwinners for their entire family.

Blatant advertisements of available whores in pamphlets containing their personal details were aimed at a potential male clientele. *The London Belles or, A Description of the most Celebrated Beauties in the City of London* (1707), *Kitty's Atlantis for the Year 1766* and *Harris's List of Covent Garden Ladies* (1788) provided thumbnail sketches of desirable women available in London at the time of issue, complete with addresses of the brothels where they could be found. Colourful pictures were painted of famous prostitutes such as Nancy Dawson, Lucy Cooper and Charlotte Hayes: 'The lively Nancy *D——n*; much alter'd for the better. I would recommend her continuance of the useful *Dublin Factor*, for she may be certain that trade cannot be well carried on without the help of those useful gentlemen or agents. *King's-street, Red-Lyon-Square*.'

Women beyond their early twenties were generally considered past their prime but Lucy Cooper managed to retain her attractions, considered 'still gay and thirty'. However, women with too much sexual experience were a risk, as was the 'bouncing Miss *Giff——d*' who worked the Haymarket and 'had layn with more men, than she has hairs upon her head' and 'seven years ago was broke down so, that there was no riding her without the risque of falling'.

Extra flesh on a woman did not put off a man, as with the comely Miss *Nug*—, then visited by a married gentleman at Russell Street, Bloomsbury: 'tho' inclin'd to be fat, I assure you she's very agreeable and entertaining, and always well drest'. Over-application of make-up, though, was frowned upon, as with 'The great Miss *Jo*——. This lady, not content with the complexion of her hair, makes use of lamp-black and oil to such a degree, that her head stinks worse than a stale fishmonger's shop; her cap, by the time she's wore it half an hour, is in a moister condition, than the paper that comes from a roasted haunch of venison.' A woman's hair colour was thought to indicate her sexual nature and therefore worth mentioning in the adverts. A redhead, it was suggested, had more vaginal lubricant, the author confessing, 'I have heard numbers say that they wou'd rather —— with a woman that had red hair, than another, for this reason, because they are always juicy; therefore you who love juice, repair to Miss *Jo*—, for I am certain a loose embrace of hers, is greasier than the carcass of a sheep, that has hung four hours in the sun in the middle of the Dog-days.'[25]

Women had to be skilled in entertaining their clients – wit, charm and convivial conversation were all highly prized qualities. *Harris's List of Covent Garden Ladies* revealed the latest whores' attributes, advising on one, Miss Br—wn of No. 8 Castle-Street, Newman-Street, who 'sings a good song, and is a chearful *bon* companion'. Meanwhile, a certain Miss B—rn at No. 18, Old Compton Street, Soho, was an 'accomplished nymph' who 'plays on the piano forte, sings, dances, and is mistress of every *Manouvre* in the amorous contest that can enhance the coming pleasure'. Similarly Miss J—ns—n entertained from No. 17, Goodge Street, where she 'sings, dances, will drink a chearful glass, and is a good companion'. An added bonus to this particular lady's talents was her sexual agility: 'She has such noble elasticity in her loins, that she can cast her lover to a pleasing height, and receive him again with the utmost dexterity.'[26]

The fifteen-year-old Miss L—v—r, of No. 17, Ogle Street, off Queen Ann Street East, went out to seek her clients 'who may put their case to her either in a tavern or her own apartments'.[27] Thus, women used public places to pick up men but gave them the choice of hiring a back room in the pub or going back to their lodgings. Personal hygiene and vaginal cleanliness were not the norm, but were well appreciated when found. Of Miss Harriette J—n—s of St George's Hotel, opposite Virginia Street, Wapping, it was said, 'A beautiful *black fringe* borders the *Venetian Mount*, and whether she pursues the Grahamatic* method from a practical knowledge of its increase of pleasure, from motives of cleanliness, or as a certain preventative we will not pretend to say; but we know it makes her the more desirable bed-fellow.'

* James Graham was a notorious quack known for his promotion of genital hygiene, his methods filtering through to his public through the dramatic use of advertising and exhibitions.

As washbasins and bathtubs were to become widespread only in the late eighteenth century, and then mainly in richer households, attention to hygiene was wanting in both men and women. John Wilkes, lamenting the lack of feminine hygiene, declared, 'the nobler parts are never in this island washed by women; they are left to be lathered by men.'[28] This might account for the scarcity of talk about oral sex, either in sex advice manuals or pornography. None the less, some women did supply it. The oral sexual skills of Miss N—ble of No. 10, Plough Court, Fetter Lane were considered admirable and she was commended for her expertise: 'She has a most consummate skill in reviving the dead . . . and her tongue has a double charm when speaking and when silent; for the tip of it, *properly applied*, can talk eloquently to the heart, whilst no sound pervades the ear and sends such feelings to the central spot, that immediately demands the more noble weapon to *close* the *melting scene*.' These particular women, the directory claimed, could be bought for anything from five shillings to two guineas, with one guinea seemingly the average charge, and two guineas the more expensive.[29]

Suppressing Lewdness

Anti-vice societies were formed in an effort to clamp down on immorality in London. Their main purpose was to suppress prostitution and close down bawdy-houses. Between 1695 and 1701 the Society for the Reformation of Manners published an annual blacklist of whores who had been successfully prosecuted. Their supporter, Judge Jeffreys, presided over the floggings of convicted prostitutes who were to be stripped to the waist, and often whipped until their bodies were bloody. By the end of the century, between 1787 and 1808, the Proclamation Society against Vice and Immorality made the enforcement of morality laws its main objective. The society, which William Wilberforce, known for his campaign against slavery, helped to found, remained small and select until his death in 1833.[30] Yet exactly how successful such societies were in suppressing vice is questionable. In his essay 'Modest Defence of Publick Stews', the satirical pamphleteer Bernard Mandeville accused its members of inadvertently contributing to vice, stating: 'It is no small addition to my grief to observe that your endeavours to suppress lewdness have only served to promote it, and that this branch of immorality has grown under your hands,'[31] the implications being that the very fact of talking about vice attracted people towards it.

With the founding of the first Magdalene Hospital for Penitent Prostitutes in London in 1758 came a change in attitude towards sex and sin: prostitutes were no longer considered to be strumpets who sinned for the sake of it, but unfortunate women who had fallen by the wayside, poor girls who might be rescued from vice. With this in mind, Robert Dingley, director of the Bank of England, and Jonas Hanaway, Commissioner of the Victualling Office, put their energies into opening the new Magdalene hospitals. These places were designed as a retreat for fallen women but, because of the severe restrictions placed on the women and girls, were in fact more like houses of correction.

The rescued prostitutes were first drilled in good behaviour. A hierarchy was encouraged in which conduct, appearance, deportment and education all counted towards a girl's status within the institution. Newcomers were kept in a separate ward for one month, then moved to an inferior ward until they had proved worthy of promotion to a better one. 'Trusties' were given an elevated monitorial status and were allowed to wash and cook for themselves. Yet, despite the benevolence of the reformers, the strict regulations imposed in the hospitals, which were ostensibly designed to rescue the women, served to contain and discipline them. Hanaway saw idleness as the cause of evil and prostitution so his aim, and that of his followers, was to keep the girls busy, thus the girls were put to work. Rules and punishments were drawn up; bed- and meal-times were set in regimental style; piety was encouraged with hymns sung every morning and evening and grace said before and after meals. Insolent or foul language resulted in confinement to one's room for six hours, public admonishment by the chaplain for the second offence, twelve hours' solitary confinement for the third, and so on. There was also a sliding scale of fines and failure to reform resulted in expulsion.

In their *Thoughts On The Plan For A Magdalen House* (1758), both Saunders Welch and Jonas Hanaway held that recruits to prostitution came not from the labouring poor but were daughters of poor tradesmen placed in domestic service. Defoe, in his *Some Considerations Upon Streetwalkers* (1701), confirmed the belief that many a poor girl had sunk into prostitution after being debauched and then discarded by her master or by the master's son. Although the Magdalene hospitals were reported to be a success, as with the anti-vice societies, it is dubious whether they achieved much. The reformers certainly promoted themselves as saviours of potential prostitutes but the statistics they gave were dubious. By 1769, over 1,000 girls were admitted, rising to 2,998 by 1795. Of these, 1,960 were allegedly reconciled to family and friends. The inquiry for the period from May 1786 to May 1790 declared that 'about two-thirds of the whole number of women admitted were permanently reclaimed'.[32] In truth, the charity boards increasingly regulated whom they admitted to the Magdalene hospitals. Those allowed entrance were more likely to have been naive young women, 'seduced' under the promise of marriage rather than selected from hard-core prostitutes, and this would perhaps account for the reformers' claims of success. Nevertheless, it was impossible to record how many girls returned to prostitution at a later date.

But, despite their philanthropical intentions and claims that the hospitals were reformative, the Magdalene houses became, in reality, a means of social control over female sexual behaviour. The treatment of these women – as criminals – ran counter to the image which the charities were trying to create: that of innocent victim. They acted more as a model for exercising authority in order to repress prostitution than out of genuine concern for the condition of the inmates, although no doubt there was some measure of genuine humanitarianism.[33] In line with contemporary thinking, the reformers, all male gentry, would have viewed women as inferior to men. These women, in particular, because they had sex before marriage, would have been viewed as even further down the social scale.[34] With no evidence of female sex reformers at this time,[35] the type of assistance the prostitutes received was therefore dependent on the ideas of a group of middle-class men and their notions of the correct place for a fallen woman.

The image of the rescued maiden permeated the whole of society. Letters were published in *The Rambler's Magazine* in March and April 1751 which opined on the need to rescue prostitutes; novels advocated the same, as seen in William Dodd's *The Sisters.** But some people did recognize that many women fell into this way of life out of economic necessity. The Revd Martin Madan in his *Account of the Triumphant death of F. S.: A Converted Prostitute who Died April 1763, aged 26* recounted the story of a poor girl whose only means of survival was prostitution. He implied that prostitution was one of the few ways by which women could support themselves and that society, not the prostitutes themselves, was to blame for their plight.

Reactions to prostitution and how it might be curtailed varied widely from the sensitive to the sardonic. The British author John Campbell (alias M. Ludovicus) believed that the establishment of foundling hospitals would prevent young girls falling into prostitution.[36] This was to come about through the determination of Thomas Coram who, after many years as a sea captain and commercial shipbuilder, combined his business acumen with his sensitivity to the plight of unwanted children. After twenty years of tireless campaigning and fund-raising, he opened the first Foundling Hospital in Hatton Garden in 1741. Four years later, this moved to purpose-built premises in Lamb's Conduit Fields, north of Gray's Inn. Here, destitute mothers would anonymously leave their children outside the doors for collection by the hospital staff. The child would then be sent to a wet-nurse in the country until the age of five, when it would return to the hospital for its education and training in a lowly occupation. Yet John Fielding, a Justice of the Peace, who was a pioneer of modern professional law enforcement, saw the large number of foundling children as being responsible for the high crime rate in London; boys became thieves and girls became prostitutes through economic necessity. Fielding was subject to criticism for his charitable attitude towards prostitutes and his education scheme. Proffering a different idea, Bernard Mandeville advocated the establishment of a hundred legal public brothels, containing two thousand women, with regular medical inspections paid for by a tax on the brothel. Lewdness could then be contained in its proper place without influencing the behaviour of other women and children. Needless

* Dodd was later executed for forgery.

to say, despite all these suggestions, no remedy was successful – women continued to make a living from their sexual activities and men continued to pursue them.

The wide range of images of the prostitute which ran simultaneously throughout this period show just how mixed were the public's attitudes towards them: the Brazen Whore was seen as the personification of unbridled lust and sin; the Seduced Maiden represented the naive maid corrupted by promises of marriage; and the Penniless Profligate was seen as a victim of poverty with no other means of making a living. The latter two were believed to be the victims of circumstances beyond their own control, and were thus considered redeemable. Yet the realities of prostitution were grim: women walking the streets in the hope of a pick-up to pay for their next meal. Some women were pretty and witty enough to claw their way out of a life of grinding poverty to become the mistresses of men with means. But their prosperity was often short-lived as their looks faded and they became riddled with venereal disease.

Despite the proscriptions on sexual morality, few new laws restricting prostitution were passed. Prostitution was not illegal. Punishments for streetwalkers were only meted out if they were found to be 'disorderly'. Although a parliamentary statute was passed in 1752, this was directed against brothel-keeping. The Vagrancy Act of 1824 allowed the use of the Vagrancy Laws against prostitutes, but it was not until the 1860s with growing concern about the spread of venereal disease that London police attempted to suppress the brothels.[37]

The Clap and the Pox

Venereal disease was rife in London, with sexual infections spreading around the city's brothels. Prostitutes were blamed for infecting their male clients, and men were blamed for infecting their wives and children. One moralist lamented, 'Many an antique gonorrhoea and even confirmed pox have they [prostitutes] transplanted, by a drunken libidinous husband, to an innocent wife, and to the blood of posterity; glorying at their chicanery, and wishing everyone as infected as themselves.'[38] Prostitutes bore the brunt of the blame, with the poorest women affected most. 'How many honest women', bemoaned Daniel Defoe in 1728, 'those of the inferior sort especially, get loathsome distempers from their husbands' commerce with these creatures, which distempers are often entailed on posterity? Nor have we a hospital separated for that purpose, which does not contain too many instances of honest wretches made miserable by villains of husbands.'[39]

Despite its seriousness, venereal disease had become so widespread in the eighteenth century that any libertine in London might expect to catch it and, indeed, many of them did. When Boswell's father shared his concerns about his son having contracted the pox yet again with his friend, Mrs Montgomerie-Cunningham, she responded casually that 'it was now become quite common'.[40] For all its familiarity, the disease was dangerous, could cause early death and, despite the quacks' recommended remedies, as yet incurable. The havoc wrought by the disease was encapsulated in Hogarth's picture of the decrepit whore in the final stage of *The Harlot's Progress* (**FIG. 8**). She lies dying with broken ornaments at her feet, symbols of her shattered dreams and her yielded virginity. Her pock-marked face is covered with fake beauty spots in a vain effort to hide the hideous symptoms of disease. Dr Rock's pills lie at her side – testimony to another quack medicine which failed to live up to its promises. Yet, to some extent, venereal disease was seen as the inevitable wages of sin earned by unruly sexual conduct. This was the fate of the sexually promiscuous, a lingering, painful death.

In the face of such adversity, one of the most curious, if not altogether surprising, reactions of VD-infected Londoners was to form a club. The 'No Nose'd Club' was formed for all those suffering from syphilis who had had their noses eaten away by the disease, the terrifying effects of which were described by Ned Ward in his *History of the London Clubs* (1709):

> A Merry Gentleman who had often hazarded his own Boltsplit, by steering a Vicious Course of Life among the dangerous Rocks of *Venus*, having observ'd in his Walks thro' our *English Sodom*, that abundance of both sexes had Sacrific'd their Noses to the God Of Priapus, and had unluckily fallen into the *Aethiopian*

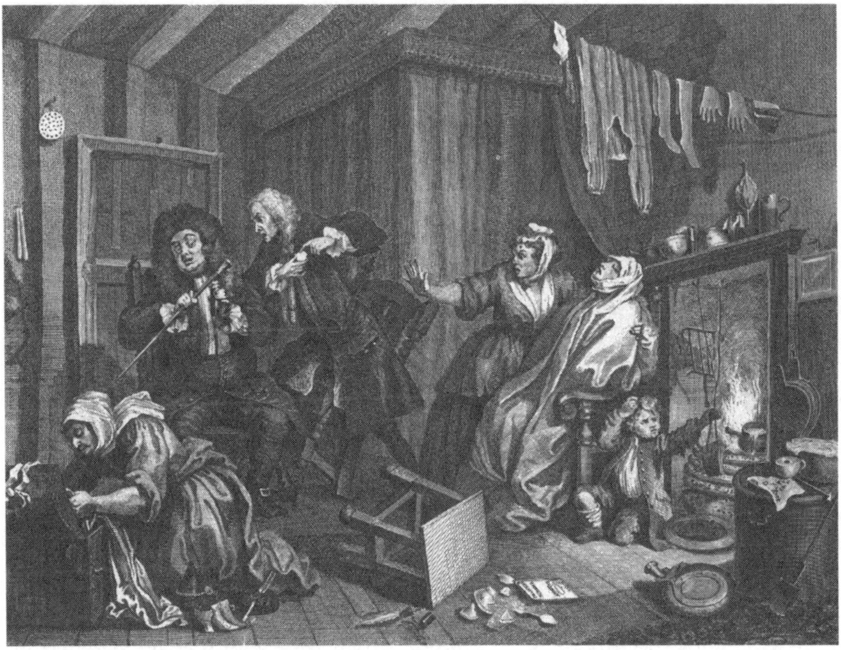

FIG. 8 William Hogarth, *A Harlot's Progress, Plate V*, 1732

> Fashion of flat Faces, pleased himself with the Opinion it might prove a very comical Sight for so many Maim'd Lechers, Snuffing old Stallions, young unfortunate Whore-Masters, poor Scarify'd Bawds, and Sallivated Whetstones, to shew their scandalous Vizards in a Nose-less Society.[41]

As yet, little was known about the spread of the disease. In his *Treatise of all the Degrees and Symptoms for the Venereal Disease* (1704), John Marten (d. 1737), one of the most prominent self-promoters and carly specialists in its treatment, cited the case of a gentleman who had approached him with a dose of the clap yet who vehemently denied having had sexual intercourse. Although his patient admitted that he had picked up a woman at the playhouse, he had merely been 'accommodat'd by her hand'. According to Marten, even such casual caresses as mutual masturbation were sufficient for the transmission of the disease: 'it was possible to get the Infection that way, and that by Friction or rubbing the *Yard* with a warm Hand, just wet with a virulent *Venereal Matter*, the *Pocky* contagious Miasms may enter into the Pores of the erected heated *Yard*, and prove infectious.'

Sodomy could also cause the clap, or as Marten more vehemently put it: 'one Man's conversing with, or having the Carnal use of another Man's Body, *viz.* B——ry [Buggery], an abominable, beastly, sodomitical and shameful Action; an action, as is not fit to be named.' Oral sex was seen as a further cause. Marten opined: 'This distemper is also gotten after another manner of Conversation, viz. By a Man's putting his erected Penis, into another Person (Man or Woman's) Mouth, using Friction &c. between the Lips; a way so very Beastly and so much to be abhorr'd, as to cause at the mentioning, or but thinking of it, the utmost detestation and loathing.'[42] Even lascivious kissing was thought to spread the disease. Marten also proffered various cures and advice on improving sexual performance and, although he could suggest remedies for those with too big a penis who inflicted pain on their wives, he could offer no cure for the man with a 'yard' which was too small.

The 'clap' and the 'pox', or gonorrhoea and syphilis, were generally thought to be manifestations of the same disease, with little distinction made between them. Pox was thought to be a more advanced stage of the clap, as the poet Alexander Pope expressed when he wrote, 'Time, that at last matures a Clap to Pox'.[43] John Burrows in his *Dissertation on the Narrative and Effects of a New Vegetable Remedy* (1780) wrote of a clap becoming 'a confirmed pox'. Conversely, a few people evidently did distinguish between the two venereal diseases. In *Thraliana*, which included her diary for 1778, the writer and bluestocking Mrs Hester Thrale retold a tale in which a tutor asked after his charge's state of health, remarking that he looked 'quite ill of late, I fear you are *Clap'd:* No Sir but I am *Pox'd* replied the Lad.' Syphilis was known as 'the French pox' and foreigners were blamed for bringing it into the country. The Earl of Rochester, Lord Bolingbroke and James Boswell were among the many who contracted venereal diseases, the latter no less than nineteen times. The satirical poet Charles Churchill, a friend of John Wilkes, and his mistress both contracted the disease in 1762–3, Churchill taking mercury as a cure.

Mercury was prescribed as one of the main cures for syphilis, either as an ointment rubbed into the skin, through injection or taken orally. The body reacted to the toxic metal by inducing a fever and causing sweating which was supposed to dispel the infection. The side-effects were horrendous: loss of teeth, foul breath, liver and kidney damage, aching joints and copious spitting. Mercury produced huge amounts of saliva in an attempt to rid the body of its poisons; a process altogether painful and lengthy, salivation did not in fact cure the disease, although it may have alleviated some of the symptoms. Some quacks tried to promote easier, less agonizing ways of taking the 'cure', as suggested by the title of William Saunders's book, *A New and Easy Way of Giving Mercury to those Affected with the Venereal Disease*. In order to boost custom, he advertised in the *Daily Advertiser* from October 1768 to January 1769. Indeed, advertisements for various potions and pills were carried in all manner of men's magazines and journals. Even respectable newspapers such as *The Times* and women's magazines such as the *Female Tatler* ran advertisements for cures for VD. According to one dated 1731, remedies for 'certain ailments' could be found at Moll and Tom King's Coffee-House where 'may be had all Manners of curious Galenic Medicines, and Chymical preparations at an easy Rate'.[44]

Quacks did a roaring trade preying on people's anxieties. One promoted Vegetable Specific Pills in 1772, while another swore by Dr Rock's Royal Patent, Velno's Vegetable Syrup or Leake's Pills. Although Boswell's surgeon, Dr Douglas, advised a strict diet, rest and internal medicine, Boswell turned to Kennedy's Lisbon Diet Drink. At a guinea a bottle a day, it was an expensive treatment, particularly galling since it did not work. One physician, Pringle, even advised a surgical procedure on his patient's bladder as a method for curing his venereal disease.[45]

Because of the very nature of venereal disease – it was transmitted through sexual activities – its treatment was often administered in secret. Dr Robert James in his *Medical Dictionary* recommended a remedy which could be taken in a drink so as not to arouse a spouse's suspicion: 'A husband can take his chocolate in the presence of his wife without her suspecting a thing: indeed, she herself can take it without realizing that she is swallowing an anti-venereal remedy; by this innocent means, then, peace and concord can be maintained in the household.'[46] One woman nearly died after her husband tried this method. The incident came to light after Martha Robinson unsuccessfully sued for divorce in 1775. Her husband had given her gonorrhoea on numerous occasions and tried to treat her without her knowledge by putting a powder in her wine. Despite this, and the fact that he beat her, she was refused a divorce.[47] The tenet of the day was that wives were expected to put up with the results of their husband's extramarital activities. Mrs Hester Thrale, on being shown her husband's swollen testicle, recalled her father's words: 'If you marry that scoundrel, he will catch the pox, and for his amusement set you to make his poultices', which she now found herself doing. Not all women, however, were prepared to be quite so forgiving. After contracting the pox from her husband in 1792, Mrs Sarah Siddons, the actress, was said to be a 'ball of resentment'.[48]

In an attempt to treat and control venereal disease, a specialist hospital for women, the Lock Hospital, opened in 1746. By 1752, the *Gentleman's Magazine* reported that 1,495 patients were being cured, 'among them several married women, children and infants, and many naked and starving'. People became benefactors – the prime minister Robert Walpole, the Duke of Bedford and the Honourable John Grey all supported the cause. Actors David Garrick and John Lacy gave benefit performances to assist the hospital's finances. Many women donated money, among them Garrick's wife, Eva Maria, the evangelical philanthropist and playwright Hannah More, and the well-loved courtesan Miss Fanny Murray. Yet the men running the hospital left a legacy of their true feeling about the female patients in *An Account for the Institution of the Lock Asylum* (1788). They laid the responsibility clearly on the shoulders of the infected women they were treating, seeing them as pitiful creatures yet responsible for personal and national destruction. 'In the mean Time their malignant Influence on Society is equally deplorable,' they lamented. 'They throng our streets and lay in wait for the inexperienced and incautious: So that a Youth can scarce walk a Mile in many Parts of this City without running the Gauntlet through at least fifty of those Temptations, which are most likely to prevail against him.'[49]

Condoms were still being purchased mainly as protection against the pox rather than to prevent conception. Mrs Philips and Mrs Perkins were leading purveyors, the former advertising in *St James's Chronicle*, the latter operating from the Green Canister in Half-Moon Street. Mrs Lewis sold condoms from her shop in St Martin's Lane in the 1740s.[50] These were made from animal membrane tied on to the penis with a small silk ribbon. Despite such barrier methods of protection, venereal disease continued to spread, along with other genital diseases such as venereal crabs. None of the disorders were easily treated and, as such, venereal diseases were part of the rigours of sexual life. Women continued to suffer from ulcerous vaginas as men endured festering penis sores.

*

Sex was pushed as the greatest diversion in town in eighteenth-century London – seeing it, doing it or talking about it. The increasing numbers of new people converging on the city from the countryside and abroad meant that the dynamics of community relationships were gradually shifting. Unleashed from traditional ties in their rural villages, new arrivals were keen to take advantage of their freedom. Morality codes enforced by close-knit family and village neighbours lost their significance in the anonymity of the towns and allowed for greater sexual exploration. London also brought with it a chance for economic opportunity. Sex was a saleable commodity. This was evident in the growing number of prostitutes, brothels and courtesans on offer. The increase in demand, in turn, brought diversification in the types of sex which could be purchased.

Gossip about scandals and intrigues was rife in the metropolis, with newspapers and pamphlets being pumped out to supply erotic entertainment – what went on in Ranelagh Gardens, who was seen with who at Drury Lane Theatre, and where a gentleman might go in order to find an attractive whore. More advanced printing methods brought with them greater choice and cheaper publications on sex.

Although moral reformers were attempting to erect barriers against the surge of such titillating reading matter, it is doubtful whether their attempts made much impact. Despite the establishment of the Magdalene houses and the Lock hospitals, prostitution and venereal disease were to become the main banes of Victorian life. Restraining the effervescence of carnally wrought desires was beyond the reach of the reformers and, for the time being at least, lascivious bodies would continue to have their way.

Chapter Two

Love, Honour and Betrayal

> Chastity is the next virtue, that is to fall under consideration; no charm can supply its place; without it beauty is unlovely, wit is mean and wanton; quality contemptible, and good-breeding worthless. She who forfeits her chastity, withers by degrees into scorn and contrition; but she, who lives up to its rules, ever flourishes, like a rose in *June*, with all her virgin graces about her – sweet to the sense, and lovely to the eye . . .
>
> Wetenhall Wilkes, *A Letter of Genteel and Moral Advice to a Young Lady* (1740)

The theological writer Wetenhall Wilkes's comments summed up the decree for an unmarried woman: she was to remain chaste until marriage, or face disgrace. Virginity, he avowed, 'is the great point of female honour, and the least slip in a woman's honour, is never to be recovered'. Such homilies were to become the mainstay of 'conduct literature' conjured up in letters to young ladies, fathers giving advice to daughters, and any amount of treatises on the subject of women's education, duties and responsibilities. This literature expressed a certain moral code based on the presumption that a woman's honour lay in her sexual virtue. For this reason, preserving a woman's chastity was seen to be of paramount importance, her reputation hinging on her restraint. As Dr Samuel Johnson pointed out, 'Consider of what importance to society the chastity of woman is. Upon that all property in the world depends. They who forfeit it should not have any possibility of being restored to good character.'[1]

In 1688, the financier Lord Halifax suggested that, once married, the best way a woman could influence her husband was through tears: 'You have it in your power not only to free yourself, but to subdue your masters and without violence, throw both their natural and regal authority at your feet.'[12] Although Halifax appears to be advocating emotional blackmail, submissive behaviour was in keeping with the image of the archetypal 'ideal' model. Eighteenth-century conduct literature defined the attributes of the perfect female: she was modest, passive, restrained, compliant, delicate and, above all, chaste. Nearly a century later, Dr John Gregory was to remind his daughter in *A Father's Legacy to his Daughter* (1774), 'One of the chief beauties in a female character, is that modest reserve, that retiring delicacy, which avoids the public eye, and is disconcerted even at the gaze of admiration.' Such writers reinforced the orthodox sexual morality emphasizing a strict code of conduct for women. Within this framework, the ideal woman was to hold a central role in the Protestant family. She was held aloft as a symbol of goodness, an upholder of moral virtue, the veritable 'Angel in the House'.

It was not only a woman's chastity which came under scrutiny in the disciplining of the female body, but also her eating habits. A woman should not appear too healthy or robust as it was considered unattractive. The weak and delicate woman, especially when combined with her intermittent fainting, was thought to be the sort to turn a young man's head. On eating, Gregory declared, 'It is a despicable selfish vice in men. But in your sex it is beyond expression, indelicate and disgusting.' Indulging in the sensual pleasures of food displayed a profligate nature and, as if to prove the point, pornography was littered with erotic depictions of men and women eating and drinking heartily together after indulging in sexual activities.

Flattery was a form of sexual seduction to which women were perceived to be particularly susceptible. In a letter to his son in 1749, the politician Lord Chesterfield warned, 'The least attentions please, the greatest charm them. The innocent, but pleasing flattery of their persons, however gross, is greedily swallowed, and kindly digested; but a seeming regard for their advice, together with a seeming confidence in their moral virtues, turn their heads entirely in your favour.'[13] Women were seen to be both intellectually weak and psychologically unstable: 'Women, then, are only children of a larger growth . . . A Man of sense only trifles with them, humours and flatters them, as he does with sprightly forward children.'

Added to these concerns about female chastity, diet and gullibility were anxieties about women's literary interests. There was a general distrust of female reading matter, particularly the romances which were thought to fill a woman's head with erotic thoughts and prime her for easier seduction. The novelist Samuel Richardson was astonished to find that his fictional rapist, Lovelace, was so appealing to his female readership and, consequently, made him more villainous in the third edition of *Clarissa* (1747–8), in an attempt to make him unattractive. In her essay *On the Religion of the Fashionable World* (1801), Hannah More, the stuffy supporter of the Proclamation Society and of the Society for the Suppression of Vice, condemned racy novels, espousing

> that the corruption occasioned by these books had spread so wide, and descended so low, as to have become one of the most universal, as well as the most pernicious sources of corruption among us.

She complained that milliners, mantua-makers, and other trades where a number of women were employed often sacrificed the labour of one girl in order that she might read these 'mischievous books' to others.[4]

Love poems posed a similar threat. The *Eclectic Review* in October 1806 warned of the dangers in Thomas Moore's love poems:

> The danger lies in dallying with sin, and with sensual sin above all other: it works, it winds, it wins its way with imperceptible, with irresistible insinuation, through all the passages of the mind, into the innermost recesses of the heart; while it is softening the bosom, it is hardening the conscience; while by its exhilaration, it seems to be spiritualising the body, it is brutalising the soul, and by mingling with its eternal essence, it is giving *immorality* to impotent unappeasable desires, it is endangering 'the worm that dieth not', it is kindling 'the fire that is not quenched'.[5]

Even worse, girls were being influenced by pornography written with the specific intention 'to debauch, poison and infect the minds of all the youths of this kingdom and to bring them into a state of wickedness, lewdness, debauchery and brutality'.[6] In *An Enquiry into the Best System of Female Education* (1809), the author J. L. Chirol noted that access to erotic fiction in boarding schools was leading girls to masturbate.[7] In 1825, the Society for the Suppression of Vice went so far as to state that boarding schools represented a substantial part of the market for indecent literature, even prosecuting some traders who were selling pornographic snuffboxes to girls' schools.[8]

Thus, sex for women was a highly circumscribed activity. A woman's position in society was inextricably linked to her sexual behaviour, especially those from the burgeoning middle classes. At all times she must appear chaste if a maid, and, if married, at the very least display modesty in her outward behaviour.[9] Yet a man's reputation was seen to be connected less to his sexual behaviour than to his reason, strength and trustworthiness. His manliness was displayed in his outward behaviour and, as the head of the household, he was expected to keep his wife, children and servants in order. None the less, sexual dalliances could still harm his reputation. A man's sexual honour, if lost, could affect the behaviour of his neighbours towards him. A vicar, Robert Foulkes, found this to his cost when his adultery with Anne Atkinson became a 'spectacle to the world'. He remarked, 'The scandal of it became so publick' that 'it burst out with a violence, like water long damned up'.[10] He was later indicted and executed for the murder of their second illegitimate child.

A woman's honour might be lost without her consent. Rape was defined as the unlawful carnal knowledge of a woman by force and against her will and carried the death penalty.[11] But this became increasingly difficult to prove, particularly between the 1770s and the 1820s when judges became less willing to accept the word of a woman against a man's. Sexual intercourse with girls under the age of ten constituted rape, but with girls of ten to twelve years was regarded less seriously. No new legislation was enacted affecting rape during the eighteenth century but there was a change based on the developing case law, rather than through statute.[12] The abduction of an heiress and her rape, seduction or marriage carried penalties but the injustice was considered to be against the injured woman's family rather than the woman herself. Sophia, sister of the celebrated courtesan Harriette Wilson, absconded with Viscount Deerhurst when she was under-age. She was gullible and sexually naive, 'innocent as an infant to the nature of seduction, and its consequences'. Having forsaken the protection of her mother and father for that of Deerhurst, 'the poor foolish girl was now put out of everyone's sight, and applications were made to Deerhurst, for a provision for her, with a threat of law-proceedings in case of refusal.'[13] For a girl in Sophia's position, the only legal plea for a provision was the claim her parents could make for the loss of her domestic services. Deerhurst settled £300 per year on her on condition that no charge of inconstancy was brought against him and, unable to return home, Sophia was placed in miserable lodgings.

As a general rule, sexual activity outside marriage was much more acceptable for a man than for a woman. But discretion was necessary to avoid loss of social standing. As Lord Chesterfield advised his son, 'There is a certain dignity to be kept up, in pleasure as well as in business. In love, a man may lose his heart with dignity; but if he loses his nose, he loses his character into the bargain.'[14] Chesterfield's salutary warning – to avoid the pox and thereby protect your reputation – might have raised fears in any young man. However, the rakes and libertines continued to indulge in immoral sexual behaviour to their hearts' content. Five years prior to his marriage in 1769, Boswell boasted to Jean-Jacques Rousseau, 'If I am rich, I can take a number of girls. I get them with child, propagation is thus increased. I give them dowries and marry them off to good peasants who are very happy to have them. Thus they become wives at the same age as would have been the case if they had remained virgins, and I, on my side, have had the benefit of enjoying a great variety of women . . .'[15] The perfect vision of the female virgin, chaste until marriage, was therefore crushed underfoot by some men intent on gratifying their own sexual desires without commitments. Ideally, however, the first step in the sexual cycle, after leading a chaste existence, would be a courtship overseen by parents which would lead to marriage.

Courting Couples

Sexual behaviour should preferably occur between a married couple, and then for procreative purposes only. This was, of course, the Protestant ideal and there were many deviations from the path of so-called sexual righteousness which supported a double standard of sexual morality for men and women. Men who indulged in fornication outside marriage did so with much more ease than women, and with fewer repercussions. They were rarely shunned in polite society for keeping a mistress or copulating with whores, although some sections of society would always openly disapprove of such activities. In contrast, a woman would invariably became a target of social outrage if she had sexual experiences outside the bounds of marriage.[16]

The period between courtship and marriage was the most precarious time for a young woman. She might choose to give up her virtue on the promise of marriage, yet the man could still renege. Hugh Kelly recognized a woman's vulnerable position in his consideration of female seduction, *Memoirs Of A Magdalene, Or The History Of Louisa Mildmay* (1767): 'of all the stages in a woman's life . . . none is more dangerous as the period between her acknowledgement of a passion for a man, and the day set apart for her nuptial.'

Among the poorer sections of the community, courtship was freer than in other classes. Sex more frequently took place before marriage, and for those who could not wait, a form of heavy petting called 'bundling' was allowed. This might include intimate conversation between the couple throughout the night and fondling half-clothed in bed, with a board placed between them or the girl's petticoats tied in a knot between her thighs. Young women sometimes consented to sexual intercourse because of a promise of marriage. Such a betrothal held significant value and was usually given with the tacit understanding that the wedding would take place sooner or later; and usually this did happen. These 'engagements' were often bound by gifts, culminating in a contract between the couples, sometimes without the consent of parents. It would then be in a woman's interest to strengthen a private marriage promise by making it public.

If a woman had sex and marriage failed to take place, she would usually be in danger of ostracism from the community, but this might vary depending on a woman's class and where she lived. In a tightly knit rural village, community pressure could be brought to bear on a man to fulfil his vow if he had had sex with a woman after promising to marry her. An exchange of vows performed by a clergyman sufficed, but elopement became more difficult after Hardwicke's Marriage Act of 1753. All marriages then had to be conducted in the church in the parish of the couple, following a reading of the banns for three weeks, and afterwards signed in the parish register by both parties. More importantly, marriages for those under the age of twenty-one were not considered legal without parental consent. Twelve was the legal age for marriage for girls, fourteen for boys, although couples generally married much later. The average age for women was twenty-two, for men, twenty-four.[17]

Courtship for the 'middling sons' or the gentry, usually meant less parental control over a choice of spouse than among the aristocracy. A man might eye a girl in public, at church, at a ball or a party, and then approach her parents and formally ask their permission to court her. Men were expected to make the first move, and women either to encourage or resist their advances. Pre-nuptial wrangling between families often stood in the way, bringing other sorts of irritations. None spelt out the frustrations more clearly than Frederick Mullins who, about to be married in 1747, complained that the trustees in charge of his marriage settlement were unnecessarily delaying the 'taking possession of the charming Phoebe', adding by way of explanation that they were not 'so eager for a fuck as I am'.[18]

Despite social pressures, some aristocratic women did have sex before marriage. The respectable Emily Lennox gave in to temptation and had sex with her beloved before their marriage. Recalling the blissful event of Christmas Day 1746 in the Earl of Kildare's empty summerhouse on the Goodwood estate, Carné Seat, some sixteen years later, she reminded her husband, 'If you are at Goodwood, and the sun shines as bright as it does here, I hope you will take a walk up to the Carné Seat, sit down in the little room and think of that you took with Lady Emily Lennox, just returned from Bognor Church, sixteen years ago, and I believe that I love you sixteen time better now than I did then.'[19] Despite her sister Caroline's view of her husband, 'The Lord Kildare is not the most clever man in the World', Emily had a long and happy marriage.

Regarding courtship with her future husband, Lady Mary Wortley Montagu (1689–1762) remarked on the dangers of sexual dalliance: 'All commerce of this kind between men and women is like that of the Boys and Frogs in L'Estrange's Fable – "'Tis play to you, but 'tis death to us – and if we had the wit of frogs, we should allwaies make that answer."'[20] Her father's choice of a peer's son was rejected in favour of her own untitled paramour, with whom she eloped. Aristocratic arrangements were strict in order to protect inheritances but she was lucky enough in that her husband made his own fortune. On their first time apart, she wrote to him, 'I Lament your Absence as if you was still my Lover', obviously missing the delights of sex. Her husband was away for long periods on parliamentary duties and they eventually parted amicably. In 1736, she fell in love with Francesco Algarotti, an Italian intellectual half her age. Her close friend, the notorious bisexual Lord Hervey, became her rival for his affections. Before Algarotti left England, he chose to spend his last evening with Lady Mary, to Hervey's dismay. Yet it was Hervey to whom he wrote first from Calais, a detail Hervey was only too glad to let her know. In his reply, Hervey told Algarotti that she had attempted 'thousands of different ways to make me talk of you', desperately trying to cover up her true feelings while becoming 'as drunk before as wine can make one, & you have added *Gin*'.[21] She eventually followed Algarotti to Venice regardless of polite opinion and Algarotti's distinct lack of encouragement. Lady Mary's behaviour was unusual for the time and made her the subject of much malicious gossip.

Companionate marriage evolved to become the aspiration for many men and women. Defoe remarked: 'I don't take the state of marriage to be designed . . . that the wife is to be used as an upper servant in the house . . . Love knows no superior or inferior, no imperious command on the one hand, no reluctant subjection on the other.' The author Hester Chapone went further, deciding that a husband must totally understand and love his wife if there were to be connubial bliss, declaring, 'I believe it . . . absolutely necessary to conjugal happiness that the husband have such an opinion of his wife's understanding, principles and integrity of heart as would induce

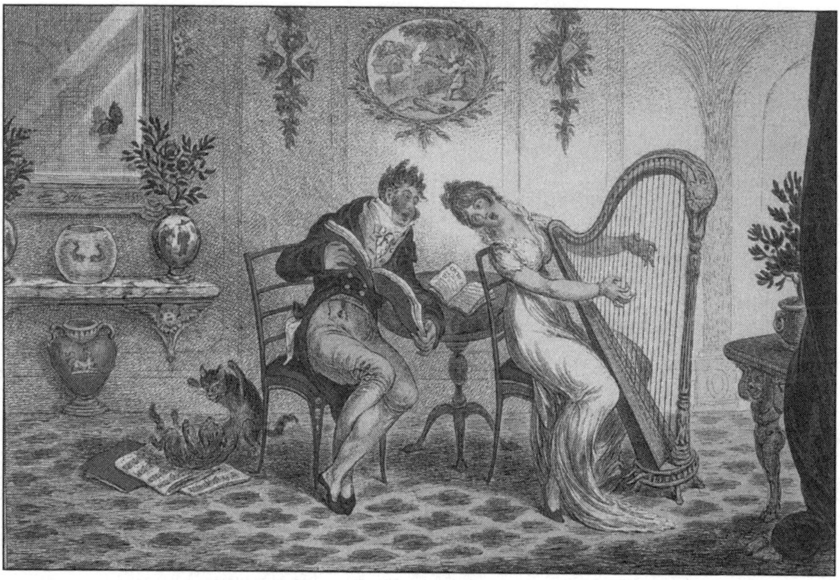

FIG. 9 James Gillray, *Harmony Before Matrimony*, 1805

him to exalt her to the rank of his *first and dearest friend.*' Dr John Gregory echoed these principles of the ideal relationship; in 1762 he opined to his daughter, 'I have always considered your sex, not as domestic drudges, or as the slaves of our pleasures, but as our companions and equals.'[22] But not everyone was to agree with these notions. Some women believed that the best way to enjoy life was to remain single (**FIGS. 9 & 10**).

Slaves to Marriage

Despite the promulgations about the benefits of sex within the bounds of marriage, there was plenty of rebellion against this ideal. In a letter to the *British Magazine* in 1748, a twenty-two-year-old woman, 'with an estate just enough to live genteelly upon', acknowledged her opposition to marriage in response to an advertisement from a lady looking for a husband. She declared, 'The acquaintance I have had among married people, and those many of them the happiest couples in the world, have given me so bad an idea of that condition in its best state, that I have no ambition to engage in it', adding, 'I am extremely happy, sir, as I am.' (**FIG. 11**)

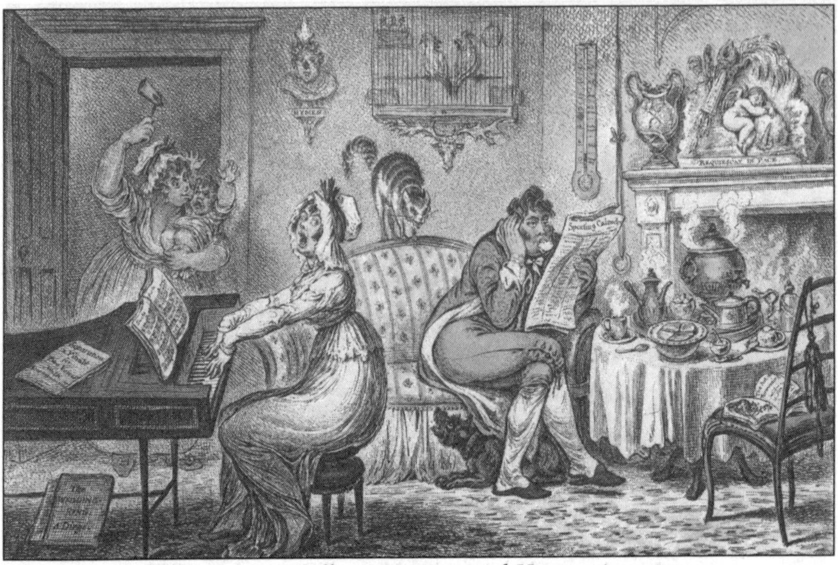

FIG. 10 James Gillray, *Matrimonial Harmonics*, 1805

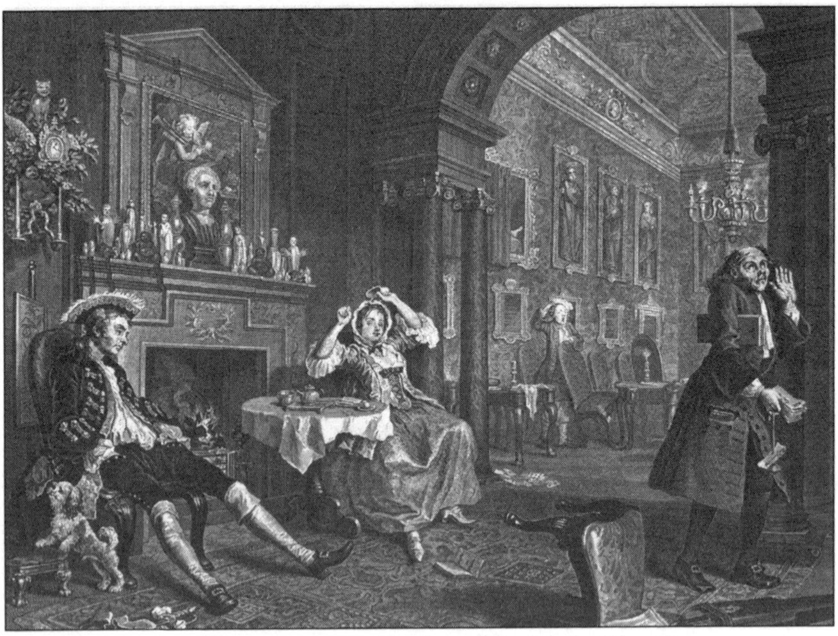

FIG. 11 William Hogarth, *Marriage A La Mode, Plate II*, 1745

In serious feminist tracts and satires alike, women advocated staying single. Lady Mary Astell, in her essay *Serious Proposal to the Ladies* (1694), argued that women were equally as capable as men. She suggested the creation of a Protestant nunnery, a female utopia where women might avoid marriage, and work and be educated together without male interference. In her *Some Reflections upon Marriage* (1700), she inquired, 'If all men are born free, how is it that all women are born slaves? As they must be if . . . subjected to the . . . arbitrary Will of Men?' Mary Chudleigh in *To the Ladies* (1703) urged women to shun the 'wretched state' of marriage; and 'Sophia' in her *Woman Not Inferior to Man; or A Short and Modest Vindication of the Natural Right of the Fair-Sex to a Perfect Equality of Power, Dignity, and Esteem, with the Men* (1739) contended that women were just as capable of holding office as men.[23] *The Female Spectator* (1744–6), a periodical edited by the novelist Eliza Haywood, took up the cudgels on behalf of women, as did Charlotte Lennox's *Lady's Museum* (1760–1) and the *Lady's Magazine* (which started in the 1770s and ran for seventy-seven years). All these publications addressed the concerns of women but perhaps none so adeptly as the *Gentleman's Magazine* (1731–1914) which frequently advocated better education for women and advised them on how to handle money matters so that they might protect themselves from swindlers or if they became widows.

Mary Wollstonecraft, in *Vindication of the Rights of Woman* (1792), criticized marriage and recognized the disparity in position between rich and poor women and the consequences of their sexual adventures: 'If an innocent girl becomes a prey to love, she is degraded for ever, though her mind was not polluted by the arts which married women, under the convenient cloak of marriage, practise.' Without monetary security, women were often left destitute after a divorce. Financially, a woman was dependent on her male kin, the estate normally passing to the eldest male heir. Women were paid less than men for all forms of work, with the higher professions barred to women altogether. In *The Female Advocate* (1799), Mary Ann Radcliffe, writer of Gothic novels, recognized that many women had little opportunity to provide for themselves, so frequently turned to prostitution. Mary herself had suffered from an unsuccessful relationship after a clandestine marriage. Her husband drank away her inheritance while she bore him seven children, two of whom died. She was forced to send the surviving children to live elsewhere and sold the family silver in order to leave her wastrel husband. She was then obliged to take low-paid work as a governess.

Mainstream fictional characters had already shown violent adverse reactions to marriage. In *Pamela* (1740–1), Richardson's heroine expressed horror at the 'strange and shocking difference' experienced by newly wed brides, when 'fond lovers, prostrate at their feet' were transformed into 'surly husbands trampling on their necks'. Similarly, Arabella, a character in the *Gentleman's Magazine*, declared: 'When she has entirely given up her fortune, her Liberty and her Person into her husband's keeping, she is immediately to become a slave to his humour, his convenience, or even his Pleasure, and that she is to expect no more Favour from him, than he in great Condescension thinks fit to grant.'

Luxury was blamed for ruining a woman's moral fibre and encouraging coquetry. Women were accused of elevating themselves above their station, making for disastrous marriage material: 'Every women with a tolerable face fancies herself a goddess or an angel, and considers it as beneath her divinity to think of man but as a slave, forced to obey, and destined to wear her chains.' Thus, ran the argument, women were no longer satisfied with men of their own rank but expected to marry dukes: 'A tradesman's daughter, who, probably, has not five hundred pounds to her fortune, will fancy herself qualified to marry a member of parliament at least.' Mothers were blamed for sending their daughters to boarding schools, which the fathers could ill afford, and then showing them off at Ranelagh Gardens: 'A few rounds of this mill of folly turns the girl's brains: She sees Lady Betty Idle coquet it with Lord Dimple; she resolves to imitate that sweet creature and longs for an opportunity to be *en famille* with a nobleman.'[24] These depictions contrast with the satirical prints of Hogarth: of young rakes marrying broken-down old hags for their money (**FIG. 12**).

Satires on marriage also came in the form of witty retorts and suggested survival tactics for sexually active women. Parodies were made of serious feminist works. *Proposal for the Erecting a Protestant Nunnery In the City Of Dublin* (1726)[25] was a bawdy parody of Mary Astell's *Serious*

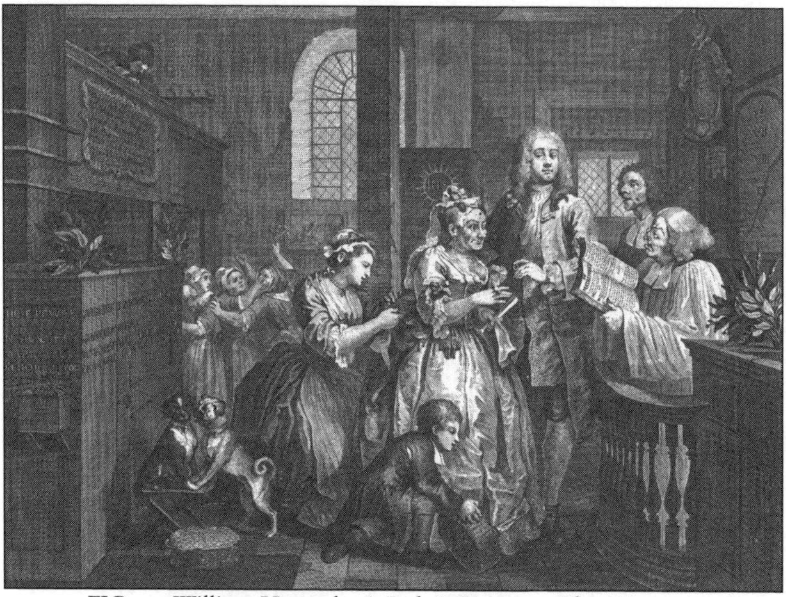

FIG. 12 William Hogarth, *A Rake's Progress, Plate V*, 1735

Proposal. Written 'by the Ladies', the six-page poem suggests a nunnery for old retired whores:

Suppose a large Cloyster, which we are debarr'd in,
That Cloyster, for walking must have a large Garden,
The Garden have Doors, each Doors have a Key,
One for the Ridotto, and one for the Play;
Take care that the Garden is handsomely wide,
To open on Both, and the Castle beside:
Some Fellow, perchance, if the Maggot shou'd bite,
May be scaling the walls, to come as it Might . . .

Such ditties also reflected the anti-Catholic sentiments held by the English about the hypocrisy of the Catholic Church. British Protestants had long mistrusted the Catholics, pointing to stories of sexual scandals in convents and monasteries. The nub of the poem's joke lay in the fact that brothels were frequently referred to as nunneries and whores as 'nuns' or 'sisters'.

Erotic poems portrayed sexually lascivious women doing their best to avoid marriage. The comedy of these depictions betrayed real anxieties which were being voiced in the wider world about ungovernable women. In these skits, the characteristics of the heroine stood in opposition to the 'ideal' image of the domesticated passive wife. The protagonist was often described as highly passionate, taking the initiative in sex. Women were portrayed as high-spirited and ready to fight to retain their single status. In *Kick Him Jenny* (1737), a young maid, Jenny, is wooed by 'Country Swain' Roger. He lusts after her, but she resists his advances, rejecting marriage and clinging to the freedom of life as a single woman. Underlying this comedy is the all too common female fear of desertion if she succumbs to a man's sexual demands.

My Lady, being in merry Mood,
Ask'd her, how Marriage-Matters stood?
Whether she 'ad pitch'd upon the Man;
She'd whispered Yes *to through the Fan?*
Young Jenny *cunningly reply'd,*
She did not wish to be a Bride;
But lik'd her present State so well,
She thought of leading Apes in Hell.

Her Lady looks on through a peephole at the comic scene of Roger's attempts at seduction, shouting 'Kick him Jenny' while her husband Sir John shouts for the lad to continue.

Mad at his Wife, he cou'd have stuck her,
Aloud cry'd, —— her, Roger, *—— her,*
Kick him, as loud, the Dame went on;
—— her, still louder, cry'd Sir John:[26]

Married characters, including titled women, did not escape public ridicule and were depicted as sexually avaricious and adulterous. One collection of saucy japes, *The Court Jester*,[27] aimed its invective at the Honourable Lady Craven. It provided 'A Plumber's Bill' to her for work done 'in your Ladyship's Water-closet'.

To mending your ladyship's cistern	020
To a man to go to the bottom	076
Easing your ladyship's waste pipe	026
To a cock put in the front	053
To a double ball ditto	076

Statements on marriage from fictional heroines in erotica frequently reflect such independent views. In one piece, *A New Atlantis for the Year 1758*, the heroine, Rocforria, announces, 'Married, a fiddle-stick . . . marriage is no argument among people of fashion and quality, but rather a convenient covering for gallantry.' In this type of material, sexual educators of young girls were frequently depicted as older, more experienced women who instil their worthiness to be worshipped rather than the concept of passivity into their wards. Rocforria demands, 'Our favourite parts ought to be venerated by those who arrogantly stile themselves our lords and masters.' She declared the enjoyment and pleasure from love and sex as life's greatest experience: 'The joys of love constitute the only perfect pleasure creation is capable of, because body and soul are emulous participants thereof, in the enrapturing momentary crisis of happiness.' She concludes that, if she is to enter into sexual intercourse with a man, she has to be wooed and demands foreplay. 'I never let any male suppliant approach the shrine of my Mecca, but after proper adoration paid; such as the burning incense, repeated genufluxions [*sic*], alternate kissing of the two collateral columns (white as Parisian marble) which leads to the blissful altar, veiled from the vulgar eyes with the fringe of Venus.'[28] Restrictions on female behaviour are vehemently opposed by another female character, Petronia. Upon her husband's death, she expresses her pleasure at being set free:

> Then what pleasure, ye gods, to be a widow, mistress of my person and jointure, free to chuse [*sic*] whom I please, and to retain him in my service but whilst he can please me. Thus shall I emulate the grand Turk, who fixes where he likes. The matrimonial yoke I never will undergo again; be no man's property, but rather make all mankind, at least all the desirable members of it, mine.[29]

Not only will she possess her own body but her own property and estate – money will bring her freedom. Such titillating fiction, along with racy tales about the adventures of well-known figures of the day, became popular forms of ribald entertainment, with eighteenth-century readers lapping up comic satires, erotica, gossip and scandal.

Adulterous Diversions

In instances where a woman was found to be committing adultery, her husband would be labelled 'a cuckold', the most shameful name a man could be given. In 1699, Stephen Seagar of Aldgate suffered the ultimate humiliation upon discovering that, while away on business, his apprentice Tarrant Reeves had cuckolded him. Even worse, his wife had become pregnant. Seagar found himself the laughing stock of the local community.[30] A cuckold man was seen as lacking the authority to govern his wife and household and this would ultimately affect his honour. In such cases, adultery was perceived as the fault of the man, unable either to satisfy his wife or to control her.

In rural communities, rituals were established whereby neighbours could show their approval or disapproval of sexual behaviour that was considered to upset the proper order of things. Premarital or adulterous sex often invited public condemnation. Reversal of the considered 'normal' sexual hierarchy, where a woman was seen as the dominant partner, was also subject to community reaction. Rituals such as 'rough music' were practised: neighbours would come from their houses clashing pots and pans, shaking kettles, banging tins and making as much noise as possible. In cases of adultery or female dominance, these rites would become more elaborate and involve 'skimmington' rides where effigies, or men dressed in drag, were put on donkeys and ridden through the village (**FIG. 13**). Such displays were intended to mock husbands who had been cuckolded or were henpecked.

Women who were considered unruly would also be targeted by local villagers if deemed to have breached the patriarchal hierarchy; shrews, scolds and husband beaters were all subject to community hostility. In one case in 1790, Alice Evans sparked a ruction in the local community after chastizing her husband,

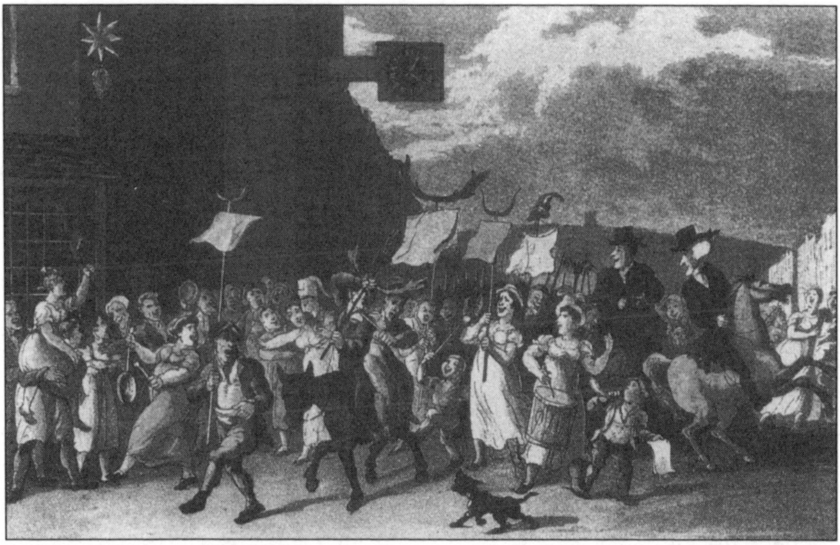

FIG. 13 Thomas Rowlandson, *Dr Syntax with the Skimmington Riders*, 1813

> This conduct [of hers] the neighbouring lords of creation were determined to punish, fearing their own spouses might assume the same authority. They therefore mounted one of their body, dressed in female apparel, on the back of an old donkey, the man holding a spinning wheel on his lap, and his back towards the donkey's head. Two men led the animal through the neighbourhood, followed by scores of boys and idle men, tinkling kettles and frying pans, roaring with cow's horns, and making the most hideous hullabaloo, stopping every now and then while the exhibitioner on the donkey made the following proclamation:
>
> *'Ran a dan, ran a dan, ran a dan,*
> *Mrs Alice Evans has beat her good man;*
> *It was neither with sword, spear, pistol or knife*
> *But with a pair of tongs she vowed to take his life.'*[31]

Among the aristocracy, family pressures rather than community reaction influenced ideas on adultery or attempted divorce, prompted by the desire to keep financial assets and inheritances intact. To this end, some aristocratic couples who entered into arranged marriages might agree to indulge in outside dalliances, accepting infidelities as part of the contract. Once again, it was the woman who would be expected to be discreet yet it was less important for a man to cover evidence of his exploits. Lord Bolingbroke conducted numerous public infidelities, including a prolonged one with Lady Coventry. His wife, Lady Diana Spencer, left him after he had infected her with venereal disease but, when she began her own affair with the wit and libertine Topham Beauclerk, it had to be conducted under a veil of secrecy.

Legally, a woman's body was the property of her husband. Indeed, everything she owned belonged to him. A woman could not sue her husband or make a contract without him and had no control whatsoever over the family property.[32] She could be charged with adultery with no provision in the law to assist her. Divorce could be obtained only by an Act of Parliament, and was usually granted to men with adulterous wives but rarely vice versa. The adultery laws were heavily biased against women: a woman could not be granted a divorce on the grounds of her husband's adultery alone but had to prove other mitigating circumstances, such as severe cruelty or sodomy. Even then, this was not always enough. The Dubliner Laetitia Pilkington (1712–50), wit, poet and protégée of Jonathan Swift and friend to the playwright and stage manager Colley Cibber, had, at seventeen, rashly married a poor parson, Mathew Pilkington. The marriage collapsed after they both committed adultery. The publication of Laetitia's memoirs, in 1748, created a scandal. Swift wrote: 'He is now suing for a divorce and will not get it: she is suing for a maintenance and he has none to give her.'

'Wife sales' were used by the poorer classes as a crude divorce procedure. A halter was placed around the woman's neck and she was sold at a market-place auction to the highest bidder. Although on one occasion a wife was sold for £100, in another, the wife was given freely for a glass of ale. The usual exchange cost between two shillings and sixpence and five shillings. On 31 August, 1772, Samuel Whitehouse, of the parish of Willenhall, sold his wife, Mary Whitehouse, in the open market, to Thomas Griffiths of Birmingham for a shilling, 'To take her with all her faults.'[33] This ritual was also used as a way out of an unsuitable marriage for a woman. In many sales, even where it appeared to be an open auction, in fact the purchaser was known and the sale prearranged. The purchaser might even have been the wife's lover or they might already have lived together prior to the event taking place, the procedure becoming merely a formality.

*

The importance invested in a woman's chastity meant that she was constantly under pressure to maintain her reputation. Yet, despite the cries of the moralists to uphold female chastity before marriage, in reality neither men nor women always adhered to the proposed protocol. Concerns about women's susceptibility to flattery were superseded only by concerns about their lascivious behaviour, while the reading of novels was considered responsible for inflaming latent female passions. On the other hand, professional men who might want to marry virgins had few qualms about enjoying sex outside marriage with women of a lower class, as with Boswell's philanderings and Chesterfield's advice to his son. As we have seen, women sometimes succumbed to their lovers' advances before marriage. Even so-called 'respectable' couples conducted sexual relations prior to their marriage if they so chose, as did Emily Lennox and the Earl of Kildare. In short, if a woman felt she was in love, and was confident that the man would marry her, there was little to prevent a couple having sex. Concerns about keeping one's chastity did not hold much consideration for some men and women when love or passion was involved.

Yet both men and women recognized the problems which might befall them during courtship, marriage and divorce. Part of the reaction to these concerns was seen in community rituals whereby marriage might be encouraged and adultery condemned. None the less, the disparity between the legal position of men and women was reflected in their treatment in court. The law consistently failed to protect women whether single, married or divorced. It was therefore left to the anti-marriage tracts, both serious and satirical, to voice concerns about just how dreadful the position of women was, often sympathizing with their desire to remain single.

CHAPTER THREE

Men of Pleasure

> Man naturally aspires and his mind is elevated, his senses grow more refined and more capable of delight. His desires are enlarged, & his wants increase with his wishes . . .[1]
>
> Nicholas Barbon, English economist (1690)

For most post-pubescent youths, sowing their wild oats was part of the process of coming of age, an activity encouraged by their peers and condoned by society. Indeed, a young man from a moderately wealthy family in the eighteenth century could make the choice to indulge himself in a wide range of sybaritic pleasures: heavy drinking, travelling on the Continent, eating to excess, as well as hour upon hour of sex. Frequent sexual activity was seen to be good for a man's health – doctors advised that sperm should be dispelled regularly to ensure the smooth running of the humours, thus keeping a healthy balance of one's bodily fluids. The quack James Graham went so far as to declare that '. . . without a full and genial tide of this rich, vivifying luminous principle [sperm], continually circulating in every part of the system, it is absolutely impossible that either man or woman can enjoy health, strength, spirits, or happiness'.[2] Although Graham was advocating regular sex within marriage, libertines also took up the advice, applying it indiscriminately and to excess. Erasmus Darwin went so far as to assert that sexual attraction was the essential cause of happiness, 'the cordial drop in the otherwise insipid cup of love'.[3]

Although initially libertines were seen to be connected with seventeenth-century French aristocracy and philosophical and religious 'freethinkers', libertinism came to be more associated with the sexual libertarianism epitomized in the activities of the eighteenth-century British rake:

> The libertine is sometimes interchangeable with, and sometimes distinguished from, the Priapean, the spark or ranter, the roaring blade, the jovial atheist, the cavalier, the sensualist, the rake, the murderous upper-class hooligan, the worldly fine gentleman, the debauchee, the beau, the man of pleasure, and even the 'man of sense'.[4]

Libertine men have been seen to be either *petits-maîtres* (or fops) or 'dangerous men'. The *petit-maître* is certain that every woman is subject to weak moments where she is more willing than she thought she ever should or could be and will succumb to him sooner or later; yet he also knows these moments are fleeting. The libertine sees a window of opportunity in the brief instance when a woman uncovers her desire, which he must snatch before she retreats, her pride unwilling to forfeit the victory of invincibility for carnal pleasures.[5] The *petit-maître* accepts with equanimity when a mistress tires of him and recognizes that he cannot take on any woman who is too risky, or who might cause him too much trouble.

The 'dangerous man', on the other hand, sees every woman as a challenge. This libertine 'measures his own ardour against the obstacles raised by the woman he covets'; he is a man more concerned with conquest and his ability to humiliate women.[6] Yet within this hedonistic lifestyle, he experiences a mixture of emotions: 'As time passes, the frustrated lover obsesses about his mistress, and thus believes that her long-awaited favours will bring him nothing less than eternal bliss. Thus, when his desire is finally satisfied, his disappointment is on a par with his wait: his fantasy, swollen with chimeras, suddenly deflated, while his pleasure, spoiled by his mind's wanderings and ridiculously high hopes, is soon transformed into repugnance.'

The degree to which eighteenth-century libertines fit these descriptions can be seen in the memoirs or diaries of three such men who wrote detailed accounts of their sexual activities: William Hickey, James Boswell and Jacques Casanova. All were libertines of their day, and all of them loved having sex with women. Yet not all libertines approached women, sex and love in the same way.

William Hickey: the Forgotten Rake

The memoirs of William Hickey (**FIG. 14**) (1749–1830) reveal a youth squandered on fast living and countless sexual experiences. Even from childhood he recalled his fascination with women, the first being Nanny Harris:

> Every night when the servant had taken away the candle, she used to take me to her bed, there fondle and lay me upon her bosom; nor shall I forget my sensation, infant as I was, at awakening one morning and finding myself snugly stowed between her legs, with one of my hands upon the seat of Love, where I have no doubt she had placed it, for she was as wanton a little baggage as ever existed . . .[7]

According to Hickey, this early encounter was to affect him in his adulthood and was directly responsible for fixing his attraction to women of 'loose and abandoned principles'.

Hickey was a plucky youth and took chances in search of adventure and

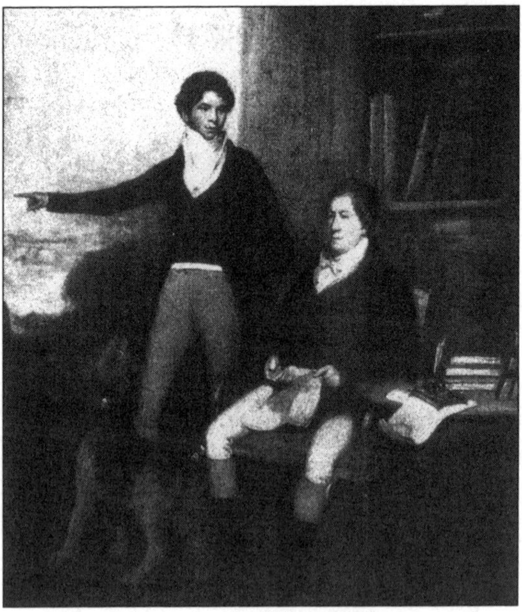

FIG. 14 Portrait of William Hickey, seated

sex. At thirteen, he accidentally discovered Nanny Harris's address. Determined to see her again, and armed with a guinea given to him by one of his father's generous friends, he went in search of her at her lodgings in Bow Street, Covent Garden. 'I told her the strength of my purse', Hickey was to recall in his memoirs, 'and proposed going out to the play, which she consented to. There was I, a hopeful sprig of thirteen, stuck in a green box, with a blazing whore.' A year later, around Christmas 1762, he had his first sexual encounter with a whore on the grass in St James's Park, in the company of a male friend. The experience was, on the whole, a disappointment but Hickey admitted that it could not have been without some enjoyment: 'I cannot easily describe my feelings upon the occasion; but undoubtedly they were not altogether unpleasant.' Later, with money dished out to him by yet another of his father's friends, he decided to retrace his steps and revisit Nanny Harris but by then she had returned to Ireland, much to his regret. He was to look her up again after her return in September 1766. She died a couple of years later from venereal disease.

Not easily discouraged, Hickey continued his search for sex elsewhere. As he wandered back to his lodgings in Westminster one evening, he was picked up by a girl of his own age in the Piazza of Covent Garden. 'You are a fine handsome boy', she said encouragingly, 'and too young to be walking in such a place alone. I'll take your maidenhead.'[8] Only too pleased, he followed her up a dark and narrow staircase to an apartment in a courtyard off Drury Lane. This was no doubt similar to the one which Dr Robert Willan* was to describe at the end of the eighteenth century, a place which only the poorest in London inhabited: 'a garret with a low roof and small windows, the passage to which is close, kept dark, and filled not only with bad air, but with putrid excremental effluvia from a vault at the bottom of the staircase'. Even the little bed was filthy but Hickey proceeded to have sex with vigour, she exclaiming all the while what a 'famous little fellow' he was. The state of the bed was typical of such hovels: '. . . persons of the lowest class do not put clean sheets on their

* The English Quaker Willan was a physician interested in skin disorders. He practised at a newly established public dispensary in Carey Street in Holborn but he made home visits to the poor.

beds three times a year,' claimed Willan, 'that even where no sheets are used they never wash or scour their blankets or coverlets, nor renew them until they are no longer tenable'.[9]

Despite his inexperience, Hickey obviously thoroughly enjoyed himself: 'In this den of wretchedness I passed three truly happy hours; and very different indeed were my feelings from what I experienced in the St James's Park scene.' He was, however, to receive a shock after seeing his shirt-tails covered in blood, unaware of the cause: 'The poor girl seemed to be in great agitation and distress, which increased my fright; whereupon she eagerly endeavoured to assuage my fears, assuring me no sort of injury would arise, that what I saw proceeded from a natural cause, though she had not been aware of it coming. She added that to avoid discovery she would wash the linen.'[10] Most likely the blood flow stemmed from the onset of menstruation. Girls such as Hickey's young whore, living in destitution, were often under-fed and generally in ill-health, resulting in erratic periods. It seems that Hickey was ignorant of the menses at this early stage in his sexual life and terrified that he might have hurt the girl.

Their encounter was evidently a success as he was to visit the girl on various occasions over several years. The two young lovers formed a casual relationship, their mutual fondness stemming from reciprocated generosity as much as from enjoyment of sex with each other. At first, the girl would not take Hickey's money, believing it was all he had. He eventually persuaded her to accept five shillings. On the occasions when she met him on the street, she would affectionately refer to him as 'her little maidenhead'. Even from this early age, women found Hickey's generous nature attractive.

By the time he was fifteen, Hickey had begun to neglect his studies and extended his sexual targets to include maidservants. One in particular, Nancy Dye, caught his eye, a 'fine luscious little jade who allowed me to take every liberty with her person, except the last grand one'. His father by this point had sent him to a boys' school in Streatham in the hope of making his son a gentleman. Here, Hickey had his own bedchamber rather than sharing a dormitory, and Nancy was able to visit him freely at night. Unfortunately, in order to reach Hickey's room, she had to pass through the dormitory where seven or eight other boys slept. One night one of the boys awoke, threatening to expose them both if Nancy would not have sex with him also. The chivalrous Hickey wasted no time in beating up his schoolmate for his impertinence. The boy exposed them anyway and, as a result, Nancy was told to leave the house despite Hickey's attempts to plead on her behalf. However, as Nancy retorted, she was about to be married and so no longer wanted their employment. Despite the fact that Nancy had a fiancé, she was happy to be fondled and take part in heavy petting with someone else, although she did not allow full sexual intercourse.

Fear of pregnancy would have been uppermost in the mind of a young girl like Nancy; if she were to become pregnant by another man, it was unlikely that her betrothed would marry her. In Nancy's case, it seems improbable that she would have been having sex with her fiancé. If she were, any pregnancy could have been blamed on him. Perhaps as well as consciously avoiding pregnancy, Nancy was saving her maidenhead for her husband. Apart from coitus interruptus and a few herbal preparations, there were few effective contraceptive methods at this time. Condoms were used mainly for the prevention of venereal disease, and sponges and douches, although popular among some Frenchwomen and higher-class courtesans, were not in common usage.[11] Hickey, on the other hand, makes no mention of any concern about illegitimate offspring. His only thought was of sexual gratification.

From these early escapades, it is obvious that Hickey loved women and saw them as equal partners in his amorous adventures. He was also not averse to showing other fellows the pleasures of the town. In one incident in 1765, after taking 'two fine West India lads' who were down from Eton under his wing, he trotted them off to London where he introduced them to two women. After an evening out at the theatre, they moved on to the Shakespear Tavern where they drank and ate their fill, only rolling back to the Streatham boarding school in the early hours of the morning.

Hickey's love of the good life extended to fine clothes. Indeed, by 1766 he had become something of a fashion victim, even acquiring the latest hairstyles. 'I was further gratified', he shamefacedly admitted later, 'by having my hair tied, turned over my forehead, powdered, pomatumed, and three curls on each side, with a thick false tail, my operator Nerot, a fashionable French hairdresser and peruke-maker justly considered the best in his line, in London. Thus equipped, I came forth a smart and dashing clerk to an attorney.'[12] No doubt, Hickey looked a picture but all this was costing money.

By the time he reached seventeen, he had cooked the books of the family firm in order to squander the money on his profligate lifestyle. After realizing funds from a substantial banker's draft which had been entrusted to him, young Hickey spent the money becoming hopelessly drunk, frittering away the remainder while keeping bad company. Predictably, in this inebriated state, he had his pocket picked. Awaking at the Cross Keys bagnio in Little Russell Street, he had no recollection as to what had happened to him:

> My first return of sense or recollection was upon waking in a strange, dismal-looking room, my head aching horridly, pains of a violent nature in every limb. And deadly sickness at the stomach . . . Getting out of bed, I looked out of the only window in the room, but saw nothing but the backs of old houses, from which various miserable emblems of poverty were displayed, such as ragged shifts, petticoats, and other parts of female wardrobes hanging out to dry. I next took up my breeches to examine my pockets; well stored as they had been the preceding day not a sixpence remained. My gold watch and appendages were likewise gone . . . I rung the bell I found in the room for the purpose of ascertaining where I had got to . . . No one answered until I had three or four times repeated my application to the bell rope, when at last a yawning man, who seemed half asleep, made his appearance, immediately exclaiming, 'Good God, how drunk and riotous you was, Sir! I never saw anything to equal it.'[13]

His adoring father was devastated by Hickey's extravagant spending and had long since despaired of his dissipated son. Hickey guiltily admitted to being 'a sluggard', keeping all hours in brothels and taverns and rising late. He regularly frequented Covent Garden, visiting his favourite eatery, Slaughter's in St Martins Lane, or one of his three favourite brothels in Bow Street. One of these, run by an old Irishwoman named Hamilton, was at the corner of a passage that led to the theatre, and another kept by a Mother Cocksedge.

Hickey's friends introduced him to Wetherby's, a lurid brothel-cum-watering-hole, notorious for its brawls. The entrance, a door heavily secured with bolts and iron bars, was guarded by a murderous-looking ruffian. To gain entrance, customers rang a bell whereupon a small hatch was opened and the ruffian rasped, 'Who's there?' Only then were customers cautiously admitted one by one. Once inside, visitors were confronted by a roomful of slovenly characters, all outrageously drunk. Recalling his first visit, Hickey described the debauched scene before him: 'I involuntarily shrunk back with disgust and dismay . . . Two she-devils, for they scarce had a human appearance, were engaged in a scratching and boxing match, their faces entirely covered in blood, bosoms bare and the clothes nearly torn from their bodies.' Here liquor was served until three o'clock in the morning, at which time Hickey and his friends would move on to another 'find', Murphy's (later renamed Marjoram's) which remained open until five in the morning.

Knowing that he was upsetting his father by this behaviour and despite vowing never to return to these dens, Hickey found himself back inside Wetherby's within a few weeks. He adjourned from the public room to a private one where he found his brother 'quite at home' with a 'poor wretch' called Blasted Bet and a singer, Burgess, entertaining them. Burgess had been one of the participants in the fight he had witnessed and so he immediately recognized her. When asked why she had become embroiled in the fray, she replied 'that both herself and her antagonist were exceedingly intoxicated, having drunk an unusual quantity of spirits, and in their cups had quarrelled'.[14] Falling further into low-life, he found two more filthy alehouses to frequent, The Soup Shop in Bridges Street, Drury Lane, and a shed in Covent Garden called Carpenter's Coffee House, also known as The Finish.

Hickey's debauched, extravagant high living earned him a severe reprimand from his father who, by this time, had decided to send him off to India in the vain hope of keeping him out of trouble. To this end, Hickey, still only nineteen, was shipped off to Madras where his father had secured him a position as a cadet in the East India Company. His mistress,

Fanny Hartford, a high-class courtesan, had done her best to steer him clear of the most disreputable characters in town, without much success. Since she was to remain behind, the two of them planned to spend their last night together. After an evening out at Ranelagh Gardens, they returned to her house in fashionable Queen Anne Street in order to enjoy a night of passion. Unfortunately for the young couple, one of Hartford's other patrons suddenly returned, expecting to find her alone. In a panic, Hickey dived into a cupboard to hide. Peeping out, he was horrified to see that her lover was a man he recognized, 'whom I knew was married to an amiable and accomplished woman, who had borne him eight children, all then living, with which wife he was on the best of terms; and they were by the world considered as a rare instance of conjugal felicity in high life'. Even Hickey, with his sexual broad-mindedness, found it disillusioning that such an apparently devoted husband might keep a mistress. He was distraught at parting from Fanny, both of them in tears at his leave-taking.

Having failed to make a success of himself in India and dissatisfied with a salary that was 'too contemptible to afford the common necessities of life', he decided to return home. Back in London, Hickey's father yet again admonished him, reminding him of how much the escapade had cost him. Unfortunately, this was not enough to prevent Hickey from falling back into his dissipated ways.

He frequented the most sordid of brothels and often chose to empty his pockets on the most pitiful and commonest wenches: 'There was an extravagant and common little harlot, named Brent, to whom I was strongly attached. She was not at all pretty, being much pitted with smallpox, mercenary in the highest degree, and addicted to drinking. Yet, notwithstanding all these failings, there was something about her which fascinated me; and often did I prefer taking her to Malby's, under the Piazza of Covent Garden, and there passing the night at a considerable expense, to partaking, as I might have done gratis, of every species of elegance and luxury, at the accommodation of Fanny Temple's, or others I have alluded to.'[15] He had known Brent before going to India and immediately picked up with her again on his return. When his father very nearly caught them together strolling along the Piazza, poor Brent, 'frightened out of her wits', insisted on returning to Malby's to avoid any further risk of detection.

After disgracing himself yet again and squandering even more of his father's money, Hickey was shipped off to Jamaica, arriving in Kingston on 27 November 1775.

Inevitably, as a result of his sexual liaisons, Hickey contracted venereal disease and was soon on his way back to England for treatment. His surgeon advocated the most common remedy of mercury followed by salivation. As a result, Hickey suffered from the awful side effects of mercury poisoning: 'my head suddenly swelled to an enormous size; my tongue and mouth became so inflamed that I could take no other nourishment than liquids.'[16] Once on the mend, Hickey had no scruples about having sex with other men's mistresses, including Madame La Tour (kept by Sir Peniston Lamb, later Lord Melbourne), and seducing those of his best friends, including Bob Pott's amour, Emily Warren, and Henry Mordaunt's mistress, Charlotte Barry. Whereas courtesans would generally squeeze every last penny from their beaux, many of these women he enjoyed without paying, mainly because of his convivial nature and his entertaining character. Hickey was a gentleman with a soft heart, a man to whom women warmed despite his rakishness. His generosity was demonstrated when he arranged a dinner for 'the distressed sisterhood' of prostitutes he knew. After hearing that the whore Lucy Cooper was in prison for debt and without a penny to her name, he organized a whip-round for her, putting down ten guineas of his own money. Other men followed and together they collected fifty pounds which probably saved her life.

But it was Charlotte Barry who was the love of Hickey's life. He proposed to her but she refused to marry him, although she consented to live with him. In 1783, they returned to India together to settle in his house in Calcutta. Soon afterwards, Charlotte's health began to decline; she became seized with 'sudden and violent pains in her chest' and, despite the doctor attending her, she continued to deteriorate and died the same year, leaving Hickey grief-stricken: 'When the cruel hand of death seized upon her, then it was I felt, oh most keenly felt, the horror of my situation and the dismal loss I had sustained in being suddenly deprived of so much excellence. Safely may I say, I truly, fondly, loved her, loved her with an affection that every new day, if possible, strengthened.'[17]

Despite this setback Hickey went on to enjoy other women. He took up with an earlier Indian lover whom he was forced to abandon after having found her in the arms of his native servant. She was followed by Jemdanee, a gentle and affectionate companion who died in 1796, followed by their son nine months later. Hickey prospered in Bengal and eventually moved back to London where he is thought to have died in 1730.

Hickey was a libertine with a sense of finesse who enjoyed mixing with the dregs of society as well as with the élite. He was just as likely to be found in low-life drinking dens as he was dining with the nobility. He revelled in the fashions of the day, parading in gaudy outfits and the latest style of wigs, but none the less had a taste for good food and fine wine. It is obvious from responses of the women he seduced – working-class harlots or higher-class courtesans – that Hickey was a bon vivant.

James Boswell: the Insufferable Lecher

James Boswell (1740–95) was another profligate whose life his Scottish family vehemently disapproved of. He ate 'of every good dish', drank 'old hock' and composed rude songs for a weekly drinking club, Soapers. A friend of Benjamin Franklin, Samuel Johnson and David Garrick, he was visited by all at his home in Half Moon Street, off Piccadilly. Boswell thought himself remarkable while also suffering from self-doubt, his insecurity contributing to displays of arrogance. His bullish behaviour was no doubt a factor in his lack of success in the art of love-making. After striving most of his life to be recognized for his literary qualities, Boswell regarded his creative output as so important that he nominated three trustees to oversee his will. The most significant of his many voluminous diaries, his *London Journal*, detailed his sexual philandering, turning up in an ebony cabinet in an Irish castle as recently as eighty years ago (**FIG. 15**).

Boswell had begun studying law at the age of seventeen, under the tutelage of his father. Lord Auchinleck had insisted upon his son qualifying as a lawyer despite Boswell's protests. Resentfully, but dutifully, Boswell buckled down to learn what he could in accordance with his father's wishes. No doubt in reaction to his smothering family, and certainly as a result of his blossoming sexuality, Boswell started to frequent the

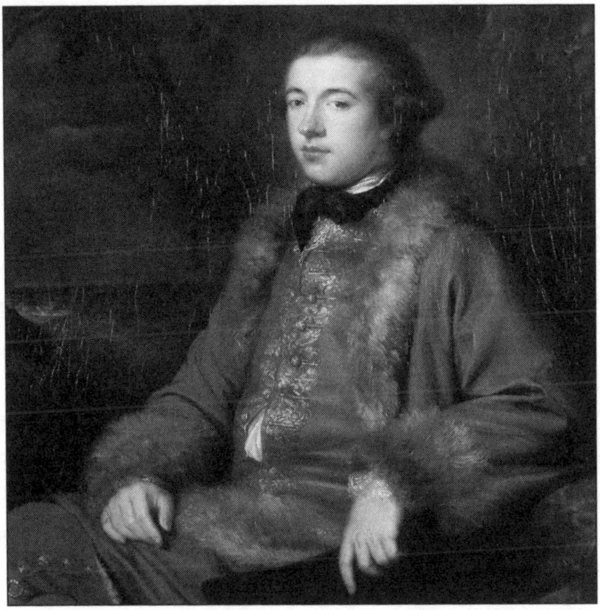

FIG. 15 George Willison, *James Boswell*, 1765

Edinburgh theatres, meeting and flirting with actresses. Here, he promptly (and unrequitedly) fell for the charms of the actress Mrs Cowper, a devout Catholic nearly twice his age. In 1759, having realized his son's extracurricular activities, Lord Auchinleck sent Boswell off to Glasgow University in a vain attempt to focus his mind on his studies.

Although mostly an energetic and happy-go-lucky youth, Boswell was frequently liable to bouts of depression and gnawed by inescapable anxieties.[18] Cut off from his entertaining friends and with little outlet for his pent-up energy, Boswell grew increasingly lonely and bored in Glasgow. In a fit of recklessness, no doubt influenced by the religious Mrs Cowper, after six months there he rashly decided to go to London to become a Roman Catholic priest. To this end, he rode non-stop on horseback for two and a half days – with four hundred miles between the two cities, this was no mean feat. Despite his intentions, no sooner had he arrived in London than he abandoned all notion of joining the priesthood. He became intoxicated with the carnal pleasures which the city had to offer and decided instead to satiate his lust. He knew that Sally Forrester, a young woman with whom he had had his first sexual encounter ('the melting and transporting rites of love' as he called it) was in London so he sought her out at her regular haunt, the Blue Perriwig in Southampton Street, Holborn.[19]

When Auchinleck discovered his son's whereabouts, he asked his friend the Earl of Eglington to take the young man under his wing. It was an ill-conceived idea on his father's part since Eglington was an unmarried rake, only too pleased to show Boswell the highlights and low-life of London.[20] The glittering scene of fashionable houses in town opened up before him as he was conducted around them and introduced to the Beefsteak Club, the hang-out of the libertines Sir Francis Dashwood and John Wilkes the politician. Still only nineteen, Boswell's head whirled with the lifestyle on offer. By the time he returned to Edinburgh, he had caught the clap and was forced to undergo a strict ten-week regime of treatment, confined to his family home and placed on a diet. Boswell was later to refer to his venereal disease as 'that troublesome companion and bar to my innocent pleasures'.[21]

Back in Scotland, during the winter of 1761–2, Boswell was indulging in various sexual dalliances. While publicly courting the respectable Kitty Colquhoun, he was also conducting a clandestine affair with Mrs Love, the wife of his actor friend James Dance (alias Love), as well as fornicating with his maidservant, Peggy Doig. Peggy was to become the first woman to bear one of Boswell's many illegitimate children. To his credit, he supported her, but, despite his seeming delight at becoming a father, he never saw his son, Charles, who died a few years later. During a jaunt to the Lowlands in 1762, he stayed at Lord Kames's house at Kirroughtrie where he thought himself in love with Kames's eighteen-year-old married daughter, Jean. Taking advantage of the fact that her husband was away, Boswell launched into a two-week affair with her. She grew fond of him despite her continuing love for her husband. Jean was able to clearly separate out her feelings for them both: 'I love my husband as a husband', she told Boswell, 'and you as a lover, each in his own sphere. I perform for him all the duties of a good wife. With you I give myself up to the delicious pleasures.'[22] Clearly a woman of passion, Jean would eventually be caught in another adulterous affair in 1772 with a young army officer.

Boswell declared himself in love with everyone who caught his eye, including a Miss Mackay, Martha Whyte, Peggy Stuart, Jean Heron and any servant that took his fancy. About Martha he wrote: 'I at first fell violently in love with her'; about Jean Heron, 'I was in love with the daughter of a man of the first distinction of Scotland'; and of a passing chambermaid, 'At supper I fell much in love with the chambermaid who served us who was a handsome girl with an insinuating wantonness of look.'[23] The shallowness of Boswell's declarations was reflected in the ease with which he dropped these women as soon as he had had his fill.

Prostitutes fell into decline at a rapid rate, many of them going out of business within a few years. Many suffered from ill-health after catching venereal disease, or sank into poverty as their looks declined. The longer they remained on the social scene, the more difficult it became to attract business as their clients sought 'fresh' girls. In November 1762, Boswell returned to London and went in search of his first love, Sally Forrester. Revisiting the brothel where she had worked, he discovered that all the women who had lived there were either broke or had died. His next call, to another ex-lover, Jenny Wells, in Barrack Street, was no more successful as she had been ruined by her own extravagance and had fled London. Boswell was astounded at the pace of the deterioration of the women he had once known: 'Good Heavens . . . what an amazing change in two years!' he reflected. 'I saw in the year 1760 these two young ladies in all the glow of beauty and admiration; and now they are utterly erased and worse.'[24] Five days later, still in search of sex, he had the audacity to try his luck with a woman he had ditched back in Scotland but she would have none of it. This was hardly surprising considering what little regard Boswell showed for the feelings of women. He had resolved not to pick up a whore, but then did exactly that.

> I picked up a girl in the Strand; went into a court with the intention to enjoy her in armour [with a condom]. But she had none. I toyed with her. She wondered at my size, and said if I ever took a girl's maidenhead, I would make her squeak. I gave her a shilling, and had command enough of myself to go without touching her. I afterwards trembled at the danger I had escaped.[25]

He had obviously expected the girl to provide 'the armour' or condoms rather than having to purchase them himself despite the fact condoms were still relatively expensive. Yet the threat of contracting venereal disease was a very real one and it would have been prudent for any man to provide his own protection, although this was evidently not the case judging from its spread in the city.

Boswell, unlike Hickey, treated the young wretches he picked up on the streets with contempt; and the disdain he felt towards women of his own class who married for money was the same as that he reserved for his whores. Of Lady Betty, who had recently married his Scottish friend Laird Macfarlane, he remarked,

> What an absurd thing was it for this old clumsy dotard to marry a strong young woman of quality. It was certainly vanity, for which he has paid very heavily. Her marrying him was just to support herself and her sisters; and yet to a woman of delicacy, poverty is better than sacrificing her person to a greasy, rotten, nauseous carcass and a narrow vulgar soul. Surely she who does that cannot properly be called a woman of virtue. She certainly wants feeling who can submit to the loathed embraces of a monster. She appears to me unclean: as I said to Miss Dempster, she is like a dirty table-cloth. I am sure no man can have the gentler passion of love for so defiled a person as hers – O my stomach rises at it![26]

Such was Boswell's attitude towards the female sex.

Out on the town one evening, Boswell and Laird Macfarlane were accosted by 'several ladies of the town' as they took a stroll through St James's Park. Boswell eyed up one woman with sex in mind: 'There was one in a red cloak of a good buxom person and comely face whom I marked out as a future piece, in case of exigency.' Boswell saw women purely in terms of potential sexual gratification; their conversation held no interest for him. Even with the women among his family acquaintances he was not moved to display any warmth. On seeing Lady Betty and her sister dressed up in their finery, he regarded them with physical pleasure: 'The ladies were in great dress; were getting into fashion and looked like the best idea of the Ladies of Kellie, daughters of a Scotch earl, descendants of the family of Mar. I did not think them vulgar but inwardly rejoiced at being in so friendly a way with them. However, after supper, they grew hot and showed a strong example of the Edinburgh women's roughness of manners, which disgusted me. They have all a too-great violence in dispute, and are sometimes put quite out of humour by it.'[27] Once women showed opinions of their own, and in strong terms, he became quite antagonistic towards them.

Instead, Boswell continued to seek out women of a lower status for sex. After an evening out at Covent Garden Theatre, when he had called backstage, he met and fell in love with one of the principal actresses, Louisa (Mrs Lewis). Louisa had lived the early part of her life dominated by over-strict parents. After absconding from her family, she made an unfortunate choice of husband, whom she then ditched for a life on the stage. Her first appearance was as the Queen in *Hamlet* at Covent Garden on 27 September 1762, later playing Mrs Ford in *The Merry Wives of Windsor*. At twenty-four, she was tall and handsome with 'enchanting languish in her eyes'. She dressed tastefully, looked genteel, had a good sense of humour and was vivacious. In order to endear himself to her, Boswell thought it prudent to tell her that he loved her: 'Madam, I can never think of having a connection with women that I don't love.' It is doubtful she believed him as she was probably accustomed to similar declarations from other suitors. He began to visit her regularly, chatting gaily, thinking, 'What delight I should have with her.' At this stage, Boswell was on a modest allowance and made it plain that he was not about to pay to have sex with her. Despite his meanness, she managed to wheedle two guineas out of him on the pretext of some debt. He boldly saw this as an open invitation to seduce her but Louisa had other ideas, skilfully parrying his advances. When he returned in two days' time she had thought up a way to confound him. 'Really, sir,' she declared, 'I have many disagreeable apprehensions.'[28] This remark was intended to throw him off balance and succeeded in that it left him uncertain about her feelings for him.

Louisa, an expert manipulator, had strung Boswell along for over three weeks. Boswell meantime was becoming increasingly agitated. During one visit to her house at the beginning of January 1763, by now extremely frustrated by his lack of progress, he forcibly barred the door of her dining-room and led her 'all fluttering' to the bedroom. Just as he was about to obtain his desire, they heard her landlady coming upstairs. By now, completely incensed, Boswell insisted that Louisa should come away for the night with him, arranging for them to stay at the inn of one of his friends, Hayward, the Black Lion in Water Lane, Fleet Street, pretending they were married. Louisa continued to be apprehensive and attempted to delay the event, 'Not', said she, 'that I have changed my mind. But it cannot be.' Boswell, in short, understood that she was referring to her monthly period, and that 'constitution forbade it'. He was of the commonly held belief that sex during the menses was not good for a woman's health.

Finally, unable to put him off any longer, Louisa submitted to Boswell's haranguing and accompanied him to the lodgings they had taken for the purpose of consummating their affair. She had employed the usual tactics used by courtesans to increase a man's desire. An occasional kiss to tantalize him was acceptable, as was the hint of something more. The most important part of the process was to ensure that he gave her as much as possible whereas she gave as little as she could in return.

When they finally ended up in bed together a month after their first meeting, Boswell was only too keen to fulfil himself. He was well aware of his success – 'my fair prize', as he saw Louisa, was 'in my possession' and about to allow him 'the full enjoyment of her person'. Smugly praising himself on his masculine prowess, he boasted, 'Proud of my godlike vigour, I soon resumed the noble game. I was in full glow of health . . . A more voluptuous night I never enjoyed. Five times was I fairly lost in supreme rapture. Louisa was madly fond of me; she declared I was a prodigy, and asked me if this was extraordinary for human nature.' She had obviously tired of sex long before he had, but he ignored her requests to stop. When she insisted that they go to sleep, he would not consent to it. He concluded gleefully, 'I really conducted this affair with a manliness and prudence that pleased me very much. The whole expense was just eighteen shillings.' Thus Boswell summed up the success of the affair with Louisa – how much sex he could obtain for as little money as possible.

As might have been predicted, from this night on, Boswell's feelings underwent a complete change: '. . . I felt my passion for Louisa much gone.

I felt a degree of coldness for her and I observed an affection about her which disgusted me.' He did at least admit to an 'inconstancy of disposition' but, unconcerned, he immediately turned his attentions to Lady Mirabel only to discover that he had contracted venereal disease. It began with the sensations he had experienced before – 'an unaccountable alarm of evil; a little heat in the members of my body sacred to Cupid . . .' He called on Louisa in order to blame her for giving him the infection. 'I have for some days observed the symptoms of disease,' he railed, 'but was unwilling to believe you so very ungenerous.'[29] It could easily have been a recurrence of the disease he had caught earlier but he found it a good excuse to divest himself of Louisa. She vigorously denied any symptoms herself, but, despite her defence, in Boswell's eyes she had become 'a most consummate dissembling whore'.

During the winter of 1763–4 Boswell went to study law in Utrecht, and while there he fell for Isabella Agnes Elizabeth Zuylen, known as Zélide, later writing rashly to his friend, William Temple, that he wanted her for his wife. During his Grand Tour through Germany, Switzerland, Italy and France, he met up with Rousseau, Voltaire and Wilkes. Rousseau had long been conducting an affair with his forty-five-year-old mistress, Thérèse Le Vasseur, with whom he had had five children, all deposited in the Foundling Hospital in Paris. Boswell had no hesitation in seducing his friend's lover, a common enough trait among the libertines of the day. After all, Thérèse had agreed to travel back to England with Boswell, so why not make use of the interlude? Boswell was, once again, delighted with his success, obsessively reporting they had 'done it' thirteen times before they reached Dover. But the compliment was not returned. Thérèse was sorely disappointed with his lack of finesse in bed, particularly with his coarse bedside manners. After their first night together, he again boasted of his prowess, to which she replied, 'I allow you are a hardy and vigorous lover, but you have no art.'[30] In Italy, Boswell was less successful; the women were not interested in him and he hypocritically condemned them as 'so debauched that they are hardly to be considered as moral agents, but as inferior beings'.[31] Instead, a pimp had to find him some lower-class 'willing girls' whom he could pay for sex. Boswell was also unpopular with some of his male contemporaries. While in Paris, he received a cool reception from Horace Walpole, although the amiable John Wilkes was to offer him a friendlier meeting.

Once back in Scotland, Boswell 'fell in love' with a gardener's daughter while beginning another affair, this time a woman from his own class, a Mrs Dodds, whose husband had deserted her. He set her up as his mistress, describing her as 'very handsome, very lively and admirably formed for amorous dalliance' while decrying her as an 'ill-bred, quite a rompish girl'. Boswell seemed unable to reconcile a woman's lasciviousness with her feminine allure, calling Mrs Dodd alternately 'a lewd minx' in jealous reference to her previous lovers, then lavishing her with affection because 'her eyes looked like precious stones'. Their affair continued on and off for some years while he continued to have sex with whores. He threw over his Edinburgh girl, Jenny Kinnaird, once he tired of her, despite having promised to live with her on his return from London; he left her with some money, but then asked his friends 'to promise to go with her and offer her a bribe to break her engagement to me'.

Boswell was an inconstant man, burning up with passion at one moment, dropping a woman like a hot coal the next. He continued whoring throughout his life, sometimes having more than one prostitute at a time. At best, his treatment of women was fickle; at worst he was a misogynist. He eventually became engaged to his cousin Margaret Montgomerie in August 1769, whom he later married. She bore him seven children, of whom five survived, and died of consumption in 1789 to his enormous grief. Boswell was to follow her to the grave some six years later, while in the process of editing the third edition of his major life's work, the biography of Dr Samuel Johnson. Like so many other libertine men of his day, although he had remained devoted to his wife, 'that valuable woman' as he called her, he was to continue his extramarital affairs throughout his life.

Casanova: the Suave Poseur

Jacques Casanova (1725–98) was very much the typical eighteenth-century man of the world. In his detailed *Memoirs*, he portrays himself as a dashing man, an intellectual with charisma and charm (**FIG. 16**). He could

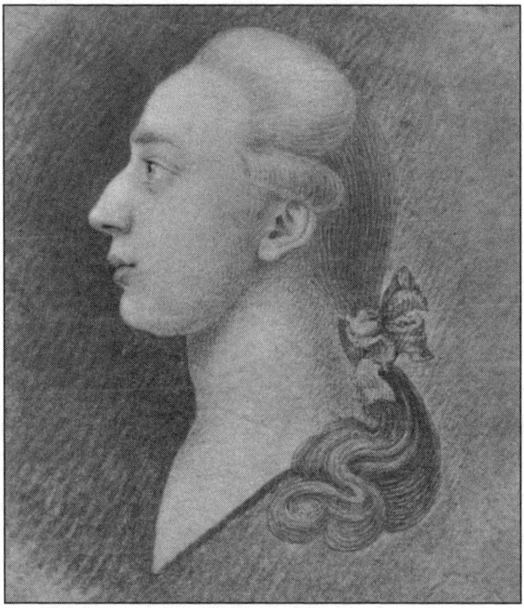

FIG. 16 Casanova

ingratiate himself with anyone; even the Pope succumbed to his magnetism to the extent that he gave Casanova a dispensation to read books forbidden by the Roman Catholic Church, which included pornography. His audacity and resourcefulness helped to get him through the ups and downs of his life and accelerated his rise into aristocratic circles. Frequently in trouble or in debt, he arranged hasty exits, climbing over rooftops and city walls, racing through ploughed fields, hopping into carriages or galloping off into the night to make good his escape. His salacious life would indirectly lead to his arrest when, in 1755, his wanton behaviour and impiety came to the attention of the Venetian Inquisition. Charged with contempt of religion, he was sentenced to five years' imprisonment. Unable and unwilling to remain confined, he made a spectacular escape from his gaol cell and continued to travel and have affairs throughout Italy, France, Spain, Germany, Holland, England, Poland, Greece, Turkey, Russia and Asia Minor.

Casanova was the opposite of Boswell – he knew how to manipulate a woman's intellect as well as her body. He knew about the psychology of sex and understood how to court women, talking to them, wooing them, and making love. He did, however, share certain characteristics with Boswell: his 'love' was passionate but short-lived; he frequently declared it but his affairs lasted only as long as his desire, or until another woman came along. 'I have always loved women', he admitted, 'and I have done my best to make women love me.' He was to bump into Boswell in Berlin but did not impress him: after the meeting, Boswell wrote in his journal for 1 September 1764, 'I dined at Rufin's, where Neuhaus,* an Italian, wanted to shine as a great philosopher, and accordingly doubted of his existence and of everything else. I thought him a blockhead . . .'[32]

Despite his reputation, Casanova was rather conventional sexually – he generally preferred his sex with a woman in a one-to-one relationship, although he did have a penchant for anal sex and occasionally enjoyed sex with two women at the same time. He attended orgies although he was not particularly interested in participating in homosexual activities. Nonetheless, Casanova would try out most things and did experience some close encounters with men. One homosexual experience took place in Constantinople with Ismail Effendi, the Turkish foreign minister, 1730–36, but Casanova, in his memoirs, is rather guarded in his description of the event. More graphically recalled was his meeting with the impotent Duke of Maddaloni. While they were examining some pornographic pictures together, Maddaloni pulled out his flaccid penis. Surprisingly, Casanova admitted that he was in the same drooping state but the unbelieving duke wanted proof and insisted on taking Casanova's penis in hand. Casanova was also known to take the initiative with men himself. When he met the beautiful Lieutenant Lunin at an orgy outside St Petersburg, Casanova was unable to resist his feminine charms and lured him into sex: 'After dinner, seated in front of the fire between [Lt. Lunin] and the French lady traveller, I told him of my suspicions [that he was a woman dressed as a man] but Lunin, jealous of the superiority of his sex, displayed the proof of it on the spot and, interested to find out whether I could remain indifferent to his beauty, he took hold of me and, believing that he found he pleased me, put himself in a position to make both of us happy.'[33]

* New House = Casanova.

Casanova's success with women lay in the attention he paid them and, to a certain extent, this was achieved through money. He believed that any woman could be bought, commenting, 'There exists no honest woman with an uncorrupted heart whom a man is not sure of conquering by dint of gratitude. It is one of the surest and shortest means.'[34] He had no compunction about bribing women with gifts in order to seduce them. While in Lyons, he encountered a pretty dancer whom he wooed with jewellery: 'The pretty Agatha had now earned her earrings. She was so gentle and so tender, and I was so much in love with her . . .' Like many other men in the eighteenth century, Casanova, was in the habit of treating women as possessions and was happy to trade them in. When a young earl, Lord Percy, fell in love with Agatha, he went to Casanova in order to bargain over her. He was aware that she was under Casanova's protection and aimed to swap his lover, Redgonde, for Casanova's Agatha. 'I know', said Lord Percy, 'that you have been very attentive to Redegonde, the pretty dancer. She is mine. Will you take her in exchange for Agatha, and what do you want over and above?' Casanova responded with mirth: 'You are as amiable as you are amusing, my dear lord, but you must own it would take a mathematician to work out this sum! How much does Agatha but value Redegonde? Redegonde has qualities, no doubt, but she is not to be compared to Agatha!' The infatuated young Percy was not to be dismissed so easily, however, retorting sharply, 'I know that, so I ask you to name your own surplus?' Unperturbed, Casanova agreed to relinquish Agatha without money changing hands, the whole affair played out as a game.

On 11 June 1763, Casanova travelled by packet boat to England where he spent the next nine months. On arriving in London, he went to the house of an old lover, Thérèse Imer, whom he had originally met in Venice in 1741 at the house of Senator Malipiero. She later married a dancer, Pompeati, and eventually became the mistress of the Margrave of Bayreuth and Prince Charles de Lorraine. In 1758, Casanova had come across her again, singing in Amsterdam under the name of Madame Trenti. By the time she moved to London soon afterwards, her fortunes had been transformed. She had become the fashionable Madame Cornelys, entertaining dignitaries at her stylish house in Soho Square. She threw twelve balls a year and continued her assemblies for over twenty years. She had borne at least one, probably two, of Casanova's children so he was deeply offended by her cold reception when he visited her in London, a rebuff for which he never forgave her. When she fell into debt, no one was prepared to offer her financial assistance. She was to die in the Fleet Prison in 1797 at the age of seventy-five.

In London, Casanova mixed with people from all walks of life. He gained his entrée to the aristocracy via an introduction to Lady Harrington; he met with the Duchess of Northumberland, Lady Coventry, Lord Augustus Hervey and Lady Rochefort, wife of the ambassador to Spain. The French cross-dresser Chevalier D'Eon introduced him to King George III and Queen Charlotte, while the twenty-nine-year-old bright spark Lord Pembroke, 'the greatest libertine in all England',[35] accompanied him to the Star Tavern in Piccadilly, a well-known brothel. He also frequented the bagnio of Mrs Welch, in Cleveland Street, where he met the notorious courtesan Kitty Fisher, covered in diamonds, awaiting her noble client. He was delighted at her extravagance and enjoyed the story of the hundred-guinea banknote she ate in a sandwich (although the amount varied from tale to tale). The London bathhouses were especially appealing to Casanova, as he could be entertained by loose women for a good price. 'In the evening', he recalled, 'I frequented the most select bagnios where a man of quality can sup, bathe and meet well-bred women of easy virtue. There are plenty of this sort in London. This entertainment only costs about six guineas, and with economy one can do it for four; but economy was never one of my failings.'[36] Despite his enjoyment of the social scene, he declared it impossible to walk anywhere in smart dress without the risk of being pelted by the mob with mud.

Having rented a three-storey house in Pall Mall, Casanova lamented that he had still not found a lover. He placed a discreet advertisement in the *Gazetteer and London Advertiser* on 5 July 1763, renting out a room where 'a small Family or single Gentleman or Lady, with or without a Servant, may be immediately accommodated with a genteel and elegantly furnished first Floor, with all Conveniences'. His intention was to reject all comers except for the prettiest young women who appeared on the doorstep. After waiting for some time, he had almost despaired of finding the perfect tenant when Miss Pauline, a beautiful Portuguese noblewoman, responded to the advert. They were to indulge in a brief but passionate affair before she returned to her own country.

But it was the ruthless Marie Anne Auspurgher, known as La Charpillon, who finally broke Casanova. 'The day I met this woman was an accursed day for me,' he rued. A young, beautiful courtesan, with a vivacious personality, Charpillon was turning the head of every man in town. 'Miss Charpillon was notorious all over London,' Casanova remarked, as she danced her way though extravagant balls, dressed up for masquerades, and paraded around Vauxhall and Ranelagh gardens. She piqued the curiosity of everyone who saw her and Casanova was no exception. He described her as 'one of those beauties in whom it is impossible to find the slightest physical defect. Her hair, of a lovely light chestnut colour, was surprisingly long and thick; her blue eyes languished and sparkled alternately. She was tall and slim, with a dazzling white skin; her bosom was small but perfectly formed; her white dimpled hands were rather longer than ordinary; her feet were tiny, and her walk graceful.' These attributes were qualities that made a courtesan popular, and small feet were found especially attractive.

Although her 'gentle face bore an expression of candour and openness', Casanova discovered she was a cunning minx in devising ways to entrance him. She refused his offer of money, saying she would only be won without bribes. 'You will obtain nothing from me by money or violence,' she rejoined. 'You may hope everything from my friendship, but only when I have found you as gentle as a lamb.'

Casanova had first met Charpillon in Paris in 1759, with the rest of the female members of her family, which included her mother and her two aunts. On a whim, he had given her a pair of expensive earrings she had admired; in addition, he had loaned her mother and aunts 6,000 francs, but both the women and the money had quickly disappeared. Back in London, he was invited to dinner at Charpillon's house in Denmark Street. Lord Pembroke was also present and he tried in vain to warn Casanova about her ruses. But by this time it was too late and Casanova was well and truly hooked. Wheedling her way into his affections still further, Charpillon went on to extract money and expensive gifts from him, while rebuffing his advances. She teased him, subjugated him and drove him to tears. In a pursuit that was driving him to distraction, she had cost him 2,000 guineas and she still would not succumb to his advances.

Worse was to come: after another visit, he was refused access by her aunt who told him that Charpillon was dying. Dramatically, he decided to commit suicide and went to the Thames with the intention of throwing himself in. Fortunately, a friend happened to walk by, spotted him and quickly talked him out of it, dragging him off for an evening's entertainment at Ranelagh Gardens. Once there, who should he see but Charpillon herself, bright-eyed and in the rudest of health, dancing the minuet. Casanova was incensed but finally realized he had been defeated. Not one to let such a rebuff go unavenged, Casanova bought a parrot and taught it to say: 'Miss Charpillon is a greater whore than her mother!' and took it out in public, much to the glee of the onlookers, everyone knowing to whom the parrot was referring. The unrequited affair affected him so much that he later admitted it was the cause of his sexual decline: 'I consider this as the end of the first act of my life.' Meanwhile, Charpillon went on to become the contented mistress of the politician John Wilkes.

Casanova sensibly recognized that he was not made for marriage, but lamented, 'If I had married a woman clever enough to direct me – to subjugate me – I should have saved my money. I should have had children and I should not be as I am today – alone in the world, and penniless!'[37] He went on to spend the remaining years of his life meandering though Europe and finally ended up as an embittered old man, employed as a librarian on a salary of 1,000 florins a year. Here, holed up in the huge chateau of Count Waldstein in Dux, Casanova scribbled away at his memoirs until his death in 1798.

*

Much has been written about libertinism as an essentially eighteenth-century masculine quality, its prominence encouraging the view of bawdiness in the Georgian era. Libertinism is thought to have been restricted to a small group of élite men, promiscuous sexual predators who followed the contemporary philosophy behind the quest for the pursuit of individual happiness. Yet the writings of the libertines themselves suggest that they were not a homogeneous group. The philanderings of William Hickey, James Boswell and Casanova show marked differences in their lifestyles and feelings.

Indeed, the only shared value between the three men is their love of sex – but they each perceived and treated women quite differently. Hickey obviously thoroughly enjoyed women's company, not merely their sexuality. He not only sought out beautiful, sensuous women but also liked to develop relationships with poor, pox-marked girls who had little education, with whom he was happy to spend an evening drinking in easy conversation. Amiable and jocular, Hickey was the sort of man who would have been agreeable and entertaining company for any woman. He was above the scheming of Boswell and Casanova and comes across as a pleasant and better adjusted individual who actually liked women.

Whereas Hickey saw his whores as friends, Boswell described the women he had sex with in cold, impersonal terms. He was boorish, conceited and displayed a lack of understanding of women throughout his life. Interested only in pleasing himself, Boswell wooed without refinement, as one of his lovers astutely pointed out, he lacked the 'art of love-making'. Self, and immediate, sexual gratification was Boswell's aim.

Casanova was a man who clearly loved women and kept many as friends throughout his life, but he also had an aggressive side. If crossed, he could be vengeful. He differed from both Hickey and Boswell in that he preferred sex with women of intellect, with whom he could have intelligent conversation. He preferred to have relationships where possible, although of course he would seize any opportunity that came along and by no means all his women were highly educated. As with his fellow libertines, he was not averse to showering women with gifts in order to gain sexual access.

Free from moral restraints, all three men sought their pleasures as the need and desire arose. More unusually, they recounted their lives in their own words and revelled in recalling their sexual experiences. Boswell, who aspired to literary fame, recorded these in his diary almost immediately afterwards and showed the entries to his friends. Hickey and Casanova wrote their memoirs many years after their sexual adventures had taken place. While Hickey wrote solely for his own entertainment (or so he claimed), both Boswell and Casanova, with characteristic boastfulness, wrote because they wanted to be remembered. Their reasons for doing so to a large extent reflect their personalities. Their fragile egos and self-importance made them particularly susceptible to manipulation by wily women, which in turn caused them to become increasingly impassioned by the teasing of actresses and courtesans like Louisa and La Charpillon. The behaviour of both men was suggestive of the libertinism of the 'dangerous man' and, whereas Hickey went on to enjoy his life, Boswell and Casanova ended up lonely and embittered.

Chapter Four

Memoirs of a Courtesan

> The following memoirs are replete with matter of serious reflection in every page, and in every line. They bear with them the internal evidence of their own authenticity. That they implicate many persons, in scenes, which they will regret to see laid open to the rude and garish eye of the day, cannot be doubted; but the editor's discretionary power did not extend further than style and construction.
>
> Advertisement for Harriette Wilson's *Memoirs*

Margaret Leeson, Harriette Wilson and Julia Johnstone were all celebrated courtesans who wrote their racy autobiographies in an attempt to cash in on their lives as the mistresses of some of the most notorious and wealthy men in society.[1] Their extravagant way of living was to find them frequently in debt, occasionally having to be bailed out by friends or lovers. No longer in the bloom of youth and their source of income drying up, through writing titillating memoirs they made a last bid to earn enough money to enjoy a comfortable retirement.

These courtesans operated within a certain social scene, connected to the affluent but beyond the bounds of 'respectability'. Their social status, their lifestyles and their working conditions were closely linked to the status of their clients. The role of a courtesan fell somewhere between that of a mistress and a prostitute. She sold herself for material benefits yet chose her lovers carefully – they should be moneyed gentlemen from the elite, for whom she felt some love or affection or, at the very least, sexual attraction.[2] Many courtesans were paid annuities by their lovers, while others had settlements made upon them, often as a result of springing requests on their lovers at moments of intoxication.[3] The mark of a successful courtesan was in obtaining a high-ranking protector and becoming a kept woman rather than merely serving clients from a brothel. Unlike lower-class whores, these women ran resplendent houses of entertainment where gentlemen went in order to enjoy sex, drinking and witty conversation.

Yet courtesans were full of contradictions: they had sex freely with whom they chose in return for money or goods, but aspired to the feminine ideal of domesticated womanhood. They refused to bow to convention, yet needed to establish a certain form of respectability. They frequently wrote diatribes in defence of their own behaviour, yet continued to feign modesty when the situation demanded. They would condemn the sexual double standard which allowed men, but not women, to have sex freely, yet they would just as easily castigate other women's promiscuous behaviour. They were ostracized from polite society but continued to mix with the elite: thus, part of the image of the courtesan was the high standard of living she maintained.

Peg Plunkett: the Vengeful Whore

> As my customers were very numerous, it was impossible for me to recollect each person in company, especially as in general they were in a state of intoxication, or at least so impregnated with generous wine as to lose their retentive faculties . . .
>
> *The Memoirs of Mrs Leeson*[4]

Mrs Margaret Leeson (1727–97), alias Peg Plunkett (**FIG. 17**), was a well-known keeper of an elite establishment in Dublin which offered entertainment and sex to members of the nobility. Her memoirs were published in three volumes between 1795 and 1797. Her clientele included a bevy of beaux, from lord lieutenants to lawyers and barristers and she led a life of luxury, overshadowed only by her inability to keep abreast of her extravagant spending. After thirty years in the profession, with her looks fading and her income dwindling, she decided to cash in her IOUs and retire, only to find them worthless. Finding herself in debtors' prison,

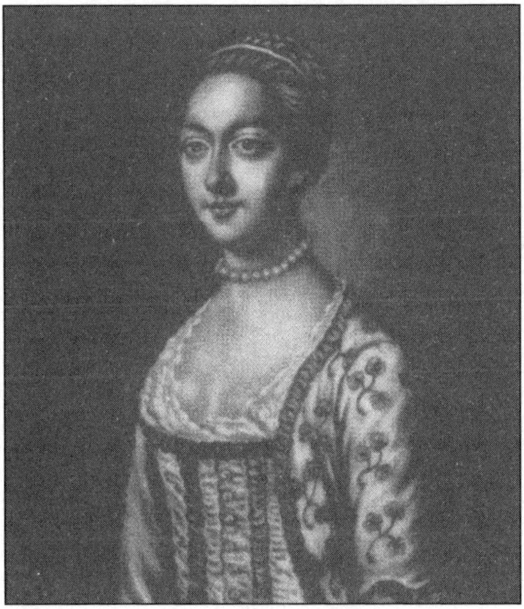

FIG. 17 Peg Plunkett

she wrote and published her memoirs in order to raise cash and to avenge herself on those who had failed to honour their debts.

At the beginning of her memoirs Peg disingenuously remarked on how virtuous they would be. She promised to be 'careful not to pen a single line or use a single expression that can excite a blush on the most refined and delicate cheek' yet enticingly suggested that her memoirs might be food for 'inordinate desires and fresh excitements', 'totally *unfit to be read* by any female of delicacy' and offered 'some *nice tit bits*, and *delicious morsels* of scandal'.[5]

Peg had had a difficult childhood; her mother died when she was still young. Her desolate father, unable to manage his own financial affairs, had passed control of the family assets to his son, a move which was to make the lives of Peg and her sisters unbearable. Her brother began squandering the estate and sometimes became violent, beating his sisters with a horse-whip on several occasions 'so that our bodies were often covered with wheals and bruises'.[6] On one occasion, Peg was so badly beaten that the sleeves of her riding habit had to be slit open because her arms were so swollen. Another time, after staying at the home of a friend after a ball, she recalls: 'I no sooner entered the door, than my brother Christopher fell on me with his horsewhip, and beat me so cruelly that I vomited blood.'[7]

In reaction to such an intolerable life, she flung herself into an affair with a friend of her brother-in-law, Mr Dardis, who set her up in lodgings, only to abandon her when she fell pregnant. Still very young and naive, Peg was at a loss to know what to do. This soon became clear when she met a Mr Caulfield who slipped her two guineas in exchange for sex. With no other offers in sight, she accepted his proposal to establish her in lodgings and she eventually bore his child. This marked the beginning of Peg's career as a kept woman. She went on to have numerous affairs and several children with various men.

In her memoirs, Peg viewed sex outside marriage as immoral and dishonourable. On contemplation of her first sexual encounter, with Mr Dardis, she equated honour with chastity, reflecting her own double standard: 'Hope was at hand, that that impudence might be amended by his marrying me, which I did not doubt his honour would prompt him to do. Yet what reliance could I have on his honour, when I had so weakly given up my own? A man's honour was in keeping his word of marriage, a woman's was in retaining her virginity.'[8] Yet despite her acceptance of chastity as an admired attribute in a woman, Peg railed against the stupidity of the notion:

> Chastity I willingly acknowledge is one of the characteristic virtues of the female sex. But may I be allowed to ask – Is it the only one? Can the presence of that one, render all the others of no avail? Or can the absence of it, make a woman totally incapable of possessing one single good quality? How many females do we daily see, who on the mere retention of chastity, think themselves allowable in the constant exercise of every vice. One woman may indulge in frequent inebriation, she may ruin her husband, neglect, beggar, and set an evil example to all her children – but she arrogates herself the character of a *virtuous woman* – truly, because she is chaste.[9]

She also accepts the premise that one fall is all it takes into the route of prostitution: 'if the smallest breach is made in the mounds of Chastity, vice rushes in like a torrent.'

After a number of affairs, Mr Leeson, whose name she was to take, offered Peg protectorship if she gave up her current circle of friends and kept company solely with him. At this time, Dublin was full of entertainment, with a nightly choice of concerts, operas, plays, receptions and balls. During a visit in 1731–2, one of Swift's female friends, a Mrs Pendarves, had recognized the fashionable pursuits that Dublin had to offer, commenting on its 'great sociableness [and] great civilities'.[10] But Mr Leeson whisked Peg away from the temptations of the city to live a relatively peaceful life far from the social whirl. Although initially contented with this proposal, in practice the life proved entirely unsuited to Peg who quickly became bored. Risking her security, she began to accept visits from two former gentleman friends while Mr Leeson was out. Although Mr Leeson had proposed marriage to her, this was not a state to which she aspired. '. . . I looked upon marriage merely as a human institution,' she revealed, 'calculated chiefly to fix the legitimation of children, and oblige their parents to breed them up and provide for them; to ascertain the descent of property; and also to bind two persons together, even after they might be disgusted with, and heartily tired of each other.'[11] Peg was contemptuous of marriage and concluded that polygamy, or a plurality of husbands for women, would not be an entirely bad idea.

Inevitably Mr Leeson discovered her unfaithfulness and cut her off. As luck would have it, a certain Mr Lawless (with whom she now realized she was in love) had come into his deceased brother's property and was able to keep her. They were to spend the next five years living happily together. During the fourth year, the affair started to disintegrate and the relationship turned violent. Lawless had started to go out to entertainments, leaving Peg at home, and both of them began to display fits of jealousy and anger. After a night out during which he had shown too much attention to another pretty women in their company, she upbraided him all the way home in the coach.

> When we got home, where we might make as much noise as we pleased, we became vociferous, in our contention till we were

> both nearly tired. I refused to go to bed, he insisted I should, which I still refused. He then cut the strings of my cloaths, and threw me into bed. I twisted from him and got under it; he, greatly enraged at my obstinacy, pulled me out, and in the struggle hurt me so much, that he was obliged to send for Surgeon Gleghorn, who found me so bad that he was forced to fetch in Mr Cullum.

Peg lost the child she was carrying, being four months pregnant at the time. In a terrible twist of fate, the couple went on to see their other five children die one by one. Later, when she found Mr Lawless drinking champagne with a Mrs Johnstone, she became livid; 'My jealousy was wound up to so high a pitch, that I screamed, trembled, and was quite beside myself. I snatched up the decanter, and was about to dash it in her face, when Mr Lawless seized and held my hands, and prevented me from murder.'[12] Finally, his finances exhausted, and their relationship in tatters, Lawless left her and sailed to America, leaving her pregnant once again. Despite his desertion, she continued to blame herself for his violence, and lamented the loss of their relationship.

Courtesans such as Peg were prey to such behaviour not just from their lovers but also from gangs of brutal young thugs prowling the streets of Dublin. Indeed, few people were safe from a group of upper-class ruffians known as the 'pinking dandies', 'deemed *gentlemen* by their birth' (another group, the Mohawks, would create similar havoc in London). Drinking until drunk, they assaulted whoever crossed their path and terrorized the neighbourhood. At night, they would rampage through the streets, attack the watch and break into people's homes. One particular night, the gang demanded to be let into Peg's house and, on refusal, they smashed all the windows, broke down the door and wrecked her furniture. Peg was assaulted and the child she was then carrying died through injuries sustained in the attack. Her other child, a little girl also present during the fray, 'was so frightened that she took a fit of screeching, and never recovered of her terror, but died in consequence of the fright'.

Peg filed a prosecution against them, in spite of threats from the leader of the gang, a Mr Balloon,* that he would shoot her. She battled on, threatening him that, 'I would keep a case of pistols in my pocket, and blow his brains out if he approached me.' The dissipated men continued to call at Peg's house attempting to intimidate her but she was successful in her case: 'At length, by paying high, I got Mr Balloon apprehended and lodged in Newgate.' His imprisonment for the murder of her unborn child resulted in a string of entreaties from respectable people, including his baronet brother, for the charges to be dropped, as it was possible that he might be hanged. She eventually agreed but embarked on a second suit for damages which she won.

Peg was the epitome of the vengeful whore. Never did she let a person off without an even or winning score. 'I seldom failed of not only resenting any affront or ill-treatment given here,' she admitted, 'but have taken the pleasure of avenging myself of enemies, in proportion to the degree of the offence.'[13] Another celebrated courtesan, Anne Catley, an actress, singer and comedienne (1745–89), was to become the object of her venom after she had slurred Peg's reputation in front of a gentleman friend. Peg resolved to confront Anne publicly at the first possible opportunity. After tracking her down at the theatre, Peg waited for her at the stage-door and, as Anne was leaving, bid her approach her carriage. She then rounded on her, calling the actress 'a little street-walking, ballad-singer, and told her I would have hissed at her every time she came upon the stage'.[14]

Peg was never deterred by a fight and took on Signor Carnavalli, the violinist and impresario who, together with musician Signor Giorgio, promoted a season of Italian opera at the Theatre Royal in Smock Alley, Dublin. He had decided to exclude women of the *demi-monde* from the performances and indeed had to some extent succeeded as some women 'like cowards submitted' and had left their seats on the previous night, at his request. Peg, scoffing at all who obeyed him, would have none of his exclusion order and went to the theatre to stand her ground. On arriving there, Carnavalli's door-keepers immediately picked her up and carried her out, fighting all the way. 'I struggled for some time and strove my way up,' she remarked, 'but he being stronger than me, took me in his arms and

* Richard Crosbie, brother to Sir Edward Crosbie, who was famous as Ireland's first aeronaut to cross the Irish Sea in a balloon in 1785 and 1786.

carried me back into the box-room, and on setting me down gave me a push. Irritated with such behaviour, I gave him a slap in the face, with my whole strength.' Her fellow courtesan was not much support but 'stood by all the time of our contention, with her mouth gaping' and not offering to give the least assistance. In order to ensure success in her revenge, Peg reined in favours from influential paramours: 'I went and consulted an eminent barrister, with whom I was very intimate; and pursuant to his advise, on Saturday morning, lodged examinations, and procured warrants against them for an assault, and for robbing me, by detaining the ticket for which I had paid.' With an entourage of bailiffs, she swept into the theatre and had Carnavalli and his two henchmen dragged off to gaol. At the end of the incident, Peg made a profound curtsey to the public gathered around, watching agog. 'Ladies and gentleman,' she apologized, 'I am extremely sorry to deprive you of the pleasure you may expect from this night's entertainment; but I have sent Mr Carnavalli, the first fiddle, to Newgate, and am now sending two of his domestics after him, lest he should want company or attendant.' And away she went, leaving them all amazed.[15]

Despite her steely determination, Peg recognized her own fallibility when it came to indulging in luxury. While living in Drogheda Street in Dublin with her closest friend Sally Hayes, she had attended an endless round of pleasures and, on coming to London, continued her path of decadence. Taking up residence in an elegant house at No. 4 Cleveland Row, she threw herself into the capital's wealth of entertainment. 'I visited every place of diversion,' she admitted, 'the theatre in winter, and in the summer I was frequently at Ranelagh, till twelve or one o'clock, and then to sup at Vauxhall, till six or seven in the morning, dancing, and drinking burnt Champagne, and sometimes even rioting. All the fine ladies and demi-reps, wondered where I got so many diamonds, and such variety of fine cloaths . . .'

A courtesan's life was a precarious balancing act between luxury and debt. All too often, a small misfortune could plunge a woman into poverty and she could easily end up in debtors' prison. This was the case with Peg – her money ran out after she had suffered an illness and her maid had robbed her. She found herself with just enough money to return to Ireland, so packed up and left, arriving back in Dublin with 'just two shillings left in the world'. Experienced courtesans were resilient, however, and Peg was no exception. Within a short time, she was again in the money, declaring, 'Living in splendour, enjoying every luxury of dress, table or shew, no matter from which source they derived, made me resolve not to quit the means of gaining an end. Thus, I went on in a circle of pleasures, one commencing where another ended.' By 1784, she was at the height of her glory, 'the reigning vice queen of the Paphian Goddess', extravagantly and elegantly furnishing her house in Pitt Street 'in the most superb and luxuriant style, with lustrous girandoles, branches, *elastic beds*, lascivious prints and paintings, and every matter that genius or fancy could suggest to the most heated and eccentric imagination'.[16]

Despite running her own flash house, she was astonished at the 'bare-breeched' love-making she encountered between a client and one of the whores, Mary Russel. Many couples kept some clothes on during sex so this couple's nakedness must have been wanton and unusual enough to mention. During their exciting entanglement the couple inadvertently set fire to the house. Peg described the pyrotechnics resulting from their sexual encounter: 'Miss Mary Russel, of Limerick, a dashing little girl, who in the height of their love feats, performed in the true Humphreys and Mendoza [well-known boxers] stile – *buff* to *buff*, forgetful of the candle, which was placed behind the arras, and regardless of the consequences, nearly perished like another *Semele* in love's flames; the bed, their wearing apparel, and all the furniture of the room, having been consumed to ashes, and they themselves, turned out of the house, like our unhappy parents without even a fig leaf to cover them . . .' (**FIG. 18**).[17]

Plunged yet again into the depths of poverty, Peg had had enough of her precarious existence. By this time, at the end of her career, she felt life had little left to offer. She attempted suicide, calling on God to help her, surviving only to suffer a fit of depression when she found herself once again in serious debt, the men to whom she had given her services having failed to honour their promissory notes and bonds of thousands of pounds. Even though her memoirs made her six hundred guineas, she continued to spend extravagantly, sharing her life and money with a companion, Betsy Edmonds, and was eventually taken to the sponging house in Angel Court.

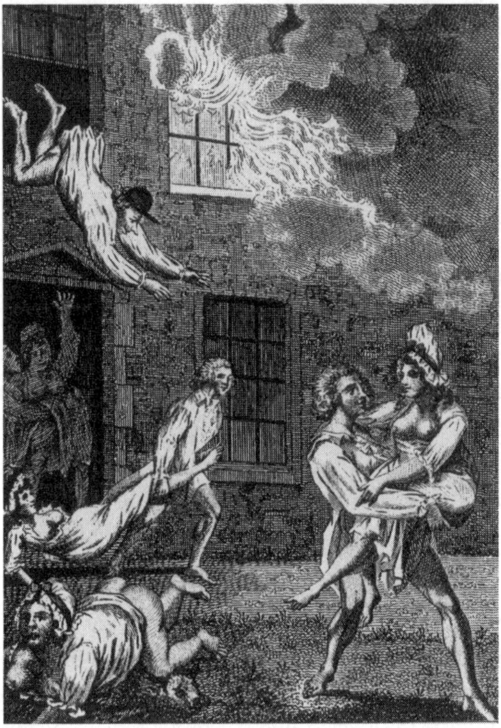

FIG. 18 *Amorous and Ludicrous Conflagration*, *Bon Ton*, vol. I, 1791

Following Betsy's death, which awoke memories of the death of her dear friend Sally years earlier, Peg was inconsolable. She eventually died on 22 March 1797 at the age of seventy.

Harriette Wilson: the Spirited Profligate

> 'Tis a pity so beautiful a casket should hold within it no gem worth picking the lock to obtain. She is all hollow as sounding brass, or tinkling cymbals – she has no heart for anything but flattery, fine clothes, and love of admiration . . .
>
> The Duke of Argyll on Harriette Wilson[18]

Harriette Wilson (1789–1846) was one of the most popular and well-known courtesans of her time. She was mistress to some of the most powerful and influential men in England, including the Dukes of Wellington, Argyll, Beaufort and Grafton. A somewhat vitriolic figure, Harriette (**FIG. 19**) published the first volume of her autobiography, *The Interesting Memoirs and Amorous Adventures of Harriette Wilson*, in 1825, with blackmail intent. Deprived of her pension by the shabby treatment of the Duke of Beaufort and with her looks fading, she was desperate for money. Her memoirs came out in sequential volumes, each issued with a warning as to what could be expected in the next, offering the opportunity for her intended victims to buy themselves out of trouble. The Duke of Wellington, on hearing that she was threatening to include a chapter on him unless he paid up, spoke the infamous words, 'Publish and be damned'.

Although some of Harriette's victims would be seen 'on the town' with their courtesans, others kept a more discreet profile, only visiting their mistresses at home. In any case, no reputable gentleman, whether married or not, would want his affair with a women from the *demi-monde* written up in a scandalous memoir. Harriette was clever in selecting her prey: all the men she included in her memoirs were wealthy and privileged. Not only did they need to keep a lower profile but also it would be easier to make money from them. Julia Johnstone, her friend and latter-day rival, criticized her, saying, 'Harriette Wilson will attack *no poor man*; for she can get nothing from him; – she will not expose many *single men*, for they need not care for her calumnies; but the wealthy and wedded, are her marks, whose money may be expected to bribe her silence, and many

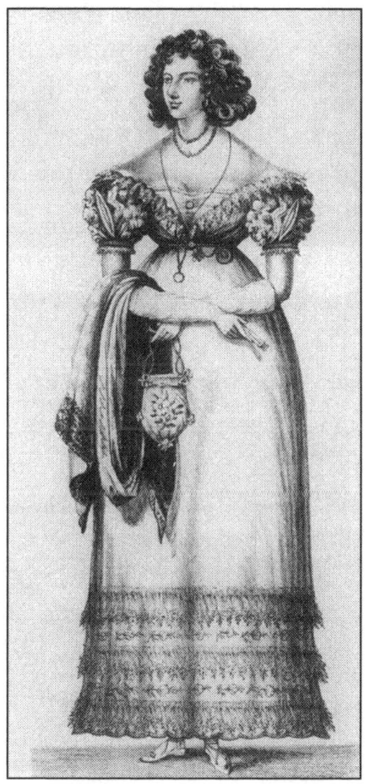

FIG. 19 Harriette Wilson

who have no more than innocently prattled with her, sooner than having suspicion sown in the minds of their wives and families, by her artificial insinuations, will, I apprehend, submit to her extortions.[19]

As a result of the publicity surrounding the books, relating high-profile characters and scandal, Harriette's memoirs went through at least thirty-eight editions and became extremely popular. ''Tis from high life, high characters are drawn' ran the publicity blurb for the thirty-third edition which sold in four volumes for 7s 6d. Her publisher, Stockdale, prefaced the various volumes with lists of the names of the men the author would be mentioning, bringing them instant notoriety. In descending order of merit, she included the King, the Duke and Duchess of York, Prince Coburg, the Dukes of Wellington, Devonshire, Argyll, Beaufort and Grafton; the Marquises of Hertford, Headfort, Londonderry, Wellesley, Worcester and Tavistock; Lords Craven, Jersey, Melbourne, Charles and Frederick Bentinck, Byron, Proby, Burghersh, Alvanley, Dudley, Palmerston, Lowther, Ponsonby, Carysfort, Bessborough, Bathurst, Deerhurst, Bective, and so on, through barons, counts, generals, colonels, doctors and ordinary folk. Yet, despite the allusions to her many sexual affairs, there is very little explicit detail in Harriette's memoirs, perhaps for fear of prosecution (although this would not stop the authorities from attempting it). Her only reference to sex itself is in her perfunctory description of her reconciliation with Lord Argyll: 'Our reconciliation was completed, in the usual way, and on the spot.'

Harriette was immensely attractive but it was her personality rather than her looks which often appealed to men. Walter Scott admired her quick wit and described her as 'far from beautiful . . . but a smart saucy girl with good eyes and dark hair, and the manners of a wild schoolboy' (**FIG. 20**). On publication of her book, he was to muse:

> The gay world has been kept in hot water lately by the impudent publication of the celebrated Harriot [*sic*] Wilson, who lived with half the gay world at hack and manger, and now obliges such as will not pay hush-money with a history of whatever she knows or can invent about them.[20]

Harriette had led the fashion in high society and was the toast of London

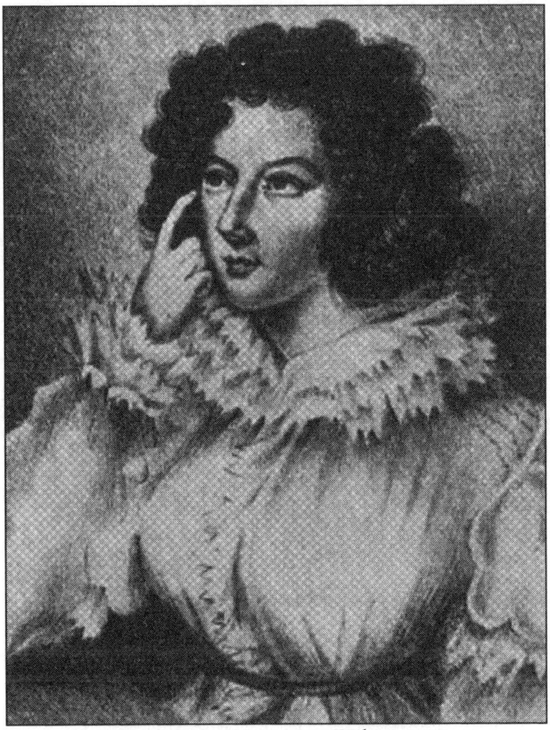

FIG. 20 Harriette Wilson

town. She held court and entertained in her various highly decorated houses and flounced her way through the ballrooms and playrooms of the rich. Julia Johnstone grudgingly admitted that Harriette 'must have possessed the *knack of pleasing* to a high degree'; she was without rival, 'supreme goddess in the temple of profligacy!'[21] Along with her sisters, Amy, Fanny and Sophia, and their friend Julia (**FIG. 21**), she threw a yearly event called the Cyprians' Ball at the Argyll Rooms in London. Over the years, Harriette led many a man a merry dance and squeezed whatever she could from her lovers to ensure that she was not left without a comfortable means of living. Tom Sheridan, son of the playwright, took a liking to Fanny, Harriette's sister, but regarded all of the sisters and their friends as flirtatious and insincere. He commented, 'Fanny is the sweetest girl on earth; but you are all a race of finished coquettes, who delight in making fools of people.'[22]

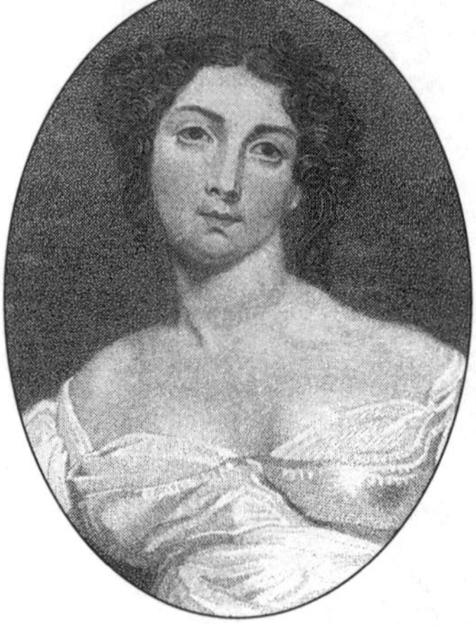

Amy

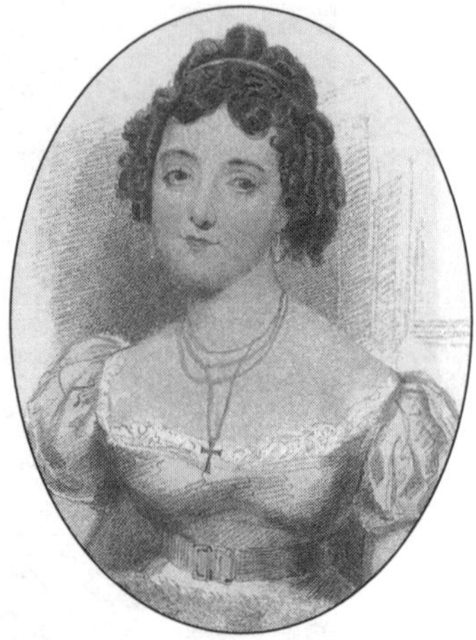

Sophia

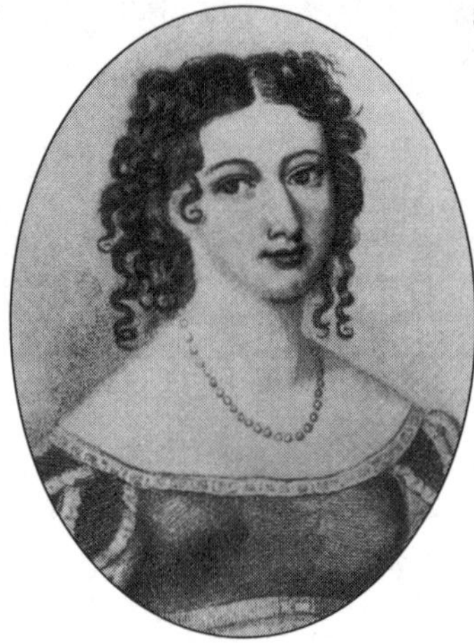

FIG. 21 Julia Johnstone

From her memoirs, we gain an insight into Harriette's background and how she first fell into the life of a courtesan. She opened with a statement about her life with her first lover, the Earl of Craven, musing:

> I shall not say why and how I became, at the age of fifteen, the mistress of the Earl of Craven. Whether it was love, or the severity of my father, the depravity of my own heart, or the winning arts of the noble lord, which did induce me to leave my paternal roof, and place myself under his protection, does not now much signify.[23]

Harriette failed to understand the initial attraction she had felt for Craven, remembering him only in a decidedly unflattering light: 'He was, in fact, a dead bore, and had no peculiar interest for a child like myself, in short I soon found that I had made a bad speculation, by going from my father to Lord Craven. I was even more afraid of the latter, than I had been of the former.'

An overbearing father might well have explained why she escaped into the arms of her lover. Certainly one sister had already fled, and two more sisters quickly followed suit. Harriette's father, John James Dubouchet, kept a shop in Mayfair and was an aggressive man; her relationship with him was poor but she was close to her mother. As one of fifteen children, Harriette always felt there had not been much money in the family, yet her parents had been able to give her a convent education and encouraged her musical skills. Their unhappy marriage influenced her decision in later life to avoid being attached to one man. 'My dear mother's marriage had proved to me, forcibly,' she remarked, 'the miseries of two people of contrary opinions and character, torturing each other, to the end of their natural lives, that, before I was ten years old, I decided, in my own mind, to live, free as air, from any restraint but that of my own conscience.' Yet, in escaping her domineering father, she made the mistake of choosing a man who was twice her age and whose fondness for drawing cocoa trees, sailing boats and wearing cotton nightcaps left her cold. Harriette was half the age of her lover and still in search of fun.

Her attentions soon turned elsewhere, this time to a younger man, Lord Frederick Lamb. On discovering her intrigues with Lamb, Craven dismissed her, not because of the affair itself but because of her lack of discretion. If she had kept them out of the public eye, Craven might have ignored her dalliances with other men. 'You might have done any thing with me, with only a little more conduct,' he told her. No man wanted to be made a cuckold, particularly by his mistress. Harriette turned on Craven, declaring that, if she had wished to deceive him, she had the wit to do so more successfully.

Although she loved Lamb and believed he loved her, he was a poor choice for he had little surplus money. For Lamb's part, he was unaware of quite what a handful Harriette was. Petulant and greedy, she demanded to be kept in the manner to which she had become accustomed, dramatically accusing Lamb in the memoirs of leaving her without means. 'I lived in extreme poverty,' she complained, 'while he contrived to enjoy all the luxuries of life; and suffered me to pass my dreary evenings alone, while he frequented balls, masquerades, etc.'

It is presumed that courtesans were outcasts yet they often dined in high society, in halls resplendent with oak panelling, portraits hung on walls over huge chimney-breasts, ceilings brightly lit with glittering chandeliers, the tables laid with china plates, lead crystal goblets and shining silver cutlery. Harriette was determined to retain a foothold in fashionable circles, and continued to share a table with titled personages, dining, along with Lamb, at Lady Holland's in Kensington. At such dinners, there might be anything from two to twenty-five dishes, with offerings including pheasant, collared pig, wild hare, fresh crayfish, other delicacies and elaborate puddings. Yet, for all the apparent glamour, Harriette was firmly entrenched in the *demi-monde*, not necessarily seen as 'respectable' but allowed to pass off as such if enough modesty was feigned. None the less, she did sometimes regret the kind of life she was living, observing, 'I thought of the youth I was passing away, in passions wild and ungovernable.'

Harriette quickly tired of the situation with Lamb and eyed up her next target, the handsome Marquis of Lorne (Argyll). She arranged to meet him in the park, flirting with him outrageously and encouraging his advances. She had the decency to tell Lamb what had transpired between herself and Argyll but, contrary to expectations, Lamb was delighted that other men found his mistress attractive. Harriette was obviously smitten with Argyll but, since Lamb had done nothing wrong, felt she should stay with him out of loyalty. She was also reluctant to abandon a man who was still prepared to look after her: 'There was a want of heart and delicacy, I always thought, in leaving any man, without full, and very sufficient reason for it.' Argyll would disagree, however, and, according to Julia Johnstone's memoirs, he declared of Harriette, 'She will try to please everyone, but him whom she ought to please most. She is one of those creatures, nature makes thousands of in a hurry; merely animates their frames with the breath of life, and then throws them upon the world, ashamed of her handy work.'[24]

In 1806, Harriette once again fell madly in love, this time with Lord John Ponsonby, a descendant of the Devonshire family (his grandmother was Lady Elizabeth Cavendish). Unbeknown to Harriette, he had been secretly watching her walking in the park from behind the trees: 'I came immediately in close contact with the stranger, whose person had been concealed by two large elms, and who might have been observing me for some time. I scarcely dared encourage the flattering idea. It made me wild.' After initially declining him, Harriette impetuously wrote to Ponsonby to encourage him. Although she had fallen in love with him because of the sexual attraction she felt for him, she saw herself as debauched, calling herself 'a poor fallen wretch'.[25] This attitude towards sex permeated the contemporary moral code, even forming part of the courtesan's philosophy. But Ponsonby was already married and, once his wife, Fanny, found out about it, the affair came to an end. Ponsonby offered Harriette a yearly annuity of £200 but, because of her feelings for him, she refused to accept it.

Harriette obviously knew how to instil jealousy in a man. According to her memoirs, Lamb nearly killed her in a passionate attack after they had talked for more than an hour about her liaisons with Argyll and Ponsonby, and his own earlier affection for her. He took hold of her hand and kissed her forcibly. She recalled:

> I resisted all his attempt with mild firmness. At last he grew desperate, and proceeded to be very rough, I may say brutal, violence, to gratify his desires against my fixed determination. I was never very strong; but love gave me almost supernatural powers to repel this very tiger; and I contrived to pull his hair out by the roots . . . he placed his hands on my throat, saying, while he nearly stopped my breath and occasioned me almost the pangs of suffocation, that I should not hurt him another instant. He spoke this in a smothered voice and I did in truth, believe my last moments had arrived.

Another lover, Captain Sir Joseph Nourse, remarked to Julia that Harriette swore like a trooper: 'Your friend Harriette is very pretty, and would make an excellent sailor's wife, she swears such good round oaths.'

Julia agreed, 'She had indeed got a knack of swearing by her maker too often, and I had often cautioned her on this silly as well as immoral habit. She thought it gave her conversation a zest, as olives do wine. Lord Petersham once said, an oath came prettily from her lips; and she has practised swearing pretty much ever since.'

Harriette and her sisters relied on each other for emotional support despite sibling rivalries and jealousies. Harriette resented her older sister Amy in particular and petulantly blamed her for her own fall from grace and that of her other sisters, Fanny and Sophia: 'It was Amy, my eldest sister, who had been the first to set us a bad example. We were all virtuous girls, when Amy, one fine afternoon, left her father's house and sallied forth, like Don Quixote, in quest of adventures.' The first person to address Amy was a Mr Trench, 'a certain short-sighted pedantic man, whom most people know about town. I believe she told him she was running away from her father. All I know for certain is, that when Fanny and I discovered her abode, we went to visit her, and when we asked her what on earth had induced her to throw herself away on an entire stranger whom she had never seen before, her answer was, "I refused him the whole of the first day; had I done so the second, he would have been in a fever."' Amy later took up with a certain General Madden who was often abroad. After the opera, she frequently gave gay evening parties 'to half the fashionable men in town'. According to Harriette, money played little part in Amy's decision as 'poor Madden had not a shilling'. Amy continued with her entertainments, often giving parties at Sydenham's house that lasted until three in the morning.

Julia Johnstone was even less flattering about Amy: 'Amy was a perfect jilt and a modern Messalina,' she remarked acidly, 'she received and dismissed lovers daily, nay, hourly, if that be all. She had neither delicacy of feeling – her sole motive for action, for debasing herself, was to amass money: in dress she was very extravagant; in her household affairs mean and pitiful; and her door was continually beset by tradespeople, dunning her for small sums, when she had probably a thousand guineas spread on her toilet during morning visits of her admirers – to let them see she was not comeatable but by prompt and large payments.'[26]

Courtesans were in a precarious position, living constantly in the shadow of poverty. Harriette pleaded ignorance in financial matters, commenting, 'I do not understand economy, and am frightened to death at debts.' After giving some money to Julia to pay off Harriette's debts, the Marquis of Lorne had remarked: 'She cannot be grateful, and would probably apply to me the saying, "a fool and his money are soon parted"; so mark me, you pay her debts yourself; if you give her the cash, she will go out and squander it on gew-gaws, and to-morrow be as miserable as ever.'[27]

A handful of courtesans were lucky enough to achieve security by finding a titled man to marry. After being seduced by Viscount Deerhurst, Harriette's sister Sophia, at fifteen, married Thomas Noel Hill, the second Baron Berwick, and became a countess, throwing off all her other lovers. Sophia's husband was to see through Harriette's extravagant ways in later days when, in debt, she asked him for twenty pounds, declaring that she had no fire in the grate and no chop in the larder. Berwick refused, remarking to Julia, 'I would have given her the cash . . . but I will not encourage her profusion; she would, in an hour, have squandered it on little shoes – little caps – little watches – little lap-dogs – and then, the little devil, when she rose tomorrow, would not have a little sixpence left, to supply her little wants for the day.'[28]

Harriette's elite clientele actively discouraged women of their entourage from entertaining the non-aristocracy. Fanny had been seen out riding one day with a 'sugar-baker', John Mitchel. Despite the fact that he had been to a public school with Lord Alvanley, the titled men in Fanny's circle were quick to tease her for mixing with 'new money'. While chatting about the incident among the women and men of their group, Alvanley discouragingly opined, 'I know who he his . . . Fanny is a very nice girl, and I wish she would not encourage such people. Upon my word it is quite shocking.' Fanny retorted that Mitchel was 'a very respectable man, of large fortune'. The men dropped some more jokes about 'the grocer', but, when the laughter subsided, the British dandy Beau Brummell added somewhat more seriously: 'But, Fanny, you will make a point of cutting this grocer, I hope?', to which Harriette retorted, 'I vote for cutting all the grocers and valets who introduce themselves into good society.' Brummell, who was a friend of the Prince of Wales, objected to this remark, pointing out that his father was a 'superior valet'.[29]

Violence was something the courtesan had occasion to deal with often, usually from lovers inflamed by drink and jealousy. Fanny was attacked by George Cooke, the tragedian, after she had been entertaining his friends by singing for them. Julia recalled, 'One evening, when she had exerted her talents in this humiliating way, the company expressed their admiration so warmly that her keeper became jealous, and actually made an attempt to cut out her tongue, and probably would had he not been prevented by others more sober. He, however, made a scar on her upper lip and cheek, which diminished greatly the small remains of beauty she had left.' Fanny and Cooke 'both drank and lived hard, and neither valued the world's opinion a rush'.[30]

None the less, these women enjoyed good relationships among themselves, drawing on each other for friendship and company. They frequently spent evenings together without the presence of male company. When Amy joined Harriette and her friend, Julia Johnstone, for dinner at her sister's house, Harriette declared, 'You are welcome . . . so that [*sic*] you bring me no men; but men I will not admit.'

'Why not?' Amy enquired.

'Why? because I am not a coquette, like you; and it fatigues me to death to be eternally making myself agreeable to a set of men who might be all buried, and nobody would miss them.'[31]

The women were happy to talk for hours together, sharing intimate gossip about themselves. Julia immediately reported to the other women when she first became pregnant by Sir Henry Mildmay; and Amy shared a tale with Harriette and Julia of how William Ponsonby came to be in her bedroom unbeknown to her and watched her undress while her mother was in bed in the next room. The women would also sometimes share the same lovers: Mildmay was to become Harriette's lover; Sophia would become the lover of Harriette's ex-lover, Ponsonby, and James Napier was passed from Julia to Fanny.

There were, however, limits to shared intimacies. A 40-year-old woman, Mrs Nesbit, who took a shine to Harriette, took her aside to show her an intimate problem she was having. With distaste, Harriette recalled: 'To prove her unreserved friendship, she took me out of the society of some very pleasant young men, into a cold, dirty bedroom, where she acquainted me with an affliction which had befallen that part of her person, which made it impossible for her to sit down without torture. I was very sorry, and duly condoled with her, of course; but I never saw the lady in my life before, and, if I had, how could I help her tremendous boils, or their very critical situation!' She added, 'I am not modest, as this woman is, thought I, according to the world's acceptation of that word, and yet I could not, I am sure do this, even with my own sister!'[32]

Frequent trips to the theatre were part of the working life of courtesans – to see and be seen was an important part of their advertising. At the theatre, Harriette, her sisters and Julia would seat themselves in a prominent position, at the front of the second circle of boxes. The two most popular ones were the Drury Lane and Covent Garden theatres. When the Drury Lane Theatre was rebuilt in 1791–4, after a disastrous fire, the opportunity was taken to create a more impressive building. With seating for three thousand people, excellent acoustics and a huge stage, exciting spectaculars could be shown using the new stage machinery to create amazing visual effects.

Harriette also rented a box for the season at the King's Theatre, one of the leading opera houses in Europe. Italian opera had become established early in the century: Handel's *Rinaldo* in 1711 was followed by English ballad operas, the most successful being John Gay's *The Beggar's Opera*. One evening while out at the opera, a certain Mr Meyler came across Harriette with Julia and one of her sisters. He meekly suggested that she might come home with him that evening so that they could spend the evening alone together, since he was off to the country the following day. This was evidently not to Harriette's liking. 'If you were going to the devil tonight,' she smartly retorted, 'I would not move till the Ballet is over. Besides which, I have twenty friends to see.'

On its publication in 1825, the first volume of Harriette Wilson's memoirs created such a sensation that people thronged ten deep and a barrier had to be erected outside the bookshop where it was on sale. Naturally, the memoirs attracted various critics because of their salacious detail. One critic declared the book not only libellous but detrimental to society: 'A more disgusting and gross prostitution of the press cannot be than the recent publication entitled "Memoirs of Harriette Wilson": it may very properly be called infamy exulting in its profligacy – or pollution seeking a retribution for the hire of its vice. This is the formidable precedent of the press! Is it not calculated to call forth the same offensive conduct in others, and to encourage them in the selection of any object for their attack, however innocent of the participation of their vice?'[33]

The book caused such a sensation that Harriette had to flee to Paris to avoid prosecution. From there, in December 1826, she wrote to her publisher Stockdale with fashionable titbits including Parisian gossip for his newspaper *Stockdale's Budget*. Commenting on the feigned virtue and hypocrisy of Parisian women, she observed:

> There, no doubt, are modest women, in Paris, as elsewhere. I only remark on those, who, while, incessantly, changing their favourites, and intriguing with whatever they meet, to their taste, are still called modest women, and mix in the first circles. As long as they will be hypocrites, in public, refusing, even, on a rainy night, to step into the carriage of the very man, whom they slyly slept with, the night before; and though these ladies are known for what they really are, they are, nevertheless, considered femmes honéttes [correct females] until they no longer affect that virtue, which they, in reality, never possessed.

A woman in France might have forty intrigues one year and not be excluded from society so long as she remained discreet. Harriette acknowledged that a similar sexual code of practice was in operation in England:

> A man who should give the slightest reason, in public, for supposing that he had intrigued with a lady, would be voted the most ill-bred, stupid, low creature, alive, though every person, in the room, had known, for years, what had been going on, between the parties. In short, though there are more points of etiquette required to be observed, in England, the neglect, or the slightest infringement of any of those, which the French might

> consider of consequence, is punished with more severity of contempt, in Paris, than in London.[34]

In later life, Harriette's past lovers clubbed together to provide a dowry to enable her to marry a Colonel William Henry Rochfort, rake and adventurer. She allegedly wrote two novels, *Paris Lions and London Tigers* and *Clare Gazul*, but it is doubtful that she had much, if any, hand in them. She returned to London to live, before dying there in 1846. Her sister Fanny, who had lived as Mrs Parker, was helped out by Lord Hertford in her final hours. Amy, having spurned Count Palmella and his £200 a month, married a disreputable musician, Robert Nicholas Charles Bochsa but her end is unknown. Sophia, who became the Countess of Berwick, survived to the ripe old age of eighty-one, dying on 29 August 1875.

Julia Johnstone: the Dishonourable Prude

> Since the appearance of that scandalous work, 'Harriette Wilson's Memoirs', I have suffered much by my own reflections and those of my friends: she has calumniated me whenever she has mentioned my name, and appears to delight in reducing all to her own disgusting level. Though I have fallen, it is not certainly beneath my own good opinion, nor am I so lost as to despise the censure, or be indifferent to the approbation of the wise and the good.
>
> *Confessions of Julia Johnstone* (1825)[35]

Julia Johnstone was Harriette Wilson's former friend and rival and, much to her chagrin, not quite as successful as Harriette. She prided herself in being more honourable than Harriette as she had fewer lovers, but in truth, she was not as sexually alluring. Alleging to have written her memoirs in response to Harriette's condemnation of her, 'because I have a character to vindicate, and a great regard for my friends', she asserts that she had been entreated by them to write the book to clear her own name and theirs. She judges herself of good character: 'my feeling shall never overpower my impartiality, nor shall the tenderest ties cause me to swerve from truth.'[36] For this reason, despite her intentions, Julia inevitably comes across as a prig.

Julia's family was not rich but she came from a well-connected background; her mother was a maid of honour to Queen Charlotte. Like Harriette, her confessions begin with a quick dismissal of her family: 'I shall dispose of my family very briefly as they disposed of their Julia in her early days . . . my father I never saw – he died abroad in embarrassed circumstances; it was a love-match betwixt him and my mother – like all early love-matches, it proved unhappy. My father most cruelly – but, no matter – at least it is no matter to the public – and over a parent's errors, however greatly a child may have suffered from them, she is bound to draw the veil of Christian charity.'[37]

Julia's mother managed to send her to a boarding school near Eton. From there, she went to a convent in the South of France where the Lady Abbess was somewhat laissez-faire in her educative principles; 'she had no religious prejudices, and paid no attention to her boarders – their morals and education were alike neglected.' Julia's description, to some extent, echoed popular images of Catholic convents and boarding schools. Both were seen to be hotbeds of vice, places where young girls might be sexually corrupted, or at the very least introduced to lascivious reading materials or the practice of flagellation. Despite the school's lack of rigour, Julia 'learnt to read novels, dance with grace and elegance – to play tolerably on various instruments – and dream of love when I knew of it no more than the name'.[38]

Julia blamed her downfall on her unsupportive parents. She believed her mother had never loved her and, after leaving home, never saw her again. She was sent to live with a Colonel and Mrs Cotton, 'abandoned to the care of strangers at the most critical period of a girl's existence', as Julia put it. Mrs Cotton proved to have a dreadful temper and a 'repulsive manner'. But her husband, Colonel Cotton, no doubt only too pleased to have an attractive young woman to show off, introduced Julia to balls and the social scene. She was sixteen and just ripe for sexual advances from the attentive colonel. Not having been shown affection before, Julia found it easy to fall in love with him: '. . . passions, though not wild as the wave, [were] certainly too strong for me to keep under control without the advice of a friendly monitor', Julia excused herself. 'I must have been more than mortal to have withstood temptation.'[39]

Julia was not so much a seduced victim as a willing partner in adultery. Unfortunately, her affair with Cotton was to ruin her reputation, leaving her with no option but to retire from polite society. Luckily, she had inherited some money and was able to support herself and rent a small cottage within reach of London where she lived 'in the closest retirement, for over eight years'. Although Cotton might have little money, he did care for her, according to Harriette. 'I never saw such romantic people,' she commented, 'after nine years and five children.' However, Julia denied this rosy picture and saw her predicament as an error of moral judgement on her part: 'I saw, in the fullest extent, the crime I was committing in living with my seducer',[40] a surprising position to take as she had been left with little alternative. Financial aspirations could hardly have played a part in Julia's choice of partner, for according to Harriette, 'Cotton had not a shilling to spare for the support of Julia's children', yet she was falling pregnant once every eleven months. She often vainly applied to her parents for financial help, as well as to her uncle, Lord Carysfort, 'who only wrote to her with reproaches'. At one stage she was so deeply in debt that, as Harriette recalled, 'Julia assured us she was, at that moment actually in expectation of being arrested; and she entreated that Fanny or I would make an application to some of her noble relations, which she promised to do.'[41]

Julia exposed herself as a hypocrite. She was more interested in relating lurid tales about Harriette than in writing about her own lovers. She questioned the reputation of both Amy and Harriette, alleging that Amy had had an earlier affair with a 'dusty miller' and that Harriette had had four lovers even before Lamb, including a liaison with a young waterman. Yet, despite her castigations of the other women for their sexual intrigues, she also railed against the double standard. 'The world is very uncharitable! man may commit an hundred deviations from the path of rectitude yet he still can return, every one invites him,' she complained bitterly; 'in sober truth, he gains an éclat by his failings, that establish him on the Ton, and make him envied, instead of pitied or despised. But woman, when she makes one false step, can retrieve it no more!'[42]

Harriette saw Julia as a detached and brittle character: 'her heart, unlike mine, was as cold as her imagination was warm.' According to Harriette,

Julia had little by way of sexual charisma. 'The men were so rude as often to suffer her to follow us, by herself, without offering their arms to conduct her to the carriage.' She was short-sighted and shy, and 'not being very young, nobody would be at the trouble of finding out what she was.' When Fanny, Harriette's sister, informed Harriette that she was to give up her own house to live with Julia, she told her forlornly, 'I would prefer living alone . . . Julia is so dull, [but] my paying half her rent will be of service to her.'[43]

In return, Julia condemned Harriette as insincere and flighty: 'her lovers she threw off as indifferently as her shoes – or trampled on them without compunction.' According to Julia, Lord Craven turned Harriette out of his house after catching her with his servant. 'She forgot to say her sudden dismissal from my cottage at Greenwich', proclaimed Julia, 'was because I caught her on the knee of my black footman, Mungo, and I bundled *black* and *white*, into the coach together to seek their fortunes.' Elaborating, Julia recalled,

> A black man frequently called with letters for Harriette, which she pretended were from her mother. I knew well that the poor woman could not afford even to hire a black servant for a day, she at that time living by grafting stockings, a business which, in her *home-days*, had often soiled the fair hands of the alabaster skinned Miss Wilson . . . She used to take this fellow of the breed of Cain upstairs; and I once heard a report in the neighbourhood, that she had been seen with him in the gardens and shady walks near Chalk Farm, but I treated it at the time with contempt. Since the explanation given me by my Lord Craven, of the reason why he dismissed Harriette so suddenly . . . I am, of course, thoroughly convinced, that a most disgusting and improper intimacy subsisted betwixt this lady of fine feelings and her Mungo. [44]

In Amy, Julia saw 'a fine woman, with a Siddonian countenance, and a masculine spirit', but Fanny was 'a poor timid, good-natured thing, capable of doing either harm or good, she scarcely knew the distinction betwixt virtue and vice'. She condemned them both as being 'without any fixed principal [*sic*], except that of self interest'. She accused Amy of being 'proud and avaricious', yet Julia lacked the independence of spirit of Harriette and her sisters, which left her jealous and embittered. She failed to spread her affections in order to ensure financial security, as other courtesans had done, relying too heavily on Cotton who was eventually to desert her. Amy had shown shrewdness when she inveigled the first gentleman she lived with to settle on her an annuity of one hundred pounds per year for life, swearing never to leave him. Julia portrayed Amy's actions as ingratitude as she described how Amy had left an old gentleman, her ex-lover, in his coach to be dropped at General Madden's door, sending back a message with the footman. 'Tell the old fool I have done with him, and shall see him no more.'[45]

Although these women conducted a series of intrigues, the sexual etiquette of the day demanded discretion. Affairs were not to be too obviously aired or too easily admitted and sexual activities had to remain hidden. Harriette adamantly denied any intrigue with Captain Nourse despite Julia's discovery of a silver-mounted penknife inscribed with Nourse's name in Harriette's bedroom. Julia's attention was directed 'to a *certain place* [the bed], where all was in complete confusion'. After checking the bed for proof of the act having taken place, and having her suspicions confirmed, she approached Harriette the next morning. Harriette was most embarrassed and annoyed that Julia had discovered her dalliance with Nourse: 'Next morning at breakfast I drew the knife from my reticule, and observed where I had found it. The lady's cheeks reddened like fire; after some hesitation, she "recollected borrowing it from the gallant captain to cut her boot lace". "I scorn your suspicions," exclaimed the fiery little meteor, "and would have you know I am the mistress of my own actions, and will not be schooled like a child."'[46]

Although some courtesans tried to escape financial insecurity through marriage, it was generally a status to be scoffed at and extramarital affairs were accepted as normal. Julia, on enquiring as to Sir Charles's lamenting references to 'dear little Mary Cox', asked:

' "Is she dead then?"

' "Worse, worse than that; she is married."

' "Oh, that ought to be no obstacle," I ventured to observe.'

The fate of the lower-class whores was often much worse, however. A female servant of Harriette's ended up in one of the Magdalene houses. 'This wretched poor woman had been on the town for a year or two, and undergone the discipline of the Magdalen charity, and got foisted by some of the members upon the public as a reformed woman,' Julia noted; 'they get into service by recommendations from the subscribers by a series of false characters. This woman had been dismissed from Brocket Hall, for stealing a cream ewer; and she met Harriette at Knight's Tavern in Jermyn-street, where she often called in disguise with some of her paramours.'[47]

Julia painted a cruel portrait of Harriette at forty-three:

> No tightening of the waist, to show *the figure* of the wearer, nor any ornament to be seen whatever. Her figure, at a short distance, might not inaptly [*sic*] be compared to a mile-stone, with a carter's hat resting on its summit. Her once little feet, now covered with *list shoes*, to defend them from attacks of desultory gout, which she has suffered by in both extremities. Her *face*, at the time I allude to, was swollen with this disorder almost to distortion. She has *no colour: le couleur de rose a disparu*, and in its place appears a kind of dingy lilac, which spreads all over her once bright countenance, and appears burnt into her lips. The *crow's feet* are wide spreading beneath her eyes.[48]

Unkind descriptions of Harriette and her sisters litter Julia's memoirs and are the liveliest part of her otherwise dull life story. Julia also shows herself to be disloyal and dislikeable in such behaviour as informing Harriette's lovers about her other affairs, well knowing that Harriette would lose her income from them. She has few excitements of her own to recall; any success she enjoyed with her writing was gained on the back of Harriette's sparkling memoirs.

*

All three courtesans explore the same themes and address similar concerns in their memoirs. They all describe their family backgrounds and their unhappy childhoods. They blame early loss of parental care or tyrannical male family members for forcing them into the arms of their first lovers. Lacking family protection, they had been placed in a position beyond their control, where they had to become mistresses rather than wives. Their fall from virtue – a matter of concern for courtesans, reflected in contemporary anxieties about 'fallen women' – led to frequent railings on chastity and condemnation of the double standard of sexual morality for men and women. All three writers wanted to make clear the reasons for their downfall and to distance themselves from blame.

Their education allowed them to reach a higher social status than would otherwise have been possible and to become companions to richer clients. They managed to present themselves as 'ideal' women while remaining sexually available. Thus the memoirs display direct contradictions: the courtesans had to project an image of respectability in order to attract their wealthy clients, while actually having sex with them in return for money or expensive gifts.

The extravagant and often passionate natures of the courtesans are illustrated by their insecure lifestyles, oscillating between luxury and debtors' prison. Yet frequently we see these courtesans putting love before money. They often left rich men for men they loved or found attractive. Peg left a wealthy Mr Leeson for Mr Lawless who was broke. Harriette left Craven for the impecunious Lamb. Julia succumbed to Cotton who was certainly not affluent. Extravagant behaviour was second nature to them and action by debtors not uncommon. All three became embittered when spurned by their true loves: Peg was deserted by Lawless; Harriette was cast off by Ponsonby; and Julia was abandoned by Cotton. Once rejected, they became increasingly cynical about men and marriage. However, unlike Julia, Harriette and Peg retained their sense of humour.

Excitement, commotion and disturbance were all part of the volatile lifestyle described in their memoirs. Men rapping violently on doors, declarations of unending love, jealous outbursts and indignant whippings were everyday occurrences. Displays of anger and denial of affairs were necessary in order to salvage a reputation. Lecherous men, seduction techniques, secret trysts, amatory advances and passionate machinations were all part of the imagery in a new genre of bestseller depicting the daring adventures of the courtesan.

Yet the most significant motive of the memoirs is that they were written out of revenge; they allowed these women to humiliate the men who had let them down, and to rail against a society that had failed them. They are full of condemnations of the double standard and vilification about the hypocrisies of men. Furthermore, unlike the memoirs of men, courtesans rarely wrote in any detail about sex. Neither do they mention their enjoyment of sex. Their chief pleasures in life were the wealth, power and independence which sex brought them.

Chapter Five

The Monks of Medmenham

Whilst Womanhood in habit of nun
At Medmenham lies, by backward monks undone.
Charles Churchill (1732–64)[1]

The libertine Sir Francis Dashwood held various important eighteenth-century political offices including Treasurer of the Chamber, Chancellor of the Exchequer to George III, Keeper of the Great Wardrobe and Joint Postmaster-General. He also established one of the most notorious hell-fire clubs of the century at Medmenham Abbey in Buckinghamshire and became renowned for his libidinous lifestyle. On the subject of Dashwood's sexual prowess, the politician Horace Walpole remarked, '[he has] the staying power of a stallion and the impetuosity of a bull'.[2] His sexual antics, along with those of his friends, became both the source and the subject of many an erotic tale, with anecdotes being frequently related and lascivious poems emanating from his circle.

From his early life, Dashwood had shown an inclination for controversy (**FIG. 22**). Between 1729 and 1731, he embarked on a Grand Tour of Europe, a standard part of any young gentleman's education, during which he managed to upset the Roman Catholic Church and terrorize its worshippers. Sir Francis was chaperoned by a strict and rather conventional tutor, Lord Westmorland, whom, it was hoped, would keep the lively young man's spirits under control. On passing through Italy, they visited the Sistine Chapel and attended Mass. Dashwood sat quietly throughout, observing the worshippers, all the while planning a rebellious outburst. He harboured a fervent dislike of the hypocrisy of the Catholic Church and a hatred of Papists in general and was waiting for the right time to make his move. The pivotal moment arrived when the priest called upon the Holy

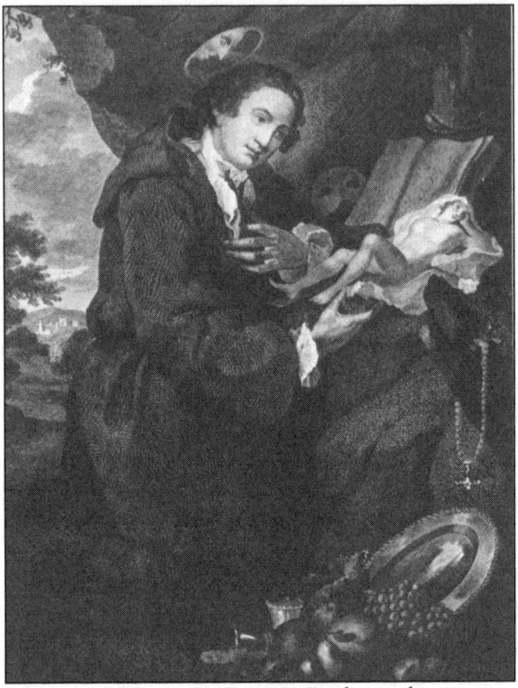

FIG. 22 Sir Francis Dashwood

Spirit. Dashwood suddenly leapt to his feet, threw open his cloak and loudly cracked a whip, frightening the praying penitents half to death. This demonstration against the Catholic practice of penitential flagellation was perhaps missed by the penitents themselves, but that did not deter Sir Francis. On the death of Pope Clement XII in 1730, he caused another furore. He set up a mock assembly, dressed up as Cardinal Ottoboni and imitated his trembling voice, incanting oremuses (liturgical prayers). These early incidents reveal Dashwood's abhorrence of formalized religion. As Walpole was to remark, 'This cursed Huguenot had a repertory of licentious songs against the Papacy.'

Sir Francis became an enthusiastic founder of clubs which revelled in the enjoyments of the flesh and the connoisseurship of food, wine, travel and art. He formed the 'Sublime Society of Beefsteaks' around 1735 for the appreciation of good food and wine, the motto of the club being 'Beef and Liberty'.[3] Here, he met with both William Hogarth and John Montagu,

Earl of Sandwich, sharing an appreciation of a thick steak and a good glass of port where ribald poems and songs were part of the festivities.[4] A love of the classical world was another defining characteristic of the richer Protestant eighteenth-century libertine and, in 1732, Dashwood's love of Rome and Greece led him to found the Dilettanti Society. Inspired by his journeys to Smyrna and Constantinople, he also started the Divan Club for those who had travelled to Turkey. Founded on 8 January 1744, at the Thatched Tavern in St James's, its members included Lord Sandwich and Lord Duncannon. All members had their portraits painted in Turkish dress, among them Dashwood, Sandwich, Fanny Murray, Dashwood's half-sister Mary Walcott, his wife Lady Sarah Ellys and the diarist Lady Mary Wortley Montagu, wife of the British ambassador living in Constantinople.[5] Fanny Murray, Mary Walcott, Lady Mary Montagu and Lady Betty Germain were also among the women reputed to be part of Sir Francis's controversial Order of the Knights of St Francis, or the Monks of Medmenham as they were sometimes known: a society replete with mock anti-religious ceremonies at which the members dressed up as monks and nuns.

Nocturnal Revels

Dashwood's most famous antics involving the Monks of Medmenham occurred during the years between the early 1750s and 1764. Approximately six miles from his estate in West Wycombe, he leased the remains of an old Gothic monastery, owned by Francis Duffield, partly still in ruins, partly restored as a three-storey house. Around 1751, Dashwood further restored the old abbey, adding stained glass and a cloister, with the intention of holding meetings for his newly established society. The staircase was lined with lurid paintings and the drawing room was dressed in a Romanesque style, adorned in green damask and ornate sofas. The library contained both intellectual and pornographic books for the pursuit of pleasures of the mind and body. The ceremonial robes which members were required to wear, hung, when not in use, on a row of pegs labelled with their names. Private 'cells' or rooms with beds were provided where members slept or entertained their sexual partners for the night. A chapter room existed for the benefit of members, its walls littered with Latin proverbs such as 'Dare O Guest, to despise wealth'. Outside was a chapel which none but the friars might enter.

The Order's first meeting took place in the George and Vulture Inn in the City of London, probably some time in the 1740s, and it continued to meet at the abbey from 1751 until 1774 or later. According to the existing papers of the club, the 'brothers', dressed as monks, met at regular 'chapter' meetings twice a year when they took part in mock-religious ceremonies.[6] Members might conduct their 'private devotions' or affairs in secret, if they so chose. Although there is no proof that he actually saw them for himself, Walpole described cells and cots next to the chapel where the 'brothers' retreated with their women, the 'nuns'. Lord Stanhope asserted that orgies took place at the abbey. Of Dashwood, he said, 'He was in truth and almost professedly what is termed a man of pleasure; an associate of Wilkes and Lord Sandwich; a partaker in the orgies of Medmenham Abbey.'[7]

The Medmenham Monks might meet up on occasions other than the full chapter meetings. Much of their time was spent reading, drinking and enjoying sexual frolics. From the Cellar Book inventory for 1762–4, it seems that they enjoyed good wine, consuming one or two bottles each. When Sir Thomas Stapleton met up with John Morton on 22 June 1762, they shared three bottles of claret and a bottle of port.[8] Yet the focus of the club was not merely on bodily pleasures; it was also intended as a place where members might conduct elevated conversation about the arts and sciences:

> The area of improvement and refinements in arts, sciences, taste, elegance, politeness, luxury, debauchery, and even vice, could not help being distinguished in the mode and ceremonies used in the devotion paid to the Cyprian Goddess.*

One of the problems in investigating Dashwood and his circle lies in separating fact from fiction in the wealth of information on the Medmenham set. Many of the anecdotes which have become firmly set in legend

* Aphrodite, the Goddess of love.

claim to be true. One such 'factional' version of the events, *Chrysal; or The Adventures of a Guinea* (1765), purports to expose the profligacy of well-known personages through the 'eyes' of a coin relating its journey and its observations. The book began as one volume in 1760 but proved so popular that it was reprinted and extended to four volumes over the following five years. Thought to have been written by Charles Johnstone,[9] an enemy of Wilkes and the poet Churchill, it contained scathing attacks on Dashwood and his Knights. Some of the scenes were evidently based on rumours about events at the abbey: 'You are astonished how such scenes of debauchery and excess could be supported, either by the fortunes of the entertainer, or the constitutions of his guests.' Some of the hearsay about the rules of the convent was grounded in truth, making any fabrication or exaggeration more easily believed:

> To prevent satiety or fatigues, these meetings were never protracted beyond a week at a time; nor held oftener than twice a year; by which frugality of pleasure, they were always returned to, with the keenness of novelty: And as for the expense of them, that was defrayed jointly by the whole community; (the superior [Dashwood] contributing nothing more, than any other member, except the first cost of the building the *convent*, which he thought himself amply recompensed from, by the honour of having struck out the plan)

the principles of the society being 'the professed ridicule of moral Virtue and religion'.[10]

Other revelations about the cavortings of Dashwood and his coterie came from a less reliable source, *The Fruitshop*. Here the author described a 'Garden of Eden', a 'happy spot whcrein flourished *the tree of trees*', a euphemism for the best and biggest penis. *Double-entendres* reveal the stallion-like sexual prowess of Dashwood (called 'St Francis of Assises'), 'a wight [*sic*] gifted with such frequent uprisings of the standard of humanity, as would do honour to any officer of the guards, young templar, lieutenant of the navy, or profest fortune-hunter of whatever denomination'.[11] The garden was described as 'a fertile source of a thousand different and celebrated conjectures, even among those who were the best qualified to devote themselves to profound researches',[12] in the dual sense of a breeding ground for scandal and a place of love-making. Although this could equally be a description of the grounds of the Medmenham Abbey where the Order met up, it was more likely to be an allusion to Dashwood's own estate at West Wycombe, the gardens of which he had had redesigned as a huge neo-classical erotic playground, with caves, grottoes and classical statues, such as that of Priapus, and temples to gods and goddesses, such as Venus and Apollo, no doubt fuelling the flames of gossip.

Another book, *Nocturnal Revels, Or, The History of King's-Palace and Other Modern Nunneries* (1779), was purportedly written by a member of the Medmenham set, 'a Monk of the Order of St Francis', and claimed to be an account of well-known people: 'Most of the Characters are taken from real life, with whom you are equally well acquainted as myself; they are, indeed, for the greatest part, truly original; nevertheless, they are not so *outré*, but that they may be traced in either the purlieus of *St James's*, *Covent Garden*, or *Maryebone*.' The author saw the establishment of the Order at Medmenham's refurbished abbey as a result of Dashwood's inventive imagination: 'A certain nobleman [Dashwood], who made the tour of Europe, and visited most of the capital Cities upon the Continent . . ., made judicious observations, particularly the different Religious Seminaries . . .; on his return to England, [he] thought that a burlesque Institution in the name of St Francis, would mark the absurdity of such sequestered Societies; and in lieu of the austerities and abstemiousness their practices substituted convivial gaiety, unrestrained hilarity, and social felicity.' Here, 'without either control or restraint', everyone could 'amuse himself, according to his own disposition'. Women were encouraged to join in the parties, especially those of a freer and happy mien 'to improve the general hilarity'. Separate spaces were given over to women to allow them to entertain themselves unencumbered by the monks, where they 'may make select parties among themselves, or entertain one another, or alone, with reading, musick [*sic*], tambour-work, &c.'[13]

According to this version, women also took part in the vows and the initiation ceremony. Monks' habits were worn by everyone who visited and those taking part were required to swear an oath of secrecy. The ceremony of admission was 'performed in a Chapel allotted for that purpose, upon the tolling of a bell, accompanied with solemn, plaintive music'. Women were supposedly active members of the society and were voted to a position within the group. Regulations deemed that women and men would not covet one another's partners, 'the former considering themselves as the lawful wives of the brethren, during their stay within the monastic walls; every Monk being religiously scrupulous not to infringe upon the nuptial alliance of any other brother.'[14]

The secrecy surrounding the order was due to its sexual nature and the need to protect its members. In order that none of the female members was surprised by the arrival of a husband or close relation, an escape route was left open so that they could leave before being recognized. They were all masked until 'all the Brethren have passed them in review'.[15] If a woman found herself in the position of recognizing a gentleman and wanted to keep her identity secret, she quickly retired 'without making any apology, or revealing themselves to any but their temporary husband'.

If *Nocturnal Revels* is to be believed, the priory was also used as a bolt-hole for women members who had become pregnant, in order to allow for a secret birth; according to the author, '. . . the Ladies, in case they find it necessary, may make a temporary retreat from the world, and assist posterity with respect to the rising generation'. Certainly, reputable women were known to go to the country to give birth to any illegitimate babies. According to this account, such children were then given protection and provided with jobs on the estate: 'The offspring of these connections are stiled the Sons and Daughters of St Francis, and appointed in due order officers and domestics in the Seminary, according to their different abilities, or by drawing lots.'

Pious Ejaculations

London's social circle was much smaller in the eighteenth century: actors, writers and poets would mix with the aristocracy and members of parliament. Enormously rich and fat, and totally dissipated, George Bubb Dodington recorded in his diary for 23 December 1760 a dinner party with Laurence Sterne, the author of *Tristram Shandy*, who, in turn, was a friend of the writer John Hall Stevenson who knew the politician John Wilkes.

Boswell also knew Wilkes and the actor/theatre manager David Garrick, both of whom dined with the Earl of Sandwich and knew Paul Whitehead, a friend of Dashwood's and secretary to the Knights' Society. Members of the Knights of St Francis were selected from the elite but included people Dashwood knew from his other clubs. Some of the members had originally met at the Beefsteak Club. As Boswell described on his visit to the club, 'Scarce a fortnight had passed since this holy Secretary of State himself [Dashwood] had been present with Wilkes at a weekly club to which they both belonged, held at the top of Covent Garden Theatre, and composed of players and the loosest revellers of the age.'[16] Lord Sandwich, 'a jolly, hearty, lively man', chaired the meeting that included Churchill and Wilkes.

Although Boswell was not known to have been a member of the Order, he mixed with those who were and probably visited Medmenham Abbey. Other possible visitors included Sterne, Hall Stevenson, Hogarth, Walpole, Garrick and the cross-dresser and French spy Chevalier D'Eon. Benjamin Franklin is said to have been a member during his visits to England in 1757–62 and 1764–75. In his essay *Advice to a Young Man on the Choice of a Mistress*, he addressed young men on the charms of older women:

> You should prefer old women to young ones. Because they have most knowledge of the world and their minds are better stored with observations, their conversation is more improving and lastingly agreeable . . . Because there is no hazard of children . . . Because through more experience they are more prudent and discreet in conducting an intrigue.[17]

Franklin was a frequent visitor to Dashwood's family estate at West Wycombe. In 1773, he wrote to his son, 'I am in this house as much at my ease as if it were my own; and the gardens are a paradise. But a pleasanter thing is the kind countenance, the facetious and very intelligent conversation of Mine Host, who, having been for many years engaged in public affairs, seen all parts of Europe, and kept the best company in the world, is himself the best existing.'[18]

Although Medmenham had other occasional visitors, there was a small core of members at the heart of the Order. Paul Whitehead, as secretary of the society, oversaw all the activities. The full membership, at any one time, was supposed to have been thirteen – Sir Francis and his twelve apostles. Over the years these included Wilkes and Sandwich; Thomas Potter, son of the Archbishop of Canterbury and possible co-author with Wilkes of the controversial *Essay on Woman*; John Tucker, MP for Weymouth; Sir Thomas Stapleton, a cousin of Dashwood's; Sir John Dashwood-King, Sir Francis's half-brother; Sir William Stanhope MP; Francis Duffield, the abbey's landlord; Sir John Aubrey, MP and magistrate; Sir Henry Vansittart, Governor of Bengal and an MP; Robert Vansittart, professor at Oxford University, and their brother Arthur, an MP; and the poet Charles Churchill.[19] Probable members also include the Earl of Bute,* George Bubb Dodington, Dr Benjamin Bates, physician to Dashwood, the Whig politician Charles Fox MP, George Selwyn, an MP and known necrophile, and his crony, the Duke of Queensberry.

The sexual nature of the club is evident from *double-entendres* in the correspondence between members. On 3 September 1770, John King wrote to Sir Francis Dashwood from Ashby in Lincolnshire, thanking him for his letter and regretting that he could not join the 'Brotherhood' as he was obliged to stay with his family

> so in the mean time must pay all Obedience to the Pillar* annex'd the present standard of mirth to the Sisterhood, who are determin'd to exert their Spiritualities there, as for their present Condition are able, for I assure your Lordship, their Spirits are willing, but the Flesh is weak—— etc . . .
>
> Most obedient FAITHFUL Humble Servant
>
> John King[20]

In another letter to Sir Francis, Paul Whitehead writes of violent inflammation caused by gout in both feet which prevented him from attending the meeting. He apologized for his absence from 'the celebration of the

* According to Walpole's memoirs, Bute had a passion for 'masquerading in becoming dresses'.

* St Dunstan's Pillar, erected by Sir Francis Dashwood as a landmark to guide travellers over the fens near Lincoln, was also an obvious joke alluding to sexual prowess.

Medmenham Rites', requesting 'the Prayers of the Chapter for a sick and weak Brother'. Similarly Stanhope sent his apologies from Brighton in September 1758, being 'greatly flattered with the kind invitation of the Chapter of Medmenham, but it is my misfortune and not my fault, that I do not accept of it, well knowing how unfit a deaf man is for such a cheerful society . . . My compliments to all your Brethren and assure them they have my prayers, particularly, that part of the Litany, when I pray the Lord, to strengthen them that do stand.'[21]

The following note was sent from a Mr Hall, from John Street, Berkeley Square, on 31 August 1761, presumably for presentation at the next chapter meeting:

> Mr Hall presents his compliments to Mr Wilkes and is still under the scourge of an invincible cholick which has induced him to such a state of contrition that he is obliged to live by the rules entirely opposite to those of St Francis, whose shrine he venerates, but dare not approach under his present incapacity; he desires ye prayers and ye congregation and hopes their Devotions may be attended with the choicest of blessings of their Patron . . .[22]

Hall Stevenson, although not thought to be a member, obviously attended some of the meetings. At one point, he alleged that Lady Mary Dashwood, Sir Francis's stepmother, was one of the 'nuns' as he sometimes picked her out in the line-ups. He promoted the idea of an incestuous relationship with Dashwood in a poem entitled *The Confessions of Sir F— of Medmenham and of the Lady Mary, his wife* (his wife was in fact Sarah Gould, so this would have been a reference either to his stepmother or to his sister):

> *Like a hotspur young cock, he began with his mother,*
> *Cheer'd three of his sisters, one after the other*[23]

When Hall Stevenson moved to Skelton Castle (which he named Crazy Castle), he made it a headquarters for a group of men called the Demoniacs, possibly inspired by the Monks of Medmenham Abbey.[24] In *Crazy Tales* (1762), he conveyed his delight in a certain breast size, most likely in reference to Lucy Cooper, rumoured to be Dashwood's mistress:

Lucy was not like other lasses,
From twelve her breasts swell'd in a trice,
First they were like cupping-glasses,
Then like two peaches made of ice.[25]

He proceeded to describe the place of sexual revelries which includes a possible reference to Dashwood's gardens at West Wycombe.[26]

In his book *Pious Ejaculations*, Hall Stevenson affectionately satirized Wilkes with a skit on the love life of friar John [Wilkes]: 'With rosy cheeks and double chin / To kiss a wench he thought no sin'. Even during his youth John Wilkes led a profligate life. He admitted to Boswell some twenty years later that, as a student at university, he was 'always among women at Leyden. My father gave me as much money as I pleased. Three or four whores; drunk every night. Sore head next morning, then read.'[27] After his Grand Tour, he returned to find that his parents had arranged a marriage match for him to a wealthy but dull woman, Mary Meade. Wilkes was later to admit, he 'loved all women except his wife'.[28] He was, however, devoted to his daughter, Polly. After separating from his wife, he took Polly to live with him, as Mary did not appear to be interested in the child. In early 1757, when Polly was very ill with smallpox, her mother had not bothered to visit her. Polly would become Wilkes's lifelong companion and provide him with the comfort of a loving daughter.

Despite a squint and a crooked jaw that Hogarth was to satirize in an unflattering print (**FIG. 23**), Wilkes was an entertaining wit who charmed his way both into bed with many women as well as into the higher echelons of society. In 1754, he had become a member of the Beefsteak Club and an active member of the Knights of St Francis six years later. He thus became party to the inner workings of the Order, including some of the odder aspects of the ceremonies. In a letter to fellow member John Armstrong of 20 December 1760, Wilkes referred to a stage in the initiation ceremony, held at the abbey, which involved shaving parts of the body. He mused, 'Well, but I hope you don't shave all – nothing below the chin – at least I trust the Sisters are excused from any ceremony of this kind.'[29] The act was probably the shaving of part of the top of the head in mock imitation of a monk's tonsure. Wilkes obviously enjoyed his sessions with

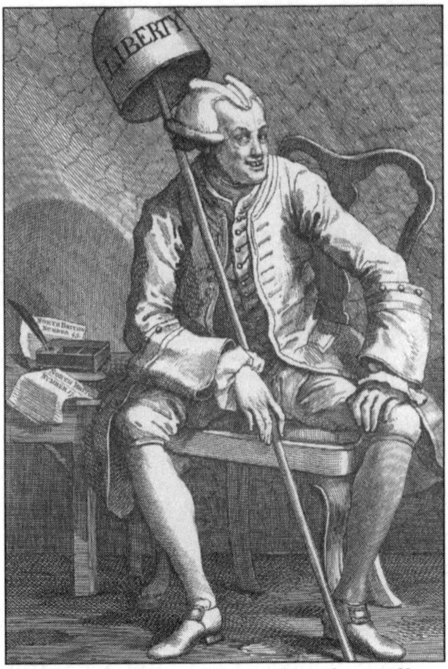

FIG. 23 William Hogarth, *John Wilkes*

the 'monks' for, in 1762, he wrote to Sir Francis declaring happily, 'I feast my mind on the day of Medmenham on Monday and hope to indemnify myself there for the noise and nonsense here.' In a letter to Lord Temple, written on his return from Medmenham Abbey, he made reference to the jovial monks of St Francis who 'kept me till four in the morning'.

The amiable Wilkes was known for his wit and repartee but his jokes did not always go down so well with those on the receiving end. In one famous encounter with Lord Sandwich, the latter remarked on Wilkes's debauchery, commenting that he would surely die either of venereal disease or on the scaffold. Wilkes famously retorted, 'That depends, My Lord, whether I embrace your mistress or your principles.'[30] Sandwich was later to fall out with Wilkes in a much-publicized stand-off which included public attacks in Parliament. Another oft-told tale related in *Chrysal* was of a jape played by Wilkes on Lord Sandwich, entailing the services of a large baboon. The night before one of the meetings of the Order, Wilkes had taken a baboon into his cell. When the brotherhood had retired after dinner to prepare for the ceremony, he dressed the baboon up as the Devil and hid it in a large chest, fastening a cord to the lock so that he could open it at an opportune moment. Thus, at the height of the jollities, Wilkes pulled the cord, and let the animal loose. The frightened creature gave a sudden spring on to the middle of the table, scaring the wits out of the unsuspecting company. The petrified baboon then leapt on to Lord Sandwich who was shocked to the core, thinking it was indeed the Devil.[31] Some accounts maintain that Wilkes was not to blame for the baboon incident. The late Sir Francis Dashwood, of the twentieth century, believed the incident was often misreported. According to the Vansittarts, it was another family member, George, a guest at the abbey, who released the baboon which Henry Vansittart had brought back from India. None the less, these stories fanned the flames of the gossip surrounding the Order.

Wilkes became a close friend of Thomas Potter, son of the Archbishop of Canterbury, as they shared a taste for debauchery. Indeed, it was probably Potter who was responsible for introducing Wilkes to the Order. He was certainly a bad influence on him, even though Wilkes was eager enough himself to engage in any lascivious activity. Tempting Wilkes away from his family and back to London, Potter wrote in a letter dated 19 October 1752: 'If you prefer young women and whores to old women and wives . . . hasten to town . . .'[32] Potter was undoubtedly a loyal friend to Wilkes, supporting him through the run-up to his election as MP for Aylesbury in 1757.

Perhaps unwisely, Wilkes ran his sexual and political lives with equal vigour and consequently they sometimes spilled into each other. In 1762–3, a row caused by Wilkes divided the Order – Wilkes, supported by Churchill and Hall Stevenson on the one hand, versus Lords Sandwich and Bute on the other. Bute had just been made Prime Minister and faced opposition from William Pitt 'the elder'. Wilkes was a staunch supporter of Pitt, whose brother-in-law, Lord Temple, was one of his patrons. The split was further exacerbated by the fact that Dashwood had become Chancellor of the Exchequer, something of a joke according to Wilkes, who saw his friend as 'puzzling all his life over tavern bills'.[33]

As part of his campaign against Bute, Wilkes established the newspaper *The North Briton* in collaboration with Churchill. Hearing that Hogarth

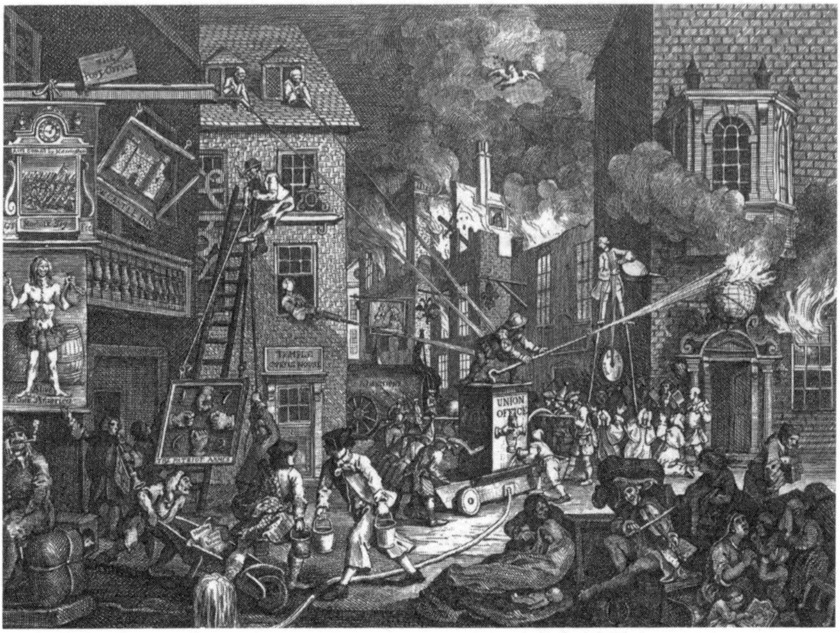

FIG. 24 William Hogarth, *The Times, Plate I*

was about to publish a satirical illustration of Pitt and Temple, he launched an immediate counter-attack: in the September edition he referred to Hogarth as a 'house-painter'. Hogarth, in retaliation, produced satires on Wilkes and Churchill in *The Times*, *Plate I* (1762), depicting Bute and the King as firemen trying to douse the flames of war sweeping Europe, while Wilkes and Churchill are in the attic aiming their hoses not at the fire but at the firefighters (**FIG. 24**).[34]

The story of the battle between Wilkes and his opponents is well known, particularly in relation to the infamous issue no. 45 of *The North Briton*, which contained accusations made by Wilkes that King George III had deliberately misled the country about the Peace of Paris and accused Lord Bute of an intrigue with the Queen Mother. Wilkes was arrested for seditious libel but was released on a technicality – as an MP he was, in fact, exempt from prosecution through parliamentary privilege. After republishing the offending issue, his house was searched under an illegal warrant and a copy of the manuscript of the bawdy *Essay on Woman* was found. As a result, Wilkes was accused of obscene libel, a legal term frequently applied by those attempting censorship of erotica. He was expelled from the House of Commons on 20 January 1764, but not before Sandwich had taken his revenge by reading the offending poem out to the House of Lords, feigning moral indignation. Some were to judge this as a hypocritical move by Sandwich, particularly in the light of his involvement with the Medmenham Monks.

As a democratically elected MP, Wilkes at first refused to accept his expulsion from Parliament. Much to his disgust, he was eventually outlawed and forced to flee to the Continent. While in exile in 1764–5, Wilkes travelled through France and Italy visiting all the fashionable places of entertainment, from opera houses to salons. In Paris he fell madly in love with a beautiful Italian dancer, Gertrude Corradini, who was pious enough to veil the portrait of the Virgin Mary which hung above her bed when she was visited by Wilkes. Wilkes established her in lodgings at Rue Neuve des bons Enfants overlooking the Palais Royal, and would divide his time between his daughter, his mistress and the French salons. Corradini obviously retained a place in his heart as he fondly mused some thirty years later: 'She was a perfect Grecian figure, cast in the mould of the Florentine Venus, excepting that she was rather fuller and had flatter breasts. Extremely delicate in person, she continued constantly attentive to every circumstance which could give herself, or a lover pleasure. She possessed the divine gift of lewdness, but nature had not given her strength adequate to the force of her desires.'[35]

At some stage, Corradini's health deteriorated so she decided to return to the town of her birth, Bologna, where Wilkes there was to join her later. This allowed him to take a trip to Naples where he bumped into Boswell and they climbed Mount Vesuvius together. In Rome, he met up with the art historian Johann Joachim Winckelmann (1717–68),[36] who was well known to other libertines with similar interests. The affair with Corradini was brought to an end by her continuing demands and fiery temper. In a calculated move, aware that Wilkes's finances were in a parlous state, she emptied his house of everything of value and disappeared.

In February 1768, Wilkes successfully re-entered British politics, intending to stand for the City of London. With popular support behind him, cries of 'Wilkes and Liberty' resounded in the streets. Signs emblazoned with the numerals 45, the number of the issue of *The North Briton* which had caused the furore, and Wilkes's insignia, a blue cockade, were displayed everywhere. Wilkes was eventually arrested but, when riots ensued, he was brought before the King's Bench judge who quashed his outlawry on a technicality. Nevertheless, he was sentenced to serve twenty-two months in prison and fined a thousand pounds for publishing *Essay on Woman* and the controversial issue No. 45 which denounced the King's speech. In 1769, he was expelled from the House of Commons three times in as many months and so prevented from taking his seat as MP for Middlesex. Finally, he was successfully elected Alderman of the City of London (1769), Sheriff (1771) and Mayor (1774), eventually returning to Parliament in 1774.

During the 1770s, Wilkes succeeded in attracting the attention of Mademoiselle Charpillon, the woman who had spurned the advances of none other than Casanova. Their affair lasted three years. He then went on to form a strong relationship with Amelia Arnold, a woman three years younger than his daughter Polly. He set up a home for her at 2 Kensington Gore and she bore him a daughter, Harriet, on 20 October 1778. Despite the difference in their ages, Amelia proved to be a pivotal part of Wilkes's life, providing him with a stable relationship that lasted until his death.

'Awake, My Fanny'

Wilkes had produced *Essay on Woman* in 1763 as an inside joke for a group of close friends but it was to create a furore which reverberated throughout Parliament.[37] Thomas Potter wrote to him, 'I have read your parody for the ninety-ninth time, and have laughed as heartily as I did the first . . . I think you exceed yourself.' Although Wilkes denied responsibility when prosecution was threatened, in 1766 he admitted to having written it.[38] Walpole thought it was a joint effort, declaring, 'Wilkes and Potter, son of the late Archbishop of Canterbury, has formerly composed this indecent patchwork in one of their bacchanalian hours.'[39] Initially, only twelve copies had been made but these were quickly followed up with reprints of pirate copies. Once the illegal raid on Wilkes's house had uncovered the handwritten manuscript, it was whisked away as incriminating evidence, along with other items belonging to Wilkes. This instigated a flurry of letters in magazines and newspapers. The *Gentleman's Magazine* of 1763 gave a full account of *Essay on Woman*, describing the work where 'the lewdest thoughts are expressed in terms of the grossest obscenity; the most horrid impunity is minutely represented; the sex is vilified and insulted; and the whole is scurrilous, impudent and impious to an incredible decree.'[40] Wilkes defended himself in an open letter to the electors of Aylesbury, his constituency, in subsequent editions of the same magazine.[41] A wit for *The Times* for 21 May provided a list of the other items allegedly found in Wilkes's home, including, 'One dozen of Mrs Phillips purses – warranted by that *useful* and *public-spirited* matron to be as *good goods* as ever came out of her shop' (Mrs Phillips was a well-known vendor of condoms).[42] A reply printed in *The Times* on 24 May 1763 declared:

> I dare say some of the *curious* articles in the inventory you published, said to have been found among Mr Wilkes's papers which were carried off to the Secretary of State, have been imported by that gentleman from France when he returned from the tour he lately made to Paris, to complete the valuable collection of that sort, which is in the saloon of the famous Convent on the Bank of the Thames, called *Medmenham Abbey*, where the Right Hon. the Lord De Despencer presides with so much Decency and Order, and has spent many a jovial day with Mr Wilkes before their late difference in politics.

Essay on Woman was dedicated to Fanny Murray (**FIG. 25**), a known member of Dashwood's Divan Club and mistress of some of the members, including Wilkes:

> *Awake, my Fanny, leave all meaner things,*
> *This morn shall prove what rapture swiving brings.*
> *Let us (since Life can little more supply*
> *Than just a few good Fucks and then we die . . .*
> *Expatiate free o'er that lov'd scene of Man.*

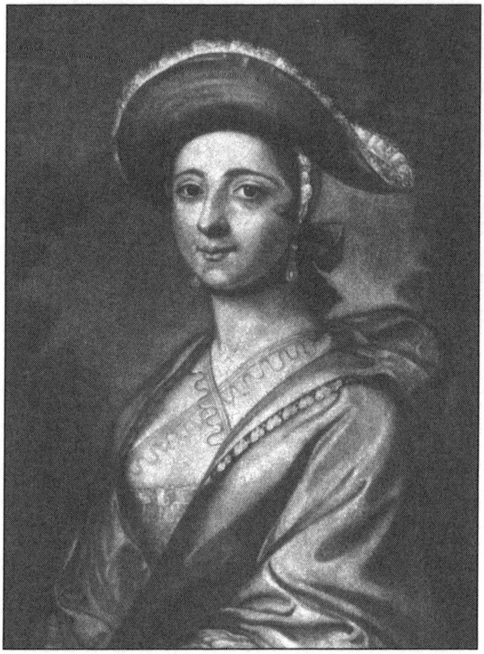

FIG. 25 Fanny Murray

Anecdotes of the celebrated women in Wilkes's social circle abounded, including Peg Woffington, the acclaimed Irish actress and mistress of David Garrick: 'Peg Woffington being asked, how it was possible that she, who had swallowed at Dublin many of the noblest Pricks of this World, yet was never got with Child. Greatly replied, *No Man ever played up to me*', meaning she thought no man worthy of her. Famed for her beauty and the freedom with which she pursued sexual activities, she was at one time elected head of the Dublin Beefsteak Club.[43]

Part of Wilkes's attack against the Scots in *Essay on Woman* included an attack on their women, especially their lack of female hygiene. In it, Wilkes remonstrates, 'It is shocking to find how much it [the vagina] is neglected, especially in the Northern Part of this Island. The Face, the Neck, the Hands, I owe are clean, but of a Whiteness which would rival Leda's lover. All the rest, alas! is hid in mysterious Sluttishness.'[44] He also satirized hypocritical figures of the Church, attributing a lewd ditty of his own to the Archbishop of York who had died in 1743:

> *Unsully'd* Virtue *my esteem demands*
> *But 'tis at* Beauty *my true Pointer stands;*
> *I grant the Dignity of wedded Love;*
> *The holy Contract first was sign'd above;*
> *Applauding Angels clapp'd their Wings and read*
> *The senseless Jargon of my Lawyer's Head.*
> *Into this* holy State *shall Lewdness enter?*
> *My pious Prick cries* no, *and will not venture . . .*

Wilkes had no doubt heard about the activities of the cleric: according to Horace Walpole, the Archbishop of York was a 'jolly old' clergyman who kept a veritable 'seraglio'.[45]

The persecution of Wilkes during the early 1760s was due as much to the political climate as to either *Essay on Woman* or the offensive issue No. 45. He had provoked the new Tory administration under Lord Bute and his declarations as editor of *The North Briton* further aggravated the situation. 'The liberty of the press is the birthright of a Briton,' he declared, 'and is justly esteemed the firmest bulwark of the liberties of this country.'[46] After the theft of the poem from his home, it was only a matter of time before the government would make use of their ammunition. The government, however, foresaw the danger in pressing charges on illegally obtained papers so Lords Bute and Sandwich persuaded one of Wilkes's printers to pass on a proof copy of *Essay on Woman* to a parson called Kidgell. Lord Sandwich was only too pleased to exact revenge on Wilkes, no doubt still smarting from having been the butt of his cruel jibes and practical jokes. As a result of his disloyalty to Wilkes in the House of Lords, Sandwich earned the nickname 'Jemmy Twitcher' (reputedly given to him by Churchill) after a character in *The Beggar's Opera* of whom the highwayman, MacHeath, declares: 'that Jemmy [a member of one's own gang] should peach me I own surprised me.' Lord Sandwich was also made fun of in *The Life, Adventures, Intrigues, and Amours of the Celebrated Jemmy Twitcher* (1770) which revelled in spurious details of his catching the clap, drugging and debauching a servant girl at his school, escaping from a ship bound for New York on which his father had placed him, his marriage and his entry into Parliament.[47]

Although the Medmenham Monks occasionally met up in other capacities, the Order of St Francis gradually went into decline. Because of the immense publicity stirred up by Wilkes, Dashwood, fearing recriminations and possible scandal, quickly stripped any incriminating evidence from the Chapter Room of the abbey, including portraits of the monks and nuns, and removed the hooks on which the brothers had hung their habits. Paul Whitehead burned all papers from the Order just prior to his death in 1774 and, although Dashwood continued to lease Medmenham Abbey until 1778, the society's activities had ended some years earlier.

Nuns at the Priory

Lady Mary Wortley Montagu was certainly a member of the Divan Club and was part of Dashwood's circle but it is unlikely, despite reputedly being a member of the Order of the Knights of St Francis, that she took part in any of their sexual activities. She was a freethinker, with sexually liberated views, and her intellect and interest in the classical world attracted Dashwood. Dashwood had first met Lady Montagu on his travels in Italy, along with other British travellers who had met up to sightsee. But although Lady Montagu was popular for her wit and amusing conversation but she was not universally liked. Having seen her in Florence, mixing with a group of English travellers which included Dashwood, on 25 September 1740, Walpole wrote:

> Did I tell you lady Mary Wortley is here? She laughs at my lady Walpole, scolds my lady Pomfret, and is laughed at by the whole town. Her dress, her avarice, and her impudence must amaze any one that never heard her name. She wears a foul mob, that does not cover her greasy, black locks, that hang loose, never combed or curled; an old mazarine blue wrapper, that gapes open and discovers a canvass petticoat. Her face is swelled on one side with a [pox], partly covered with a plaister, and partly with

> white paint, which for cheapness she has bought so coarse, that you would not use it to wash a chimney. In three words, I will give you her picture as we drew it in the *Sortes Virgilanæ** – Insanam vatem aspicies [mad sorceress]. I give you my honour we did not choose it; but Gray, Mr Cooke, Sir Fr. Dashwood, and I, and several others, drew it fairly among a thousand for different people.[48]

Lady Montagu came from one of the richest aristocratic families in England yet had eloped with a man of her own choosing, rather than marry the peer's son picked by her father. She was a prolific writer, had taught herself Latin and Italian, and counted among her friends some of the more sexually abandoned characters of the eighteenth century, including Sarah, Duchess of Marlborough, Lady Skerrett and the bisexual Lord Hervey. Although smallpox later ruined her looks; she famously promoted vaccination with cowpox, having discovered its use in Turkey. She rebelled against any form of social control, particularly if it enforced women's inferior position, and she was one of the first to popularize the East with her epistles of Turkish harems. In middle age, she shocked her contemporaries by starting a love affair with the Italian Franceso Algarotti.[49]

Lucy Cooper and the well-known courtesan Kitty Fisher are more likely than Lady Montagu to have been involved in the events at Medmenham Abbey since the former was Dashwood's mistress and the latter was mistress to Lord Sandwich, while simultaneously carrying on an affair with Lord Mountford. Cooper had also been kept by Sir Orlando Bridgman, an old debaucher, and by Dashwood's brother-in-law, whom she had refused to marry. He allowed her, nevertheless, a very handsome maintenance and supported her in an elegant house in Parliament Street. He also kept a carriage for her, which would often be at the door of the debauched drinking den, Weatherby's, for twenty-four hours successively.

When Bridgman died, Cooper fell upon hard times and ended up in court on charges of debauchery and intemperance. In serious debt, she

* *Sortes Virgilanæ* was a prophetic game played by dipping *ad hoc* into a great work – Virgil's *Aeneid* and the Bible were used – and picking out words or phrases to account for something or someone.

wrote a letter to Tomkins, master of the Shakespear Tavern, stating that she was a prisoner of the King's Bench and 'was almost naked and starving, without a penny in her pocket to purchase food, raiment, or a coal to warm herself'. It was then that William Hickey and his friends came to her assistance with a gift of fifty pounds while another friend put her up in her house in Bow Street. When Cooper later died of the pox[50] she was eulogized in various poems and ballads, including *The Gentleman's Bottle Companion* and *The Meretriciad* (1770), the latter declaring her 'Lewder than all the Whores in Charles's reign'.[51]

Fanny Murray, one-time mistress to a number of men including Beau Nash, John Wilkes and reputedly John Montagu, also became part of Sir Francis Dashwood's circle and was a member of his Divan Club. She was so popular that she had her portrait painted at Dashwood's expense, and songs were written especially for her, such as 'A Song Wrote by Mr Boyce on Sight of Fanny Murray'. Born in Bath in 1729, she was brought up by her father who played the fiddle for a living. According to *Memoirs of the Celebrated Miss Fanny Murray*, she was a budding beauty by her fourteenth year:

> Fanny's person, which already began to testify to marks of womanhood was extremely beautiful, her face a perfect oval, with eyes that converted love, and every other feature in agreeable symmetry. Her dimpled cheeks alone might have captivated, if a smile that gave it existence did not display such other charms as shared the conquest. Her teeth regular, fine and perfectly white, coral lips and chestnut hair, soon attracted the eyes of everyone.[52]

She was seduced by the rakish Jack Spencer, grandchild to Sarah, Duchess of Marlborough, but he cast her aside after only a few weeks, leaving her homeless and penniless until the kind and generous Beau Nash took her under his wing. Murray led a life in and out of debt, common to many a celebrated whore, but shared some of the revelries and riches of Dashwood's circle.

Dashwood's mistresses, Elizabeth Roach and Agnes (sometimes known as Mary) Perrault, also became 'nuns' of the Order. Perrault had worked for the pornographic bookseller Edmund Curll, taking over much of this clientele after his death. She and Dashwood may have met through the latter's purchases of erotica for his library at Medmenham. The more notorious fashionable women known to Wilkes and his friends, among them the courtesan La Charpillon and the actress Peg Woffington, also appear to have been involved in the activities at the abbey.[53] The revelation of an intrigue between Peg and Sir Hanbury Williams was part of the reason why Garrick refused to marry her or, as he put it, to be 'noosed in the connubial knot'.

The Medmenham Monks also had 'nuns', including young virgins supplied by the prostitute Charlotte Hayes for a night's entertainment at the abbey. Lord Sandwich said admiringly of her, 'She keeps the Stock Exchange supplied with real, immaculate maidenheads.' With a little skilful preparation, she passed off the likes of young harlots Kitty Young and Nancy Feathers as untouched virgins. Hayes was referred to as Abbess or Mother Superior, titles frequently accorded to procuresses or bawds who ran brothels:

> Every Sister who is a Candidate for the Veil, must be either young or handsome . . . She must not have been very intimate with the World, nor the World with her, and if she has seen abroad, the Abbess considers her as still more worthy of being admitted among the Sisterhood. She must not be married, or have any favourite Lover . . . As the Brethren of the adjacent Seminaries are so kind as to visit this Sisterhood, and in a most friendly and loving manner, as is suitable to their characters, bring them to confession, and administer comfort; the Sisterhood must, upon all such occasions, open their *bosoms*, and conceal *nothing* from these worthy Brethren.[54]

One of the girls of Hayes's 'nunnery' was so fatigued after entertaining an old male client, Sir Harry 'Flagellum', that she begged a small respite from work in order to recover her spirits: 'Two long hours, said she, have I been with this old Curmudgeon; and I have had as much labour to rouze the Venus lurking in his veins, as if I have been whipping the most obstinate of all mules over the Alps.'[55]

By 1766, according to the whores' directory, *Kitty's Atlantis*, the 'inimitable' Miss Hayes had had to move home as she fell into debt, a common problem among women in the sex trade. 'The *Meretriciad* moved her from confinement to a convenient place near the Park by the benefit of the late Insolvent Act,' the directory informed, 'but I can assure my reader, that she's now in keeping, and rides in a stately coach; and those who love a fine motherly woman, may find the best entertainment in her company.' Even a ditty was composed for her,

See Charlotte Ha—, as modest as a saint,
And fair as ten years past, with little paint.[56]

Despite her financial problems, Hayes obviously managed to turn her business around as she became renowned for producing first-class 'nuns'. Dressing them in the highest fashions, she charged a high price for the gowns and accompanying buckles and trinkets to keep them in debt and prevent them absconding. If they tried to elope, she put them in a lock-up house until the debt was paid or until they returned to her charge. One of her tricks was to take an apartment and hire a young girl as a nurse to sleep in the same room as a female bed-ridden client, who would then, unbeknown to the girl, be substituted by a male client. Not only did Hayes's business cater to debilitated peers, impotent aldermen and rich merchants, but her brothel was also a place where one could go to seek revenge: one lord whose wife was having an intrigue with his gambling opponent requested a girl who would give his rival the pox for thirty pounds.

Another mistress of the Earl of Sandwich, Martha Reay, had started life as a milliner's shopgirl. Half his age when she became his lover, she was to bear Sandwich at least five children. Sandwich's wife had by this time gone insane. Yet Sandwich continually refused to make any financial settlement on Reay and the insecurity of her status caused her concern. If he were to die, she would be in the precarious financial position of trying to bring up her family alone with no income. In support of her case, a friend of Sandwich's advised him, 'she is a fine woman whom you debauched very young who you tell me had lived with you eleven years. I see she still possesses your fondest wishes.'[57] Although they were a close couple, each had affairs elsewhere. While living under his protection, Reay was wooed by the Reverend Hackman, an indulgence which ultimately cost her dear.

According to *The Case and Memoirs of the late Rev. Mr James Hackman*, Reay had met Hackman when he was a young army officer in Huntingdonshire. After falling in love with her, he decided to give up his military career to become a clergyman in the hope of enticing her to a country vicarage and offering her the security of marriage. Some say she refused Hackman's advances altogether, but this tale states differently: apparently Sandwich's Otaheitean servant, Omiah, had frequently observed the familiarities between the lovers and, although mute, reported the events in gestures and signs to Lord Sandwich who then threatened to cut her off. Despite promising that she would no longer see Hackman, Reay continued the affair. Reay probably did love Hackman but she needed the protection of Sandwich more, particularly since she had his children to look after. She refused to run off with the impoverished Hackman and, after this final rebuff, he shot her in the head. Hackman was convicted for her murder and hanged in 1779.[58]

After many years, the ageing Dashwood's final mistress, Mrs Barry, gave birth to their daughter, Rachel Frances Antonina, in 1774. As Dashwood lay dying, it is said that the ghost of Paul Whitehead – the Order's old secretary – haunted the grounds of West Wycombe. Family members reported seeing Whitehead's ghost beckoning and signalling, calling Dashwood to his grave. Sir Francis died soon afterwards in 1781.

*

Although eighteenth-century libertine societies were associated with a hedonistic lifestyle and a programme of pleasure, many displayed the new philosophies of the Enlightenment and took an interest in neo-classicism and science. Yet, for all their camaraderie and fellowship, they were essentially exclusive and elitist clubs that served the more serious purpose of bonding together men from the political world.

Another *raison d'être* of the libertine clubs was the breaking of moral taboos. Indulging in anti-religious satirical jibes, enjoying a night's drinking and revelling in carnal activities were all part of the fun. Dashwood and his friends took the joke to the limits with the formation of a 'secret' society in which members dressed as monks and nuns and took part in travesties of religious ceremonies. As with his other clubs, the Order of the Knights of St Francis was more an outward expression of Dashwood's interests than anything more sinister. None the less, because its activities caused so much gossip, they were inevitably exaggerated in the process and a source of scandalous material for publishers. In spite of the difficulty of distinguishing between fact and fiction, there is enough surviving documentation in St Francis' private papers to confirm the existence of the Order and its sexual nature. The evidence suggests a hearty, jovial and vivacious club which pandered to its members, fulfilling both the demands of the intellect and the more lascivious bodily pleasures of life. The very fact that the Order stimulated so much rumour is indicative that it was considered controversial by contemporaries yet bore all the hallmarks of its era.

CHAPTER SIX

Scottish Secret Sex Societies

We meet in secret – doubly sweet,
Oh! Castle Dreel! our bower to greet.
With Nature's gift of youth and health
We pine and long to come by stealth.

Alas! how easily things go wrong!
A C—t too moist or a P—ck too strong:
Yet who from F—king would refrain
Let things be never the same again?

Anon., *The Supplement to the Records Of The Most Ancient And Puissant Order Of The Beggar's Benison and Merryland, Anstruther* (1892)

In 1745, John McNaughton, Collector of Customs and current elected Sovereign of the Beggar's Benison, wandered through the narrow streets of Anstruther, a small fishing village to the north of Edinburgh famous for its smugglers, to a local tavern at the foot of the ruins of Castle Dreel. It was a chilly night and as he made his way towards one of his regular meetings of the Brethren he looked forward to the familiar scene which would greet him. The current members of the society, all men, would already have gathered in the main meeting room they hired, dressed in the sashes and medals that bore the insignia of the society, awaiting his arrival.

That evening, a new member was to be initiated and McNaughton was looking forward to the ceremony. The novitiate would already be there sitting in the annexe trying to obtain an erection while waiting for the call into the main room where the rest of the members would be standing in a circle. The breath-horn would be blown four times as a summons. On entering the room, his penis would be placed on the test-platter and covered with a napkin; the assembled Brethren would then touch his penis with their own, one after another. Thereafter, a special glass with the society's insignia would be filled with port and the health of the newcomer would be toasted. After reading from the Song of Solomon, the novitiate would be adorned with his sash and medal and the Beggar's Benison pledge declared: 'May your prick and your purse never fail you.' This would be followed by a celebratory banquet with special songs and toasts written for such occasions. At other meetings, Beggar's Benison members would masturbate on silver platters and invite local girls to exhibit themselves naked.

McNaughton had founded this unusual society with thirty-two members, all wealthy Scottish lairds, in 1732, and it would run until 1836. Anstruther was an important port, central to sea-trading (hence the strong nautical theme in the artefacts used by the society). The Beggar's Benison had at least two branches, Anstruther with its insignia represented by an anchor or ship and Edinburgh, represented by its castle, established in 1752, but more likely there were branches all over Scotland. By 1775, the Wig Club, an offshoot, was also formed in Edinburgh and, although less is known about the sexual element of this particular club, members certainly drank to excess and enjoyed expensive dinners.

Although some members of the Beggar's Benison came from the merchant class, most of the men of the Wig Club were Scottish dukes, earls and knights. The insignias, medals and sashes of the club all point to a jovial parody of freemasonry; one of their poems 'The Lady Freemason' was an obvious lampoon on the freemasons' lodges in the vicinity. More importantly, the club served as a brotherhood uniting these men in order to further their business interests. Although the club's overt strategy was to offer entertainment in the form of wining, dining and women, its intimate nature ensured a strengthening of ties for members who were otherwise less closely connected.

Knights of Castle Dreel

According to the legend of the Beggar's Benison society, its origins supposedly date back to the fourteenth century when a group of men met at Castle Dreel under 'Fisher Willie', The Earl of Anstruther. These men owned a small fleet of armed fishing vessels which guarded the sumptuous fishing waters around the Firth of Forth and the Isle of May against English and Flemish poachers.[1] King James IV, who ruled Scotland between 1488 and 1513, had visited the monks on the island and supplied money to assist with their upkeep. Here, so myth would have it, he received the blessing of the monks which the Beggar's Benison would adopt as one of their mottoes: 'Be fruitful and multiply'. These words were to be engraved on the medals worn at meetings of the Beggar's Benison over two centuries later.

Legend also helps to date the founding of the society, the Knights of the Beggar's Benison of Dreel Castle, to around 1530. The meaning of 'Beggar's Benison' was attributed to the next king of Scotland, James V (1513–42), who liked to travel around the country disguised as a beggar in order to acquaint himself with his subjects. At Anstruther, while masquerading as a travelling piper, he was helped over a burn by a kindly young maid. As a reward, he gave her a golden crown and she in turn gave him the beggar's 'benison' or blessing:

May your purse naer be toom
*And your horn aye in bloom.**

The Beggar's Benison members shortened this to 'May your prick and purse never fail you'. Hence, money as well as sex was of central importance to the activities of the Beggar's Benison society.

Charles II was said to have visited Castle Dreel at Anstruther during his reign (1660–85), where he was entertained by the Earl of Moray, a known member of the Beggar's Benison. Here he allegedly gave the knights a wig made from the pubic hair of his mistress. Although the Beggar's Benison knights never added to the wig, new members of the later Wig Club were supposed to add a pubic hair to it from their own conquests on initiation into the Order. This suggestion is thought to have originated from George IV (1820–30) (then still the Prince of Wales) when he allegedly became a member. He, in turn, presented some of his current mistress's pubic hair to

* May your purse never be empty, and your penis always be erect.

the Order in a snuffbox. It is more than likely, however, that these myths were made up in order to provide a flamboyant history that would validate the club's existence.[2]

The original meetings of the society were said to have taken place at Castle Dreel, an old haunt of smugglers and Jacobites, but it is more likely that the eighteenth-century members met in various taverns around the town. They later gathered in a panelled room in a hostelry owned by the treasurer, Andrew Johnstone, which survived until 1871 when it was replaced by the town hall. Castle Dreel eventually fell into ruin and its owner, Sir John Anstruther, gifted it to the city in 1808.

Mention of Beggar's Benison appears in Tobias Smollett's novel *The Expedition of Humphry Clinker* (1771). In it, one character, Mr Jerry Melford, writes a letter to Sir Watkin Phillips about the entertainment at Leith, where a fraternity gave a dinner and a ball 'to which they formally invite all the young noblemen and gentlemen that were at the races; and this invitation was reinforced by an assurance that all the celebrated ladies of pleasure would grace the entertainment with their company.' The events were enjoyed by eighty people including lords, courtesans and 'cawdies' (young fellows) who mingled 'as the slaves and their masters were in the time of the Saturnalia in ancient Rome'. One character, Mr Fraser, proposed a toast to 'the Beggar's Benison'. The toastmaster 'had taken care that all his brethren should appear in decent apparel and clean linen; and he himself wore a periwig with three tails, in honour of the festival'.[3] Such a wig was known to have belonged to the Beggar's Benison and used later by the Wig Club.

Members of the Beggar's Benison consorted with bawds in order to supply the meetings with women for entertainment and sexual pleasure. The eighteenth-century courtesan Mrs Leeson, alias Peg Plunkett, mentions the Beggar's Benison in her memoirs, noting that a certain Mrs H wrote a series of racy poems including 'Guide to Joy' which was apparently a favourite of members. No copy of the poem is known to have survived.[4] The authoress, most probably Mrs Robert Hill, whom Leeson refers to as 'the fat Sappho of Drumcondra', appears to have been connected with the Beggar's Benison, although there is no listing of a Mr Hill in any of the existing records. According to Mrs Leeson, the poem was distributed to new members. She believed the society to consist of around five hundred members, to whom she supplied 'nymphlings' or whores. For her services, she was given the freedom of their 'commonwealth', presumably Merryland, and presented with a parchment in a beautiful silver box 'with all the emblems of the beggar's benison handsomely carved on it'.[5]

From this, the society would seem to have been a large and dispersed brotherhood rather than a mere club. The silver box, as mentioned by Mrs Leeson, appears to have been given as a gift to all new members for the safekeeping of their certificates of membership.

Sex on a Platter

The nature of the Beggar's Benison society can be seen through its members' employment and personalities. They were all connected with the sea or with agriculture or from the nobility and all shared a penchant for a good song, a hearty meal and a lusty wench. William Ayton was one of the last lairds of Kinaldy and was noted for his joviality. Sir Thomas Erskine, writer of boisterous songs and bawdy poems for the Order, was the chief party organizer. Most of the members had connections with trade: David Row was Comptroller of Customs at Anstruther; John McNaughton was a Collector of Customs there, then Inspector General at Edinburgh where he set up the Beggar's Benison subsidiary. Charles Wightman, David Leslie, James Grahame, Philip Paton and Robert Cleland, son of the laird of Carnbee, were all merchants. Some served as magistrates: Robert Hunter was magistrate at West Anstruther as well as Clerk of Customs; Robert Waddell was chief magistrate at Kilrenny and a shipbuilder; David Aitkenhead became chief magistrate at West Anstruther. Some, including Thomas Oliphant of Carnbee and John Couper, were wealthy landowners or farmers; Alexander Miles owned considerable property. David Anstruther, whose father, Sir Alexander, had been stripped of his lands, had providentially married an heiress, granddaughter of the first Lord Newark. There was at least one medical man among the members: Thomas Nairn, a surgeon at Anstruther.

At first glance, it would appear that the aims of the society were to share raucous entertainment, but in fact there was an obvious link with sea trade and the law as well as with agriculture. Prior to Scotland's union with England and Wales in 1707, the country had made little economic progress, mainly because its million inhabitants were widely dispersed, with poor communications and inferior transport links. But gradually, throughout the eighteenth century, trade picked up, particularly with America. The coastline between Anstruther and Edinburgh had long been a haven for smugglers. Indeed, some of the society's members were involved in smuggling, which flourished whenever taxes were high on luxury goods such as spirits, silks and tobaccos. Scotland was particularly hard hit by the Act of Union of 1707 when the English customs duties, which had previously been kept low, were applied to Scotland. Smuggling became widespread as the population reacted with determination against the increased taxes, a sentiment endorsed by those higher up the social scale. There is plenty of reason to suspect that the Beggar's Benison, with customs officers, magistrates, merchants and landowners among its members, had come together for questionable business reasons. At least one member, James Grahame, along with Sir Alexander Anstruther of Newark and a ship's captain, was caught smuggling a cargo of brandy through a tollbooth in Edinburgh. Other nobles were involved in kidnapping the witnesses.[6] Forming a close-knit club was a sure-fire method of establishing commitment between members in order that they might continue smuggling and protect their commercial opportunities while evading the law, or at the very least maximize the group's own financial interests.

All members were given diplomas inscribed with the 'Codes of Institutes', the rules of the society, which had been devised by McNaughton: 'Having nothing more sincerely at Heart, than the Happiness and Prosperity of our Well-beloved Subjects the Inhabitants of our Celebrated Territories of MERRYLAND and the encouraging of Trade, Manufacturing and Agriculture in that delightful Colony'.[7] The 'Merryland' to which the diploma referred may have been a skit on an erotic book, *A New Description of Merryland*, a jovial piece of erotic writing that played on the image of a woman's body designed as a country, with its own creeks, bays and 'inlets'. Alternatively, the book might have been written or inspired by the Beggar's Benison. There could also have been a connection between the Beggar's Benison and Maryland in America, the so-called 'Free State'. One of the artefacts used at the ceremonies, the test-platter, has references to success in America and 'Merryland'. At the beginning of the eighteenth century, Maryland was home to about thirty-thousand people, many of whom were planters of tobacco, a major export crop and primary source of income for the colony. In 1689, they fought for the rights of Maryland to appoint its own officials and approve laws rather than come under Royal Protection from England. Later, the state's elite effectively challenged the power of the royal governors and continued to defend their interests under the restored proprietorship, and there would be continuing battles against those trying to collect taxes.

Certainly, there were definite parallels with Maryland in the dictates of the diploma of the Benison. The society's intention to encourage free trade – 'without payment of Tolls, Customs, or any other Taxes or Impositions whatsoever' – indicated that members wished to conduct their dealings without interference. If the members of the Beggar's Benison were involved in importing goods from America, or indeed from anywhere else, then it would be in their interest to avoid paying taxes. Over a century later, in 1897, Charles H. Krumbhaar, an attorney-at-law, wrote from Philadelphia to the Mayor of Glasgow after coming across some family papers relating to his ancestor, Andrew Ramsey. One parchment was a diploma of admittance as a Knight Companion of the Order of the Beggar's Benison and Merryland, with a seal of the Order attached, and dated 'at the Beggar's Benison Chambers of Anstruther upon the 30th Day of April 1765'. All diplomas had continued to originate from the main Order in Anstruther so Krumbhaar's relation had probably been a member of the Beggar's Benison in Scotland, the family moving to America some time later.

Members paid three guineas (£3 3s) for initial enrolment and the cost of the diploma. They were also required to purchase a medal, a compulsory accessory to be worn on St Andrew's Day, for which they paid one guinea (£1 1s), the same amount as their annual subscription. The society held a Bible inscribed with the twenty-nine coats of arms of current members and in which certain passages relating to sexual matters were listed and marked

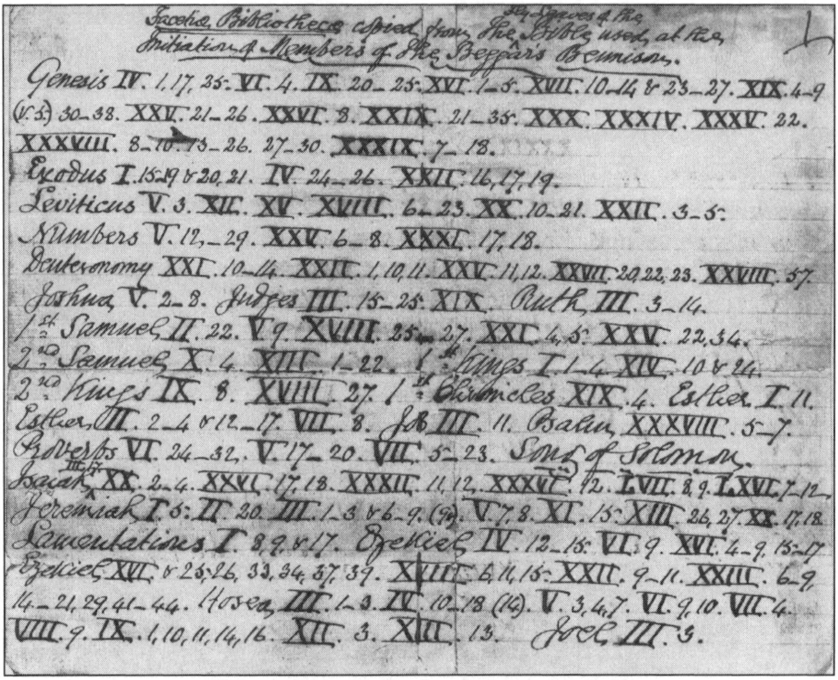
Facetiae Bibliothecae copied from the 24 Leaves of the Bible used at the Initiation of Members of the Beggar's Benison.
Genesis IV. 1, 17, 25: VI. 4. IX. 20–25: XVI. 1–5. XVIII. 10–14 & 23–27. XIX. 4–9
(v. 5) 30–38. XXV. 21–26. XXVI. 8. XXIX. 21–35. XXX. XXXIV. XXXV. 22.
XXXVIII. 8–10. 13–26. 27–30. XXXIX. 7–18.
Exodus I. 15–19 & 20, 21. IV. 24–26. XXII. 16, 17, 19.
Leviticus V. 3. XII. XV. XVIII. 6–23. XX. 10–21. XXII. 3–5.
Numbers V. 12–29. XXV. 6–8. XXXI. 17, 18.
Deuteronomy XXI. 10–14. XXII. 1, 10, 11. XXV. 11, 12. XXVII. 20, 22, 23. XXVIII. 57.
Joshua V. 2–8. Judges III. 15–25. XIX. Ruth III. 3–14.
1st Samuel II. 22. V. 9. XVIII. 25 .. 27. XXI. 4, 5. XXV. 22, 34.
2nd Samuel X. 4. XIII. 1–22. 1st Kings I. 1–4. XIV. 10 & 24.
2nd Kings IX. 8. XVIII. 27. 1st Chronicles XIX. 4. Esther I. 11.
Esther, II. 2–4 & 12–17. VII. 8. Job III. 11. Psalm XXXVIII. 5–7.
Proverbs VI. 24–32. V. 17–20. VII. 5–23. Song of Solomon.
Isaiah III. 17 XX. 2–4. XXVI. 17, 18. XXXII. 11, 12. XXXVI. 12. LVII. 8, 9. LXVI. 7–12.
Jeremiah I. 5: II. 20. III. 1–3 & 6–9. (9). V. 7, 8. XI. 15: XIII. 26, 27. XX. 17, 18.
Lamentations I. 8, 9 & 17. Ezekiel IV. 12–15: VI. 9. XVI. 4–9. 15–17
Ezekiel XVI. & 25, 26. 33, 34, 37, 39. XVIII. 6, 11, 15: XXII. 9–11. XXIII. 6–9
14–21, 29, 41–44. Hosea III. 1–3. IV. 10–18 (14). V. 3, 4, 7. VI. 9, 10. VII. 4.
VIII. 9. IX. 1, 10, 11, 14, 16. XII. 3. XIII. 13. Joel III. 3.

FIG. 26 Beggar's Benison Bible references

(**FIG. 26**). This was kept locked up with two keys, the lock engraved with two vulvas.[8] A second seal was engraved with a drawing of Castle Dreel, for use by the subsidiary group in Edinburgh.

According to the minutes of the society, on various occasions, mainly to celebrate Candlemas and St Andrew's Day, the men paid local girls to entertain them by exhibiting their vaginas. For Candlemas 1734, 'One Feminine Gender, 17, was hired for One Sovereign'; to celebrate St Andrew's Day 1734, 'Betty Wilson, 15, was hired but a bad model and unpleasant'; and the following year for the same festivities, 'A girl of 15 appeared nude for a few minutes: she shewed herself satisfactorily and was engaged for next assembly.' On St Andrew's Day 1735, Jane Bowman 'behaved well' and was described as 'a capital form of humanity'; and at Candlemas 1737, 'Two girls, 16 and 17, posed, exhibited, and danced nude.' Two 'nymphs' of eighteen and nineteen exhibited for St Andrew's Day 1737 and the gathering read *Fanny Hill*, its proper title being

Memoirs of a Woman of Pleasure. It is possible that a relation of the author, John Cleland, had managed to lay hands on a manuscript copy since the book was not published until 1749.[9] According to the minutes, all present ejaculated on to the 'test-platter', the special plate provided for that purpose.

The last meeting of the club took place on 30 November 1836 when all the members except one accepted the proposal that the society be disbanded because membership and attendance had declined to the point when it ceased to be worthwhile continuing.

Various objects held at the Artefact Museum in St Andrews relate to the society and its later offshoot, the Wig Club. These include a pewter test-platter, a punchbowl, the breath-horn, members' certificates, seals, sashes, medals, a silver snuffbox, phallic glass drinking vessels and a wig box (**FIG. 27**). However, the dating of some of these artefacts is questionable. The test-platter is thought to date from the 1780s, not the 1730s as the

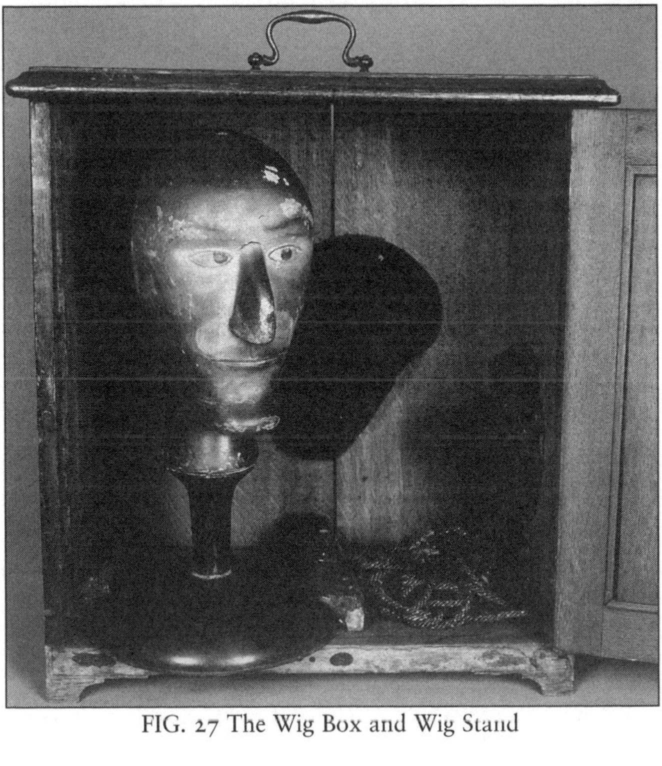

FIG. 27 The Wig Box and Wig Stand

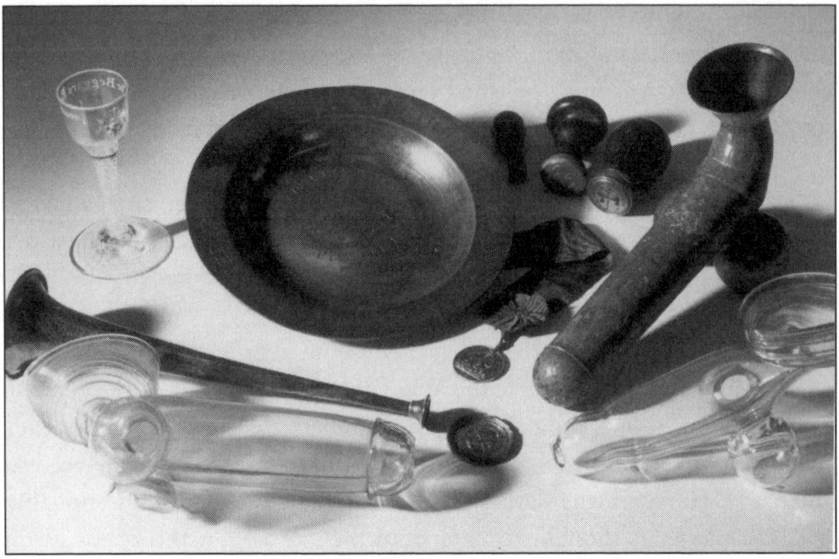

FIG. 28 The Artefacts

engraving indicates, because the maker's mark at the base of the platter is that of a Glasgow pewterer, James Graham & Robert Wardrop, which was not operating until the later date.[10] Although one of the embroidered green sashes is of hand-made silk, the other is machine made, dating it to the nineteenth century. Both are of similar design but the older one does not appear to be as old as early eighteenth century. The wine glass with the 'Edinburgh' emblem (anchor, castle and phallus) was a type that was popular *c.*1760–70. The date of the snuffbox, although engraved 1822, according to G. Dagliesh, a Scottish specialist in such artefacts, is more likely to be mid- to late-nineteenth century.

The Artefacts (FIG. 28)

1. **Test-platter.** Members allegedly masturbated into this pewter bowl. It has inscribed around its rim 'Beggar's Benison Anstruther 1732'; on the inside is an engraving of a large penis inserted into a hairy vagina with the words: 'The Way of a Man with a Maid – Test-Platter'. The erect penis has a small purse tied around it, indicative of the commercial interests of the group.
2. **Punchbowl.** Decorated with a couple of wreaths of flowers with the legend 'The Beggar's Benison' and with the Order's insignia: an anchor above a horizontal

phallus with testicles, with a purse tied on with ribbon but no maker's mark. The purse design on both the platter and the punchbowl indicates a clear connection with finance.

3. **Breath-horn.** Used to call the novices into the main gathering at initiation ceremonies, dated 1739. Engraved with a diamond-shaped panel enclosed in a vulva and the legend 'My breath is strange, LEV × 5, 16, 17, 18 1739 BB. A', giving a biblical reference. Oddly, the quote does not come from Leviticus but from Job 19:17 – 'My breath is strange to my wife'. The references on the horn might be a code of some sort but so far it has not been deciphered.
4. **Diplomas.** Two membership certificates of the Beggar's Benison still exist. One is blank; the other, handwritten in ink, bears the membership details of Andrew MacVicar:[11]

> Craving nothing more sincerely at Heart, than the Happiness and Prosperity of our well Beloved Subjects, The Inhabitants of our Celebrated Territories of Merryland, and the encouraging of Trade, Manufacture and Agriculture, in that delightful colony, and as whereas we are fully satisfied that Andrew MacVicar Esquire of Edinburgh, has all manner of Inclination, as well as sufficient abilities, and other necessary Qualifications, for promoting the noble and laudable purposes, and willing that such Bold adventures should have all suitable Encouragement, We do hereby Create, Admit and Receive him a Knight Companion of the most ancient and puissant order; of the Beggar's Benison and Merryland by the Name, Stile, and Title of Sir Andrew MacVicar, to be used and enjoyed by him in all time coming with our full Powers and privileges of Angress, Egress and regress from and to, and to and from, all Harbours, Creeks, Havens and commodious Inlets, upon the Coasts of our said Extensive Territories, at his Pleasure, and that without payment of Tolls, Custom, or any other Taxes or Imposition whatsoever.
>
> Done at the BEGGAR'S BENISON Chambers of Anstruther, upon this thirtieth day of the month known to the Vulgar by the name of November,
>
> *Witness, I the Recorder, John Graham*

5. **Seals.** Six seals imprinted with phalluses, one inscribed with 'RECTUS INS MAI 1818', another smaller one with 'ANSTRUTHER BEGGAR'S Love Cave BENISON'. One of the seals was used by General Scott, a member of the Anstruther Order, dated 1816. Two pelicans feed from a vulva inscribed *Ins: Mai* or Insular Mai, the Isle of May. This island, which is situated approximately seven miles from Anstruther, was owned by Scott, and then by his daughter, the Duchess of Portland. Legend has it that tragedy struck, in 1791, when the lighthouse failed to show light. The weather was so bad that no boat dared to sail to the island. On the third day, when the storm abated somewhat, a crew in a boat made the journey to the lighthouse. When they arrived at the door, they smelled the strong odour of sulphur. On forcing an entry, they found the keeper, his wife and five children all dead from suffocation, and a sixth still feeding at its mother's breast.

6. **Sashes.** Two green sashes embroidered with 'SOVEREIGN BEGGAR'S BENISON'; and five medals, some of different designs of a mould of Adam and Eve in various poses, bearing the quote from the Bible 'BE FRUITFUL AND MULTIPLY' with the words 'LOSE NO OPPORTUNITY' on the reverse. A cutting from a catalogue indicates the sale of a similar medal 'sold by auction in Dowell's Edinburgh on 15th April 1898'.
7. **Silver Snuffbox.** Packed tightly with ginger hair, it carries a note inside: 'Hairs from the mons Veneris of a Royal Courtesan of George IV. His Majesty was introduced to the sovereign and Knights of the B.B. when he visited Scotland and arrived at the Pier of Leith, for the first and last time.'
8. **Glasses.** Various glasses were made in phallic and vulvic shapes; a small port glass enamelled with the Edinburgh Benison badge, the legend, anchor, castle and phallus with purse attached; another with both anchor and castle, probably insignia for Castle Dreel. George IV, then Prince Regent, was supposed to have visited the Order and been presented with a glass bearing the Beggar's Benison insignia.
9. **Wig Club artefacts.** Three phallic drinking cups complete with testicles, one of these in sheet metal, two in glass, both with the drinking piece in the shape of a vulva; and one 'ballot' box including a mannequin head for a wig stand. The wig box appears originally to have been in the possession of the Beggar's Benison. The wig was allegedly of hair made from the 'Privy – hairs of the courtezans'. The Earl of Moray gave it to the Wig Club in 1775.[12]

Kissing the Wig

On 6 March 1775, eleven members gathered for the Wig Club's first official meeting at Edinburgh's Fortune Tavern in Old Stamp Office Close in the High Street. Although twenty-five knights had signed up, fewer than half were in attendance: Alex Stuart Esq., the Earl of Moray, the Earl of Haddington, Colonel Robert Campbell, Hon. John Gordon, Sir James Baird, Captain Gray, Captain Alexander Campbell, John Scott, Captain Stuart and Sir Henry MacDougal.[13] Unlike the Beggar's Benison, where lower-status members had been allowed to join, the Wig Club was made up exclusively of the nobility. Lord North was appointed 'cady' to the Wig; in other words, engaged to look after it.[14]

By the following year the club was expanding, with existing members proposing their friends for membership: Sir John Whitford proposed Lord Glencairn; Sir John Sinclair proposed Captain Stuart, and Sir William Maxwell was put forward by Mr Cheap.[15] These new members were in turn allowed to make their own proposals for new members: Captain Stuart proposed the Duke of Hamilton; Sir William Cummingham was suggested by Lord Haddington.[16] By 19 January 1778, there were fifty members of the Wig Club.[17]

The split between the Beggar's Benison and the formation of its offshoot, the Wig Club, occurred as a result of a quarrel between Thomas, Earl of Kellie, who had been elected Sovereign of the Order, and the Earls of Moray and Aboyne. Kellie resigned and Moray and Aboyne left to start the Wig Club in Edinburgh. The rest of the members do not seem to have taken sides as some belonged to both clubs.[18] Moray laid claim to the wig, two drinking glasses and an ivory statuette of Venus and took them with him to the new club. When the daughter of General Scott of Balcomie, the new Sovereign of the Beggar's Benison, was about to marry the next Earl of Moray, it was hoped that the two societies might be rejoined but the impending marriage had the effect of refuelling the old quarrel. Even worse, an argument broke out over ownership of the wig and the matter had to be referred to George IV to resolve. It was said that he decided in favour of the Beggar's Benison but, nonetheless, the Wig Club refused to give up the wig.

The most notable remaining evidence of the Wig Club is *The Minutes of the Wig Club 1775*, bound in leather and containing copious minutes of meetings up to 1792. The book itself appears to be quite old, possibly eighteenth century, yet the minutes are all written in the same hand. It is possible (if unlikely) that the same secretary was in charge (and present at every meeting) for seventeen years; more probably, the minutes were copied at a later date. The book contains an elaborate hand-painted frontispiece (**FIG. 29**) followed by the rules of the club: 'The Club to meet once a fortnight during the Winter session, Monday to be the day of the Meeting. Candidates must be put up to the Meeting before they are balloted for, with the Members' Names who propose them.' The wig was used as part of the initiation ceremony of new members: 'Each Knight when Admitted is to Kiss the Wig Standing and to wear it afterwards during the Ceremony of Drinking the Wig, and the new Knight's Health. As it is impossible to suport [*sic*] the Honor [*sic*] of the Wig, if Drinking to excess Prevails, it is agreed that after each Knight has had one Bottle of

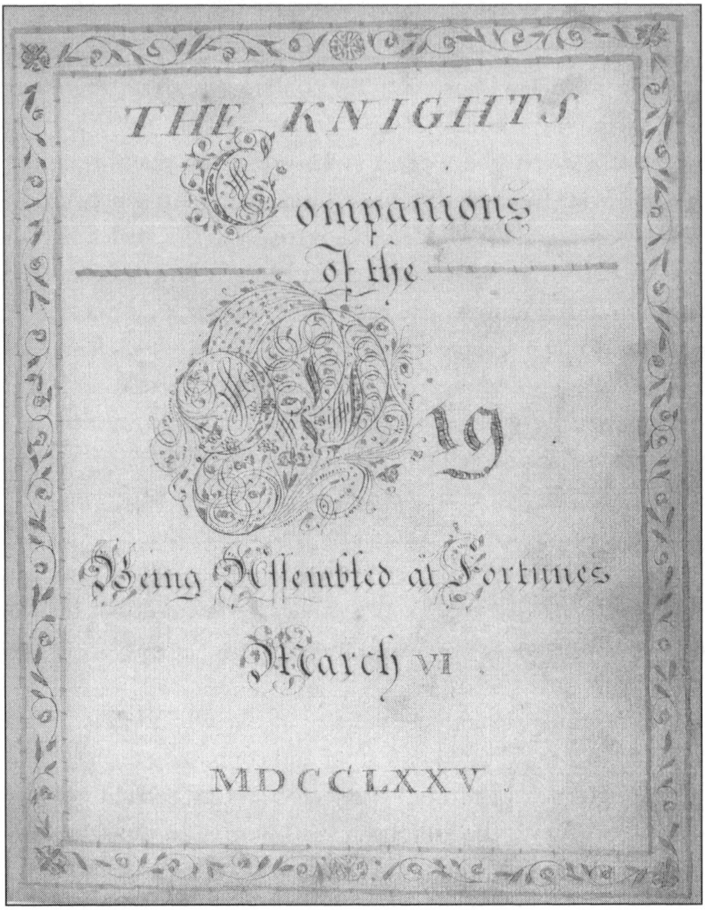

FIG. 29 The Book of Minutes for the Wig Club

Wine, the President is to call for a Bill, and the Wig is to be put in its Box, one Key of which is to be left with the President for the next meeting.'[19] Thereafter, he became a fully fledged member and a 'Companion of the Wig'. Although the wig itself no longer exists, the wig box and the wig stand, a *papier-maché* head on which it stood, is part of the collection of artefacts. It was in use at the meeting on 5 February 1776 but the original stand for the wig was not. Orders were given to Mr Wilson to make a new one immediately.[20]

The significance of the wig is now lost but there is a possible connection with the fact that George III, on ascending the throne in 1760, upset the peruke-makers by refusing to wear a wig. The *Gentleman's Magazine* and *London Magazine* put forward their case, 'setting forth the distress . . . from the decline of the trade occasioned by the present mode of men in all stations wearing their own hair'. Prior to this event, it had been common for men to shave their heads and put on some form of powdered wig, usually made of either horse or human hair. These were worn curled or straight, sometimes with a pigtail or bound with ribbons. Around 1765, it became the fashion for younger men to refrain from wearing wigs and keep their own head of hair.[21]

One of the oaths of the Wig Club forbade any knight from coveting another knight's wife, or 'cheating at hazard', a card game. While the society was totally against sodomy, drinking to excess was permitted and even encouraged. Phallic glasses were used, made out of a tube of glass complete with rounded scrotum. In keeping with this penis veneration, a day was set aside for its celebration. At the same meeting at which members had ordered a new wig stand, they unanimously agreed 'that the first Monday of every February (which is to be called St Pego's Day), the Club is to meet and drink to the Wig out of the prick Glass and on which they are to pay their Subscription.'[22]

A shared love of good food was a priority in the society, with one of the main activities of the Wig Club 'to prepare a Dinner at Half a crown a head for the Members in Town'.[23] Members usually paid ten shillings, 'being charged in the Bill for Officers, and Waiters'. However, at some meetings only a few members turned up, so a proposal was set down that in such circumstances only a shilling each should be paid. There were evidently problems regarding the collection and payment of bills, no doubt due to the inebriation of some members. It was therefore suggested 'whether it would not be better that the Members present should Pay half a Crown for their next Dinner, the mode of Collecting that Money afterwards being uncertain and Troublesome'.[24]

Plays were also a feature of entertainment for members. On 14 February 1780, it was agreed that they should book a play for the next meeting: 'The meeting having come to the Resolution to bespeak a Play they have chosen Wednesday se'en night the 23rd for the Night, the secretary is desir'd to bespeak the Comedy of the Clandestine Marriage and Fortunatus.' Written by George Colman the Elder and David Garrick, *The Clandestine Marriage* was first performed at Drury Lane in 1766 and remained popular during the latter part of the century. The second play referred to was most likely Dekker's *Pleasant Comedy of Old Fortunatus* (*c.*1598). Fortunatus was a hero of medieval legend (from Eastern sources), a beggar who chooses riches from among the rewards offered by Fortune in the shape of an inexhaustible purse and a wishing cap.[25] The joke for the members would have been the implied connection between Fortunatus the beggar and his items and the purse of the Beggar's Benison and the wig of the Wig Club. Drinking to excess would continue to be a main activity of the club: 'The next meeting to be on Tuesday the 24th Jan. 1792. The hardest drinker of the company in the Chair.'[26]

At the end of that year, there appears to be have been a hiatus in the club's activities, as the minutes abruptly cease for a period of nine years. Then a new set of minutes appears: handwritten scrappy pieces of loose, white, folded foolscap paper dating from 1801. At this stage, admission cost two guineas for six regular meetings, with no strangers allowed. Attending the revived club's second meeting were Captain Hamilton, Lord Elcho, Lord Down, Sir John Whiteford, Mr Oswald, Mr Douglas and Mr Murray. The minutes for the earlier club sessions seem to have been mislaid:

> Mr Douglas informed the meeting that he had received no answer from Gen. Stuart informing him that he had none of the old Books or minutes of the Club, the meeting therefore referred the consideration of the Rules of the Club but appoint the present members why there is Reason to meet, inspect the existing Rules and Report to the General Meeting upon St Pego's Day . . .[27]

Regardless of attempts being made to revitalize the club by introducing new members, overall attendance continued to decline and meetings became sporadic.

The reformed club was clearly struggling from the start. The minutes report few club activities, merely listing members in attendance and dates of future meetings. Following the third meeting, on 18 July 1801 (a Saturday during the Race week, when it should have been well attended) a disappointed secretary noted: '. . . finding no Person at the Dinner Hour but David McDonald Grant Esq. and have (by Consent) adjourned the meeting to the 2nd Saturday of Jan. 1802.' However, an attempt to revive the group appears to have been in vain. By the fourth meeting, held on 9 January 1802, Lord Elcho the chairman sadly reported: 'No member attending on – this – Day – I have only to regret their Loss of Power – to do Justice to the Wigs and resign the Keys of the Box and the Precious Jewells it contains into the Hands of Lord Downe – The Rightful Heir to this Valuable Property.'[28]

By the sixth meeting, efforts to revive the club were at last paying off but this had taken three years. A heartier gathering had turned up for the meeting held on 20 March 1805, with about ten people in attendance. New members were optimistically being voted in; those balloted for and admitted included the Earl of Dalhousie, Lord Stephenson, Sir Charles Douglas, Sir John Hope, Sir John Meron Maxwell, Mr Campbell of Blythwood, Captain Oswald, Lord Montgomerie, Hon. Mr Maule Major McLean Ardgour Mr R. Oswald and Hon. Mr Dundas of Melville Castle for D. H. Blair.[29]

By the seventh meeting three weeks later, the company had again dwindled to only three people: Lord Doune, Mr Douglas and Mr Oswald. It was the latter's inaugural meeting and he was taken through the ceremonial procedure as prescribed by the rules of the club, thereby allowing him to take his seat. Lord Errol was then proposed by Mr Douglas and seconded by Mr Oswald.[30] Despite the poor attendance, those present still managed to raise enthusiasm: 'Lord Doune Bets Mr Oswald a Dinner for six X 2 that he produce a Bottle of Port from Mr Ewing better than Mr O shall produce from Mr Kinlogh.' Meeting places shifted from the Royal Exchange Coffee House to Mr Ewan's Tavern, also taking in Fortune's Tavern in Princes Street, and the Maecenas Tavern. The meetings ceased to be minuted at this point but the Wig Club appears to have continued as there is evidence of a meeting on 31 July 1823 and a list of sixty-two members at December 1827. There had been about one hundred and fifty-five members during the life of the club,[31] but it would fold soon afterwards.

*

The Beggar's Benison and the Wig Club, jovial societies for the entertainment of libertines, served as systems of male bonding during the eighteenth century. Although the basis for the formation of these societies was, on the surface, a shared interest in sex, it is apparent, considering the backgrounds of the men involved and the references in the rules and diplomas, that the underlying link, at least for the Beggar's Benison, was tax evasion and the support of free trade. The fact that the Beggar's Benison was founded in Anstruther confirms the town as significant port at this time, with a need to protect the economic interests of the local elite. The Edinburgh branch was also important because of its trading value as a capital city.

From Peg Plunkett's estimate of over five hundred members, it is probable that the Beggar's Benison extended beyond Anstruther and Edinburgh. It is hardly surprising that evidence for other branches is lacking, considering the secrecy which surrounded the societies, but these are likely to have been established in trading areas where business links had to be reinforced by the organized membership of a club. What is most remarkable about the two clubs is that so many artefacts, as well as some of their records, have survived to shed light on their clandestine activities.

*

Apart from the manuscripts and the artefacts held at St Andrews University, there is a main source detailing the history and activities of the Beggar's Benison, divided into two sections. The first part, *Records Of The Most Ancient And Puissant Order Of The Beggar's Benison and Merryland, Anstruther*, was published as a history and records the strange phallic and vulvic artefacts belonging to the Beggar's Benison; the second is the *Supplement* to the first part called the *Historical Portion*.[32] These were originally produced as two separate booklets in 1892 by Leonard Smithers, a notorious publisher of pornographic works.

The *Historical Portion of the Records*, or the history of the Beggar's Benison, was allegedly taken from copies of a scrapbook purported to have belonged to the Order. According to the *Records*, a copy was made at the closure of the Order in 1836, when the scrapbook was burned by Matthew Forster Connolly, the town clerk of Anstruther and the last surviving member who died in 1877. Several books from the society were said to have been stolen or destroyed by various officials. As well as outlining the history of the society, the *Historical Portion of the Records* described various artefacts used by the members during their meetings.

The *Historical Portion* contains what are supposed to be some of the remaining minutes of the Order from the 1730s, reprinted along with songs, toasts, poems and essays that were sung and read at the meetings. Essays included detailed descriptions of genitals and of the act of sexual intercourse. Because Smithers was such a notorious fabricator of erotica, the 'facts' presented in this book are not reliable. He frequently concocted tales to make money. The minutes are the most dubious records connected to the Beggar's Benison, although the *Historical Portion* appears to be based on fact.[33]

Notes on 'The Records of the Beggar's Benison Society and Merryland of Anstruther, Fife, 1739–1836' are held at St Andrews University Muniments.[34] This claims to be a typewritten copy of a short history written by a member of a revived version of the Order in the late nineteenth century, but it looks more like proofs, with additions, of Smithers's edition of the book. The main information about the Wig Club comes from the remaining minutes of their meetings which are kept at St Andrews University library.

CHAPTER SEVEN

Sodomy: 'A Monstrous Sin Against Nature'

> If lust present, they want of women's aid,
> Each buggers with content his next comrade.
>
> Earl of Rochester, *Sodomy, or the Quintessence of Debauchery* (1684)

In the seventeenth century, sodomy was regarded as a 'monstrous sin against nature'[1] and was seen to incorporate three sexual activities, all considered abnormal. These involved anal intercourse between men, anal intercourse between a man and a woman, and any intercourse with animals. Sodomy was therefore regarded as a crime of which anyone could be capable, like murder or blasphemy. Yet a subtle shift in attitudes occurred in the following century, when sodomy became more closely associated with sexual activities between two men. It also came to describe a particular type of individual rather than the act itself.

Because the British considered sodomy abhorrent, they chose to distance themselves from it. The spread of the vice was therefore blamed on foreigners, and commentators voiced concern that it was creeping closer to home. As early as 1663, the diarist Samuel Pepys noted that a couple of his acquaintances had remarked that 'buggery is now almost grown as common among our gallants as in Italy, and that the very pages of the town begin to complain of their masters for it'.[2] According to one erotic account, *The Wandering Whore* (1660), men preferred having sex with boys but would resort to women if necessary; that men would 'fayn be buggering some of our wenches, if the Matron could get their consent, but had rather be dealing with smooth-fac'd 'prentices'.[3] The following century, the British envoy in Italy, Davenant, informed his counterpart in Paris: 'I have met with a very dirty piece of business upon my arrival here . . . Mr Cresswell was arrested by an order of a Deputation of the Senate, which has the inspection in cases of sodomy. They call them here *il Magistrato dei Virtuosi*. He was immediately carried to the prison of the palace, with a young Genoese boy he had lately dressed up, and nobody is admitted to see him.'[4] Two accounts, *Hell Upon Earth: or the Town in an Uproar* (1729) and *Satan's Harvest Home: or the Present State of Whorecraft, Adultery, Fornication, Procuring, Pimping, Sodomy and the Game at Flats** (1749), blamed the influx of effeminate sodomites into Britain on the French, the Dutch and the Italians. Boys could now easily be picked up in London and Paris, so much so that whores were complaining it was ruining their trade.

Sodomites were the main targets of early religious attacks. One tract, *A Flaming Whip for Lechery: or the Whoremaster's Speculum* (1700), defined its intentions 'as a *Caveat* and *Warning* to those who are guilty of that reigning Sin of *Uncleanliness*, to repent and reform'. Furthermore, sodomites were blamed for turning women into whores whereby 'the *lewd Conversation* of the Sodomites had before-hand infected the minds of those Damsels'. The condemnation of these '*unnatural villainies* practis'd by the Sodomites' and their '*Vile Lusts*'[5] echoed contemporary reaction to such activities. Indeed, in most early writings there is an obvious aversion to sodomy. Another book, *The Priest Gelded: Or, Popery At The Last Gasp Shewing* (1747), attacked the Catholic Church for more easily accepting sodomy and adultery than clerical marriages, grumbling, 'the Tax for Eating Eggs in *Lent* is greater than that for *Sodomy;* and the Penalty upon a priest that marries is greater than upon those that commit that monstrous and unnatural Villainy.'[6] Marriage between a man and a woman was considered the one true path, the prime aim of such couplings being propagation of the human race. The fact that sodomy was not procreative was part of the reasoning for its being perceived as against nature. Not only were sodomites deemed unnatural but they were

* 'The Game at Flats' referred to lesbianism: two women rubbing the flat parts of their pudenda together.

considered brutish even when classed as effeminate. A letter to the *London Journal* for 7 May 1726 from 'Philogynus' (women-lover) denounced the current 'effeminacy', suggesting that these men 'despise the Fair Sex', and concluding that they were 'brutish People . . . hardn'd in Inquity'.[7] According to the newspapers of the day, there were more cases of sodomy than of any heterosexual crimes. Even the theatre took up the cudgel against sodomy. In the same year, in *The Stage Defended*, John Dennis raged, 'Let fornication be ever so crying a Sin, yet Sodomy is a Crime of a thousand times a deeper Dye. A Crime that forc'd down a supernatural Fire from heaven, to extinguish its eternal Flames . . .'

On sodomy, playwright and essayist Hester Thrale noted, 'there is a strange propensity for these unspeakable crimes.' The explanation for its spread was given in *Plain Reasons for the Growth of Sodomy in England* (1728), printed as a twenty-four-page pamphlet selling for sixpence. The blame was thrown at the door of new schools, particularly those which taught dancing as part of a boy's education. Although old schools like Westminster and Eton could still produce a manly man, it was claimed that some boys educated elsewhere were spoiled and mollycoddled by their mothers. These women turned their sons into 'milksops' by encouraging them to drink too much tea, eat too much food, as well as feeding them quack medicines. Other causes included 'early Intemperance, sitting up late Nights, eating *Meat Suppers*, and drinking Wine and other strong Liquors . . .'[8]

Effeminacy of dress and manners turned boys into fops, according to the author of *Plain Reasons* who condemned the preposterous fashionable dress of these 'pretty fellows' with their silver buckles, fancy breeches and silk waistcoats. Worst of all were the coiffures: '. . . what renders all more intolerable is the Hair strok'd over before and cock'd up behind, with a *Comb* sticking in it, as if it were just ready to receive a Head-Dress.'[9] Indeed, some of the top beaux-about-town went so far as to make themselves look like women, and had even taken to using make-up. More distasteful still were the open displays of affection between men, now grown to such a proportion that the practice needed particular discouragement. The author disparagingly remarked, 'of all the Customs *Effeminacy* has produc'd, none is more hateful, predominant, and pernicious, than that of Men's *Kissing* each other.' Again, Italy was blamed for initiating this practice, and France for following suit: 'The *Fashion* was brought over from *Italy* (the *Mother* and *Nurse* of *Sodomy*), where the *Master* is oftener *Intriguing* with his *Page*, than a *fair Lady*. And not only in that Country but in *France*, which copies from them, the *Contagion* is diversify'd.' But nothing was so bad as seeing two grown men '*Slavering* every Time they meet, *Squeezing* each other's Hand, and other *indecent Symptoms*'. (**FIG.** 30).

Criminal Couplings

Sodomy was not a crime in common law until 1533 when the 'Act for the Punishment of the Vice of Buggery' was introduced. Buggery remained a capital offence in England until 1861, the last execution taking place in 1835.[10] The very least an exposed sodomite could expect was a stint in the

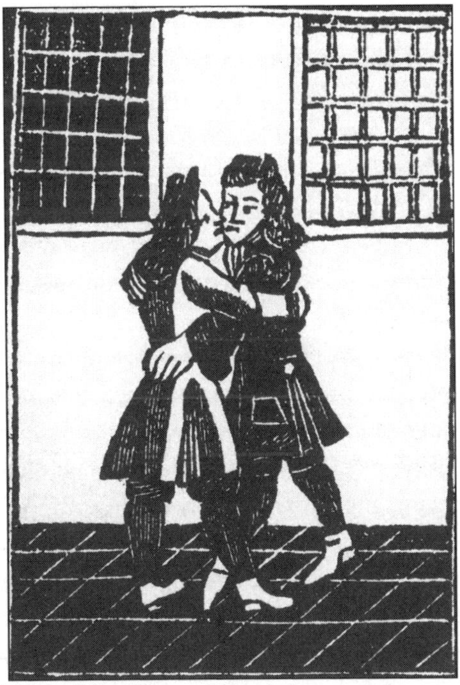

FIG. 30 *The Women-Hater's Lamentation*, 1707

pillory, a hefty fine and a prison sentence of a couple of years. The pillory in itself was often a form of death sentence as people rarely came out of it unscathed. It was an occasion of spectacle for which the mob collected rotting food, stinking fishbones, putrid eggs, and dead rats and cats to throw at the victim. The overwhelming avalanche of missiles could take out an eye, or leave the prisoner maimed. The *Gentleman's Magazine* in 1762 tells of an assault on a sixty-year-old man who had been placed in the stockade for attempted buggery. The crowd stripped him bare, splattered him with mud and left him hanging.[11]

In canon law, sodomy was a reason for legal separation between man and wife. However, this was difficult to prove and, although two test cases were brought in 1793 and 1824, they were not successful and merely a cause of embarrassment for those involved. In one case, the wife accused her husband of sodomy with a boy but, because the offence was not proven, the husband was convicted only of attempted sodomy or persuasion to consent to it. This was a cautious legal response compared with the often violent reaction of the public to sodomitical acts between two men.[12] Many of the sodomy cases were made known through the publication of pamphlets which related the trial reports and were sold as reading fodder for the inquisitive reader. The notorious pornographer Edmund Curll published a catalogue of such pamphlets in *Curlicism Display'd* (1718),[13] including *The Tryal and Condemnation of Mervin, Lord Audley Earl of Castle-Haven*, a seventeenth-century case of buggery and rape which continued to attract interest throughout the eighteenth century.

A series of trials came to the courts as a result of investigations by the Society for the Reformation of Manners which had been formed in the 1690s with the prime intention of suppressing vice. Judging by the number of prosecutions taking place during this period, one of the society's main activities was exposing and prosecuting sodomites. In April 1727, Charles Hitchen, a former cabinet maker in St Paul's Churchyard, and current Under Marshal of the City of London, was charged with committing sodomy with one Richard Williamson. Hitchen was an active member of the Society for the Reformation of Manners yet, according to Williamson's testimony, was a sodomite himself. Hitchen had invited him for a drink at the Royal Oak in the Strand but Williamson had gone off to do some business in the Savoy Hotel, leaving his hat as a pledge to return. When he came back they went together to the Rummer Tavern for two pints of wine where Hitchen made attempts to seduce him. Williamson recalled, he 'hugg'd and kiss'd me, and put his Hand ——'. The two men went on to the Talbot Inn where Hitchen ordered a bed to be made up for himself, drank another pint of wine and requested a couple of nightcaps; they then went to bed and had sex together.[14] Eventually, Hitchen was caught in the act in a Charing Cross tavern and sentenced to the pillory for attempted sodomy. Despite covering himself in armour and bribing his cronies to provide a blockade to hold off the mob, his armour and clothes were torn off and his life hung in the balance until reinforcements were called in. Hitchen was married and had at least one child. After the incident, his wife petitioned the courts for relief.[15]

In 1780, William Proctor, a grocer, and Thomas Readshaw, an undertaker, were both caught in an indecent situation. Proctor had approached Readshaw with the question, 'What do you think of a good prick?' The answer came, 'I don't do much in that Way, but when I do, I have five guineas, but as I have taken a liking to you, I'll oblige you for two.'[16] In another case, a twenty-four-year-old Derbyshire labourer, Joseph Bacon, along with a thirty-six-year-old Leicester labourer, Richard Briggs, were taken to Newgate Prison for the crime of sodomy. At their trial in January 1790, both were sentenced to be pilloried at Hay Hill in the Parish of St George, and again at Charing Cross, followed by two years' imprisonment. The Register of all the Prisoners of the Gaol of Newgate at 28 September 1793 includes the names of repeat offenders: James Harrison, a Manchester blacksmith (his second case in three years), and William Green, a London butcher, were both accused at the sessions in January 1793 and sentenced to twelve months in Newgate.[17] Despite the risks involved, these men were determined to pursue their sexual preferences. Although they knew that they would be subject to the pillory and possible imprisonment, even to risk their lives, they would continue to seek out other men.

Rum, Sodomy and the Lash

Cases of sodomy were also to be found in the army and the navy. One infamous case was that of Captain Rigby: he and a gang of sodomites at Windsor were arrested and placed in Newgate Gaol in 1698. Rigby had been captain of the *Mermaid* in 1693 and then of the *Dragon*, a man-of-war. In this instance, he had been caught attempting to seduce a young man in a park. Despite being acquitted, he was later entrapped by Thomas Bray, a member and informer of the Societies for the Reformation of Manners. The bait consisted of a nineteen-year-old servant, William Minton, whom Rigby had met in St James's Park on Guy Fawkes' Night. He had taken Minton's hand, squeezed it and 'put his Privy Member Erected into Minton's hand; kist him, and put his Tongue into Minton's Mouth'.[18] They arranged to meet up in the George Tavern in Pall Mall where, unfortunately for Rigby, a constable and his two assistants lay in wait in the next room. Rigby was found guilty and sentenced to stand in the pillory, followed by one year's imprisonment. Captain Rigby's plight had an effect on other sodomites; one Dutch merchant, known as the Queen of Sheba, on hearing of Rigby's fate, absconded to Germany.[19]

At the beginning of the century, life in the army left a lot to be desired. The *London Spy* was to write, 'A Foot Soldier is commonly a Man, who for the sake of wearing a Sword, and the Honour of being term'd a Gentleman, is coax'd from a Handicraft Trade, where he might live comfortably, to bear Arms for his King and Country, where he has the hopes of nothing but to live starvingly.' An ordinary private foot soldier would earn about 8d per day, 1s 6d in the Dragoons and 2s 6d in the Horse Regiment. Out of the 8d a day, 2d would be withheld for clothing and expenses, the balance – the subsistence pay – covering food, drink and necessities.[20] Uniforms would be provided, complete with coat, gloves, and boots. Unlike the navy, the army did not impress, or force people to join, but was largely made up of poor drunkards who had been encouraged to join up by a jovial recruiter plying them with ale. The reporter Ned Ward was to overhear the jolly conversation of some ships' masters drinking in a tavern. 'Cheer up, my lads,' said one, 'pull away, save tide. Come, boys, a health to Moll Biscuit, the baker's daughter, that swore a sea-chest was as soft as a feather bed.'[21] None the less, despite such references to women, there was a recognized penchant for buggery at sea. 'To my knowledge,' one officer was to report, 'sodomy is a regular thing on ships that go on long cruises. In the warships, I would say that the sailor preferred it.'[22]

One man on the receiving end, John Twyford of St Clement Dane's parish, related the incident at his trial in July 1745, having been indicted for 'the detestable sin of buggery'. While in a tavern, he had fallen into conversation with a sea officer who admitted that 'he loved a soldier as he loved his life', which might have been something of a clue for Twyford as to what was to come. They started drinking together, meandering on to the Plough Tavern by the Fleet Market. Twyford was to inform the court:

> He would not let me pay anything; he said he was going to the Talbot Inn in the Strand to a particular acquaintance of his, and desired I would go with him; after much persuasion I went; he asked me to lie there; I told him I must go home, but he pressed me to stay, and he agreed for a bed for one shilling; he persuaded me to go to bed; I was very uneasy, and pretty much in liquor, and growing sleepy, I went into bed, and when he thought I was asleep he began his tricks upon me; I am almost ashamed to tell – he put his —— into my fundament, and pushing so hard it awaked me. I asked him what he was at, and said he was not a Gentleman; then we began to quarrel, and I being stronger than him turned him off, and then fell o' beating of him, and we were both carried to the watch-house.[23]

Another incident of sodomy by a soldier was reported in the press in 1747: 'Last Friday Morning a Soldier was haltered [*sic*] on the Parade in St James's Park, after which he received 500 Lashes, and was drummed out of the Regiment, quite to the Admiralty Gate, for being found guilty of Theft, and Sodomitical Practices, a Paper with those Crimes written thereon, being fixed upon him.'[24] The seriousness with which this sexual practice was viewed was reflected in the severity of the punishment, both in the number of whippings and the public humiliations. The situation became even more dangerous after 1749 when a law was introduced in the navy decreeing that sodomy was to be tried at court martial and was punishable by death.[25] Even so, in some cases, courts were reluctant to prosecute. In 1757, Henry Brock was accused of buggering twelve-year-old John Booth. The boy gave evidence, stating, 'On Saturday night he came into my hammacoe [*sic*] when I was asleep and unbuttoned his breeches and put his private parts into my arse four times in my hammacoe that night and twice in this ship.' Even when this was supported by the testimony of another shipmate, Edward Gauble, who had seen them together in the hammock and had heard the boy cry out, the court was unwilling to impose the death sentence and ordered Brock to suffer five hundred lashes and be discharged from the navy.[26] In 1764, the *London Chronicle* reported that sixteen soldiers had been charged for buggery when a sex club among the footguards was uncovered.[27] In 1772, Captain James Roberts was sentenced to death for sodomy, having buggered the son of a merchant in London. He was lucky enough to receive a Royal Pardon and escaped to France. Buggery in the armed forces continued to be perceived as a prevalent problem throughout the eighteenth century and offenders were severely punished, often through death by hanging.[28]

Clerical Cravings

One of the reasons for the attack on sodomy lay in the Bible: 'If a man also lie with mankind, as he lieth with a woman, both of them have committed an abomination: they shall surely be put to death' (Leviticus 20:13). Any eighteenth-century Protestant would be familiar with St Paul's concerns, that those 'giving up natural relations with women, burn with lust for another; males behave indecently with males . . .'

As with the trial reports of offending soldiers and sailors, pamphlets about sodomitical clergy would serve as titillating erotica for publishers. William Dugdale, another notorious pornographer, published an attack on the military Order of the Knights Templars in *Monasticon Anglicanum*, alleging that they urinated upon the cross and 'Kiss'd one another's Mouth, Navels, bare Bellies, and in the *Anus*, or the Back-Bone. That sometimes on the Members, or Yard. That they told the Brothers they receiv'd, that they might have carnal Copulation with one another. That it was lawful for them to do so. That they were to do this to one another, and to be passive.'[29] For the most part, despite the fact that French pornography was replete with sodomizing clerics, pornographic material in England was more likely to feature real cases of sodomy rather than indulging in erotic fantasies.

One such case was reported in the fourpenny pamphlet *The Infamous Life of John Church, the St George's Preacher* (1817). Church (**FIG. 31**) was brought to trial as a result of his sexual relations with adolescent boys. He had been found as a baby on the steps of the parish church in Holborn and taken to the Foundling Hospital. His sexual predilection surfaced early after a complaint was made about him at the age of nine, indicating he 'was addicted to improper and disgusting practices'. After trying his hand at various jobs, Church married and took up preaching, teaching at Sunday school in Tottenham Court Road. He managed to make a living as

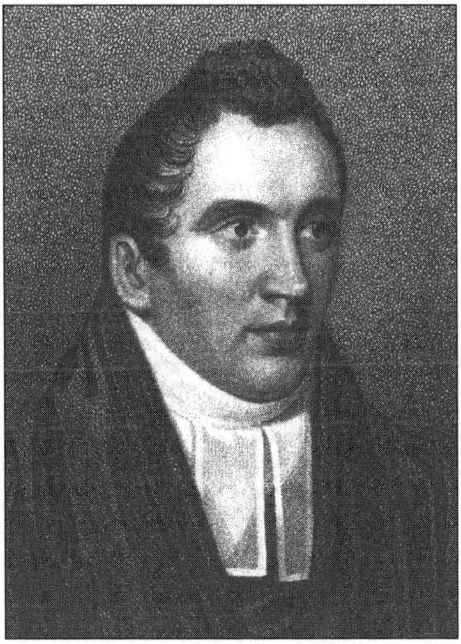

FIG. 31 Rev. John Church

a preacher in Banbury but was chased out of town when it was discovered that he had made several attempts on young men, leaving behind a wife and six children. He then became minister of the Obelisk Chapel in St George's Fields, which was frequented by a 'gang of miscreants' who nominated him as the chaplain of their mock marriages.

A further pamphlet, *The Trial and Conviction of that Infamous Hypocrite John Church* (1817), provided details of Church's molestation of one of the apprentices, Adam Foreman, in the house of Minster Patrick the potter where Church was staying as a guest. It was usual for apprentices to be bound for seven years, most often to men who ran a trade. They lived in their master's house to learn a vocation and were given the dogsbody work. It would therefore not have been extraordinary for the young apprentice to have been left to sleep downstairs. Foreman related, 'I was awoke by someone putting his hands under the bed clothes, and caught hold of him, and asked who he was.' Church had apparently visited the apprentice in the night and had put his hands on the young man's crotch. Thomas West, who also worked for the potter, gave evidence at the trial held at Surrey Assizes in Croydon on 16 August 1817. West related how he had come to check the kiln that night, which Foreman had kept burning for him, and heard about the assault that had just taken place from Foreman. Church was found guilty and sentenced to two years at Newington Gaol.

A list of the names and crimes of offending members of the clergy was printed in *The Crimes of the Clergy* (1823). Among them was the well-known Bishop of Atherton who was executed in Dublin on 5 December 1640 for seduction and sodomy. His partner, John Tithe, was also hanged for sodomy in the same year. The Reverend Cooper, rector of Ewhurst in Essex, was accused of sodomy and perverting the minds of his pupils by showing them plates from *Fanny Hill*; and John Fenwick, the vicar of Byall in Northumberland, escaped to Naples in 1797 after being accused of rape, swindling and sodomy. In July 1822, a further scandal erupted over Percy Jocelyn, Bishop of Clogher, who was caught with his breeches down at the White Hart Tavern in St Alban's Place, London, *in flagrante* with a soldier called John Moverley.[30]

Schools of Sodom

Some young men, school pupils and college students became involved in criminal actions against their seducers. In May 1730, Isaac Broderick, a teacher at St Dunstan's School, Stepney, was tried for attempted sodomy with Edward Caley, a boy of ten. He was also indicted for the same attempt on another young boy, William Ham. Stepney then was an area mainly of meadows and marshes with the parish church of St Dunstan's a local landmark. The school had been established by the Company of Coopers as a charitable institution for the education of boys. Another such institution was the Merchant Taylors' School, set up by city merchants, which would have operated on a similar basis. Some of the pupils attended free of charge, others paid a token fee of around 2d per week. These schools taught mathematics and navigation to between twenty and hundred boys to equip them to be seamen. Francis Place recalled being taught in a summer school by a master and three 'ushers', two looking after the younger boys who 'taught or neglected them as they pleased'.[31] In St Dunstan's case, the master, Broderick, was a learned man, a bachelor of arts who made a habit of molesting young boys. As his victim Caley related, 'He presently followed and locked me into the room, and took a bit of Rod and bid me down with my Breeches. Then he felt all about me, and gave me a gentle Stroke or two, and bid me not cry out, for he would not hurt me —— and then he put —— between —— and ——.' The boy eventually told his father and the case came to court.[32] Broderick was sentenced to the pillory, fined two nobles and sent to prison for three months.

During 1739, public attention rested on a case involving activities at Wadham College, Oxford. The all-male college had been founded over a century earlier and its warden, Robert Thistlethwayte, was responsible for one of the most notorious cases of sodomy of the period. His infamy inspired a poem:

There once was a warden of Wadham
Who approved of the folkways of Sodom,
For a man might, he said
Have a very poor head
But be a fine fellow, at bottom.

The Wadhamites, A Burlesque Poem pointed out the dangers of deviation from the natural course of heterosexuality.[33]

The scandal began when a student at the college, William French, accused the warden of making a sodomitical attempt on him. On Saturday, 3 February, French had been sent for by Thistlethwayte's servant, after which he was not seen by his friends for several hours. When he finally emerged, they observed him to be in a very dishevelled and uneasy state. His friends tried to find out what was troubling him, but he would give nothing away. Later that evening French complained of feeling ill and, during a violent fit of vomiting, called the warden the worst of scoundrels and villains. George Baker, another student, was among those who breakfasted with French the following day and he warned him to be more cautious in what he said as he could be expelled for such accusations. He suggested instead that his friend should take the matter up with the magistrates. During dinner with another student, Baker was told by his companion that he had heard rumours that 'the Warden did not love Women'.[34] When the warden learned that French was about to take him to court, he tried to bribe him to prevent him from telling the story. Soon afterwards Thistlethwayte jumped bail, absconding to Boulogne.

The scandal did not stop there. French's friend, Baker, accused the Revd John Swinton, also of Wadham College, of sodomitical practices after hearing of Swinton's behaviour with a servant boy, Bob Trustin. Bob told Baker that Swinton 'used to put his Cock into my Arse Hole and that I felt something warm came from him, and he sometimes made me wet between my Thighs'. In response to Baker's allegation, the proctors and heads of houses decided to call a general meeting on 21 March to discuss the charges. After some deliberation, the Master of Balliol College, Dr Leigh, accused Baker of having 'cruelly injur'd' the reputation of the Reverend Swinton. The college authorities forced Baker to place a written retraction in the newspapers, including the *Daily Advertiser* and the *London Evening Post*, or else he would face expulsion.

Not to be outdone, Baker went on to write his own account of what had happened in 'A Faithful Narrative Of The Proceedings' and successfully sued Swinton at the King's Bench for libelling him. On coming to court, it was revealed that a bevy of young men had had sodomitical attempts made on them by the warden of Wadham, Thistlethwayte. The most damning evidence was given by Robert Langford, the college butler who had been invited to supper with the warden five or six years previously. After sharing a bottle of wine, Thistlethwayte began to talk and act 'in a beastly Manner', endeavouring to kiss Langford and attempted to put his hand down the butler's breeches. The warden told him to be quiet and continued to persist 'in a very violent Manner'. On another occasion when the warden had tried to caress and kiss him, the butler told him that he wondered why 'Gentlemen of his Fortune did not provide themselves with Women, or Wives, and not act in so vile and beastly a Manner'. The warden responded that he would not give a farthing for the finest women in the world, and that 'he loved a Man as he did his Soul'.

Thistlethwayte then went on to molest the college barber who, while shaving him, found something tickling around his breeches. At first he thought that it might be the effect of the warden's gown not fitting properly, so he adjusted it and went on with his task. But no sooner had he resumed his work than he immediately found the warden trying to introduce his hand into his breeches. Thistlethwayte assured him, 'There is no Harm in this my Dear', but the barber swore that he would never shave him again.[35]

Dulwich College also proved an attraction for sodomites after young boys. The school was surrounded by fields, common land and wooded hillside and became, according to William Blake, 'the Gate into the world of vision'. It had both a charitable and an educational purpose, allowing access for twelve poor scholars, aged between six and eighteen. Richard Branson, a labourer, was tried in Southwark on 18 January 1760 for assaulting a schoolboy, James Fassett.[36] He stood accused of beating Fassett so severely that the boy feared for his life, with the intent to commit 'that most horrid, detestable, and sodomitical Crime (not among Christians to be named) called Buggery'. Fassett was a pupil at the old college, which had been built in 1619 by the celebrated actor Edward Alleyn, owner of the Fortune Theatre.

Fassett had met Branson the previous August when he had sent a message with a twelve-year-old fellow pupil inviting Fassett for a drink in the pub across the road. Fassett initially refused but Branson later asked him in person, so Fassett accepted. After a drink, Branson suggested going for a walk. At this stage, two other youths were with them but Branson turned them back. 'A little before we got to the Grove Gate,' Fassett told the court, 'he asked me, if I never got any Girls, or if I never fucked them; I answered no; I was not old enough, and I had no such Thoughts. He said I was old enough.' They continued their walk, arm in arm, until at half past nine in the evening they came to a private place in the Grove. It was here that Branson made his move, pouncing on Fassett, putting his arms around his neck and kissing him. 'He then kiss'd me again,' Fassett elucidated, 'putting his Tongue into my Mouth; and sucking his Lips, tried to thrust his Right Hand into my Breeches.' Fassett felt Branson's hand on his groin endeavouring to grope inside his breeches but they were interrupted by two men on horseback. Finally, Branson agreed not to molest him against his will and the youth went back to school, relating the incident to the gardener who then told one of the masters. 'I did not attempt to get away from him when in the Grove because I was afraid he would kill me,' Fassett explained when asked why he had not tried to escape.

Interestingly, other witnesses who had seen them together noted that Fassett appeared neither afraid nor intoxicated. One of these, Susannah Wells, a barmaid at the Bell pub where they had been drinking, reported: 'I saw Fassett, and he did not seem frightened after the walk.' Under cross-examination she added, '[I] don't believe he was in liquor before the Walk.' Richard Miller, who was a barman at the Bell, supported her story: 'I did not observe him in liquor 'till after the Walk, when he seemed very fuddled, and they all drank together . . . the Boy was not frightened, but very merry and I heard him drink Mr Branson's Health.' Despite their testimony, and the probability that Fassett had started off as a willing accomplice, Branson was found guilty.

Mollies: 'All Manner of Effeminacy'

Prowling through the sexual subculture of the London underworld in the early eighteenth century, Ned Ward stumbled upon a group of men called mollies. In *The History of the London Clubs* (1709), he wrote unflatteringly, 'There was a particular Gang of *Sodomitical* Wretches in this town, who call themselves the *Mollies*, and are so far degenerated from all masculine deportment, or manly exercise, that they rather fancy themselves women, imitating all the little vanities that custom has reconciled to the female sex, affecting to speak, walk, tattle, curtsy, cry, scold, and mimic all manner of effeminacy, that ever has fallen within their several observations.'[37] More influential men than Ward held this low opinion of the mollies and, in a few years, all those who could be identified as such were to suffer persecution to the fullest extent of the law.

Mollies often met together in the back rooms of taverns and private houses to enjoy sex and conduct rituals which involved mock marriages, births and christenings. They held 'Festival Nights' at which they performed a highly stylized ceremony of childbirth at which one of the mollies was delivered of a wooden doll:

> Not long since they cushioned up one of their Brethren, or rather Sisters, according to Female Dialect, disguising him in a Woman's Night-Gown, Sarsanet Hood, & Night-rail who when the Company were men, was to mimic a woman, produce a jointed Baby they had provided, which wooden Offspring was to be afterwards Christened, whilst one in a High Crown'd Hat, I am [t]old old Bedlam's Pinner, representing a Country Midwife, & another dozen up in a Huswife's Coil for a Nurse & all the rest of an impertinent Decorum of a Christening.[38]

Similar rituals were still being played out in 1728 when the street robber James Dalton witnessed mollies holding lying-in ceremonies. The mollies had created a complete birthing chamber in which one of the men was placed on a chair while the rest of the group attended him with towels and basins of water. Susan Guzzle, a gentleman's servant, stood in as the midwife, delivering a jointed doll, the 'baby', from under the birthing chair on which the man sat. Local bawds assisted and were in attendance at the ceremony, acting as gossips.[39]

By the 1720s, one of the most infamous molly-houses was run by Mother Clap who let out private rooms to male clients where they could have sex undisturbed. The Society for the Reformation of Manners had already begun to investigate the molly-houses and Clap's establishment was under surveillance. The place was eventually raided and she was brought to trial in July 1726. Unbeknown to Mother Clap and the mollies, Samuel Stephens had been at the house acting as an undercover spy on behalf of the Society of the Reformation of Manners and gave evidence against them. On 14 November he had gone to Clap's house in Fields Lane, Holborn, where he had found forty or fifty men making love to one another, 'as they call'd it'. 'Sometimes they would sit in one another's Laps,' he reported, 'kissing in a lewd Manner and using their Hands indecently. Then they would get up, Dance and make Curtsies, and mimick the Voices of Women. *O Fie, Sir! – Pray, Sir – Dear Sir – Lord, how can you serve me so? – I swear I'll cry out. – You're a wicked Devil – and you've a bold Face. – Eh, ye little dear Toad! Come buss!* – Then they'd hug, and play, and toy, and go out by Couples into another Room on the same Floor, to be married, as they call'd it.' A man called Eccleston would stand on guard to warn them in case anyone came, while Mother Clap went out to fetch the liquor.

Police Constable Joseph Sellers's deposition supported Stephens's statement, adding that he believed there were above forty sodomites taken from that house and committed to prison in one night. In her defence, Mother Clap denied any interest in what went on under her roof and said, 'I hope it will be consider'd that I am a Woman, and therefore it cannot be thought that I would ever be concern'd in such Practices.' Since the authorities had so much evidence against her, and nobody appeared as a character witness, the jury found her guilty. She was sentenced to the pillory in Smithfield, a fine of twenty marks and two years' imprisonment.

By the time Mother Clap's case came to court, William Griffin had already stood trial for sodomy along with thirty-year-old Thomas Newton (another informant). The same Samuel Stephens gave evidence: 'I went to Clap's House and found about a dozen Mollies, there, but before I came away, the numbers encreas'd to near forty. Several of them went out by Pairs into another Room, and when they came back they said they had been married together . . . He kiss'd all the Company round, and me among the rest. He threw his Arms about my Neck, and hugg'd and squeez'd me, and would have put his Hand down my Breeches.' Griffin was found guilty and hanged at Tyburn on 9 May 1726. He had been married to 'a good virtuous Wife, who had several Children',[40] although they were now separated.

Other charges of sodomy were brought at this time, all associated with the same group of people. In April 1726, Gabriel Lawrence was accused of sodomy with the informer Thomas Newton, who admitted frequenting Mother Clap's house which 'bore the publick Character of a Place of Rendez-Vous for Sodomites'. She provided beds in every room in the house for the convenience of her customers. As others had testified, she usually had thirty or forty clients a night, with Sunday nights being the most popular. Newton related, 'I was conducted to a Bed up one pair of Stairs, where by the persuasion of Bavidge, who was present all the while, I suffer'd the Prisoner to ——. He and one Daniel have attempted the same since that Time, but I refused, tho' they buss'd [kissed] me, and stroked me over the Face, and said I was a very pretty Fellow.'[41]

Generally, these men were unmarried and lived in lodgings or, if they were apprentices, at the premises of their masters.[42] Three of the accused in the 1726 cases were long-time widowers; one was separated from his wife and only one man still lived with his wife. Those who did marry may have been bisexual or may have felt forced to accept the conventional role, marrying and having children, in order to protect their reputation and avoid detection.

George Kedger, Thomas Wright and George Whittle were indicted in the same onslaught against the mollies. One day in July, Kedger had gone to dine at Cook's shop in St Martin's Lane where he took a seat in the back room in the yard. Eighteen-year-old Edward Courtney was one of the servers and gave evidence against Kedger: 'When I went to fetch away the foul plates, he squeez'd my Hand, and kiss'd me, and took me in his Arms, and asked me to let him ——, to which I consented, and he put — and ——.' Courtney later went to live with William Orme, a silk dyer who kept a molly-house and sold drink in private back rooms. Kedger responded that Courtney had asked him to 'do it' but he had refused. Thomas Newton again gave evidence, this time against Wright whom, he attested, sold ale to the mollies but did so privately. There seems to have been a surreptitious enterprise whereby men and women would lease out private rooms where mollies could have sex. Generally, as in this case, ale was served as a sideline, the landlord fetching drinks from other taverns for a slice of the profit. Joseph Sellers gave evidence of how, at Wright's house, he found 'a Company of men fiddling, and dancing, and singing Bawdy Songs, kissing, and using their Hands in an indecent Manner'. The other defendant, Whittle, also kept an alehouse with private back rooms for mollies.

In another incident, Constables Willis and Stevenson had visited the alehouse in Moorfields, a known cruising place. They took Thomas Newton with them as bait. It was agreed that he should go ahead and pick up a man while they would hang back and watch. That particular night, William Brown, a forty-three-year-old furniture maker, passed by. He stood against the wall as if to urinate, at a little distance from Newton. Slowly he edged his way forward and started his chat-up line. ''Tis a fine night,' he declared to Newton. 'Aye, so it is,' Newton replied, upon which, according to Newton, Brown seized his hand and guided it down his breeches 'putting his Privities into it'. Reacting quickly, Newton caught hold of him and hurriedly called his companions over to help him take Brown to the Watch-house. Brown was indicted for assaulting Newton with intent to commit sodomy and appeared in court on 11 July 1726. On being asked why he had made such an attempt on Newton, Brown replied, 'I did it because I thought I knew him, and I think there's no Crime in making what use I please of my own Body.'[43] He swore that he had gone across the fields merely in order to urinate. Despite the fact that several men and women testified that he had been married for twelve or thirteen years and that he was 'an honest man, a kind Husband, and one that loved the Company of Women better than that of his own Sex', the jury found William Brown guilty.

In a short space of time, three men – Griffin, Lawrence and Wright – had been hanged at Tyburn; Mother Clap had been pilloried, fined and imprisoned, and two other men – William Brown and a young orange-seller Martin Mackintosh – had been condemned to the same fate. George Whittle was acquitted and Kedger was reprieved but many other men were forced into hiding. This particular drive against the mollies had resulted in increased vigilance by the Society for the Reformation of Manners which was determined to bring as many men as possible to court.

Bride Maids and Bride Men

James Cook was the landlord of the White Swan in Vere Street, which was to become the centre of another court case at the beginning of the nineteenth century. As well as free consensual sex, the services of male prostitutes could be bought at the tavern. In the upper part of the house men hung around waiting for casual customers. These came from all ranks; even so-called 'respectable' men could be seen wallowing on the beds with 'wretches of the lowest description'. Some of the men took on women's names: Kitty Cambric was a coal merchant; Miss Selina, a runner at a police office; black-eyed Leonora, a drummer; pretty Harriet, a butcher; Lady Godina, a waiter; the Duchess of Gloucester, a gentleman's servant; the Duchess of Devonshire, a blacksmith; and Miss Sweet Lips, a country grocer. A bargeman, a coal-heaver and a deaf tyre smith had taken on the names of the well-known prostitutes Fanny Murray, Lucy Cooper and Kitty Fisher.

The house was kitted out with all amenities, with four beds in one room, another fitted up as a ladies' dressing-room with a toilette 'and every appendage of rouge', and a third room called the Chapel. As with Mother Clap's mollies, mock marriages took place and 'were solemnized with all the mockery of *bride maids and bride men*; and the nuptials were frequently consummated by two, three, or four couples, in the same room, and in the sight of each other!'[44] James Cook's establishment ran for only six months before it was raided.

Little had changed for the mollies – they were still being persecuted and Cook was to be accused of running a disorderly house, although he avoided being charged with sodomy. The fact that the men had continued their illegal sexual activity at risk to their very lives shows just how important it was to them. Robert Holloway, the lawyer involved in the case, reported the affair in a pamphlet entitled *Phoenix of Sodom, or the Vere Street Coterie* (1813), written in defence of Cook, his client. He had hoped that, by revealing the names of the noble and wealthy men who frequented the White Swan, his client might obtain a lighter sentence, 'for there is scarcely any description of men, but some individual is comprehended in the associations of this vice; even men in the sacerdotal garb have descended from the pulpit to the gully-hole of breathing infamy in Vere-street, and other places for similar vice.' It failed to work, however, and Cook was sentenced to the pillory.

Holloway thought 'many of these wretches were married'. Indeed, Cook himself claimed to be heterosexual; his wife ran another tavern, the White Horse in Long Acre. In any event, according to *The Times*, eleven men were convicted with sentences ranging from one to three years' imprisonment, depending on whether or not they had a previous conviction, and a stint in the pillory each. Holloway himself was eventually indicted for the libelling of a man called James Stewart referring to him as 'a libidinous immoral lewd and debauched person' and a sodomite and was imprisoned in Newgate for eighteen months.[45] Cook, who gave evidence at the trial, was eventually imprisoned for two years in Newgate in 1812.

Male Sodomy in Erotica

Although the trial reports of cases of sodomy made titillating reading, the exploitation of sodomy for solely pornographic purposes was not as yet actively pursued. When mentioned in erotica, it was presented as a perversion, rather than as a sexual activity with which the reader would want to identify. When later pornography became more explicit and included anal sex, it was frequently depicted between a man and a women, rather than between two men.

One of the earliest pieces of erotic literature, the seventeenth-century play *Sodom, or the Quintessence of Debauchery* (1684), has been ascribed, perhaps spuriously, to John Wilmot, Earl of Rochester (1647–80), who was known for his drunken excesses.[46] Bishop Burnet said of him, 'that, as he told me, for five years together he was continually Drunk: not all the while under the visible effect of it, but his blood was so inflamed, that he was not in all that time cool enough to be perfectly Master of himself.' He wrote the play to be performed before Charles II and his court but it enjoyed popularity throughout the eighteenth century. A satire full of jokes about sex and buggery, part of its humour lay in the names of the characters: Bolloxinion (King of Sodom), Cuntigratia (Queen), Fuckadilla, Officiana, Cunticula, Clitoris (Maids of Honour) and Buggeranthus (General of the Army). King Bolloxinion makes the following proclamation:

I do proclaim that bugg'ry may be us'd
Through all the land, so cunt be not abus'd
That's the proviso. * * * *
To Buggeranthus let this charge be given,
And let them bugger all things under heaven.

The proclamation was decreed a success, and the soldiers were satisfied. However, although buggery might be used for satire in plays, it was generally condemned in straightforward erotic prose.

In the introduction to *A New Atlantis for the Year 1758*, the narrator makes his abhorrence of sodomy clear: 'As men of morality, we have long been displeased at the illicit pursuit of pleasures *a posteriori*; which are not only unnatural, but also inconsequential' – a reference to the fact that it does not bring forth children. Another character in the book, Rocforia, also decries sodomites, remarking, 'The number of men who have not a passion for our sex, is very considerable, commonly despised by their own, and consists of fellows, whose sluggish souls have never known the kindling of sentiment, or any delicacy of thinking.'[47] The perception that men who prefer their own sex have no sensibilities is perhaps surprising given that sodomites were often seen as effeminate men, usually condemned for taking on the attributes of women, such as being sensitive and over-emotional.

Sodomitical scenes in the first edition of *Memoirs of a Woman of Pleasure* were the cause of the arrest of John Cleland in 1749[48] and these were edited out of subsequent versions. Fanny is described watching two young men 'romping and pulling one another about'. At first she believes this to be innocent horseplay, but soon it develops into something more: 'For now the elder began to embrace, to press and kiss the younger, to put his hands into his bosom, and give him manifest signs of an amorous intention, as made me conclude the other to be a girl in disguise . . .' Fanny knew that what they were doing was dangerous for them, pointing out that it was 'at the risk of the very worst consequences' – the death penalty. The excuse Fanny gives for continuing to watch is her intention to ensure that they are caught: 'The criminal scene, I had patience to see to an end, purely that I might gather more facts and certainty against them in my design to do their deserts instant justice.' She reports the incident to Mrs Cole, her bawd, who thinks the less said about it the better, yet even she condemns the men as 'the most worthless and despicable that could be, stript of all the manly virtues of their own sex, and fill'd up with only the worst vices and follies of our own'. She blames these 'unsex'd, male-misses' for loathing and condemning women while at the same time aping their manners. John Cleland was ostracized when his predilection for sodomy with males became evident.[49]

Even jocular songs like *The Honest Fellow, Or Reveller's Memorandum-Book* (1790) referred to sodomy as 'unnatural' sex:

But in these vicious days great Nature's laws
Are spurn'd; eternal VIRTUE, *which nor time*
Nor place can change, nor custom changing all.
Is mock'd to scorn; and lewd ABUSE *instead,*
Daughter of night, her shameless revels hold
O'er half the globe, while the chaste face of day
Eclipses at her rites. For man with man,
And man with woman (monstrous to relate!)
Leaving the natural road, themselves debase
With deeds unseemly, and dishonour foul.[50]

Sodomy is, once again, not seen as a British depravity but as 'this foreign vice; it grows not here'.

Although skits on buggery might be used in satire, it was usually depicted negatively in erotica. The more serious message – that sodomy was not a sexual activity which was to be enjoyed – was the point forced home. However, before the middle of the century an interesting development occurred with the publication of a strange tale, *A Spy On Mother Midnight*. This marked the first tentative venture into pornography for mollies.

The First Gay Porn

A Spy On Mother Midnight, Or The Templar Metamorphos'd, Being A Lying-In Conversation with a Curious Adventure (1748) was the first homoerotic novella.[51] Written as a letter from a young country gentleman to his friend in town, it forms an account of his experiences disguised as a woman in order to woo a young girl by infiltrating a group of women in a lying-in chamber. Although this can be read as an unusual transvestite heterosexual scenario with suggestive overtones of lesbianism, it is more likely to be the beginning of material intended for homosexuals. The contemporary market was still mainly directed at heterosexuals and thus featured heterosexual couples. However, reading between the lines and comparing it with the information we have on the activities in the molly-houses, such as the birthing ceremony on 'Festival Nights', it becomes clear that the book was merely masquerading as heterosexual erotica.

The story runs as follows: The male protagonist devises a plan of dressing as a woman in order to gain access to the woman to whom he is attracted. From merely looking at her face, he knows that despite her outwardly prudish behaviour she has had sexual experience. He can tell by her features that she will be easy to seduce: 'A moist Palm, a pretty prominent Nose, and a leering Eye, for all it's devout Aspect, were all Symptoms which promis'd me Friends within the Fort'. To this end, he dresses in his sister's hat with feather, a periwig and a blue riding habit. The fact that he obtains an erection as he dresses up in women's clothes indicates that the story is not a straightforward heterosexual account: 'In short, the very Idea of a Petticoat, especially the Inside of one, put that companion of mine into a mighty Fume, and it was some time before I could persuade him that, at present, it was there, and his Business to lie down.'

He finds the object of his affection acting as hostess in the inn where she has gone to help a friend during her lying-in period. While still disguised as a woman, he is invited into the room where the hostess is in bed about to go into labour. The details of the lying-in scene, although not erotic in themselves, are meticulous and exhaustive, displaying an obsessive interest in the subject matter. This attention paid to the birth echoes the rituals in which the mollies were interested. For women, the birthing ritual was used as a means of establishing intimacy among themselves. Similarly, the rituals, even though made in jest, provided a focal point to bring the mollies together within their socially excluded group.

The majority of the book is devoted to the birthing room, the conversation of the women and their bawdy talk. Only on the final page does the protagonist act decisively to seduce his intended paramour. He concludes with a telling explanation: 'I must acquaint you, that I am still in Petticoats, and have had more than one Affair with the Females of this Part of the World; nay, and have done some Execution among those of my own Sex.' This very last sentence turns the previous scenarios upside down. It suggests that he did not dress in petticoats to seduce a woman, but in order to seduce men.

The dressing-up as a woman and the attention paid to the birthing ritual in *A Spy On Mother Midnight*, along with the narrator's pointed admission of having sex with men while wearing petticoats, marks it as the first venture into homosexual fictional erotica for men.

*

In the eighteenth century, sodomy was seen as the most detestable of all vices, to the extent that particular individuals and groups of men having anal intercourse or taking part in all male sexual activities were blamed for corrupting the morals of the nation. An avalanche of material attested to the belief that sodomy was 'creeping nearer to home'.

Male sodomy was a matter of increasing concern for the British public, having been brought to their attention by the zealous performance of the reforming and anti-vice societies. As a result of the swathes of men being brought to court, the public were made aware of their sexual pursuits and fear of the spread heightened. The extent of negative publicity surrounding the mollies and the Vere Street coterie ensured that these men would be hounded by the mob. This antagonism found its release in the unprecedented number of prosecutions for sodomy at the beginning of the nineteenth century, the result of a greater persecution of sex between men.[52]

As well as enjoying sex in the molly-houses, individual men were picking up other men for sex in the streets and fields. There is less evidence that men were living together as couples. Indeed, as yet there is no evidence of a man dressing up as a woman to live with another man in order to pass as a married couple. The dressing-up and gender swapping seems to have occurred most often within secret group activities in 'safe' houses. Perhaps, because of the harsher penalties inflicted than on women, it was deemed too unsafe for a man to risk trying to pass as a woman and live as a couple.

The impression given in early erotica was that the less said about the practice of sodomy, the better. Most references to homosexuality were condemnatory. Just enough was mentioned to assure the reader that this sort of behaviour was distasteful and to be discouraged. Yet, through the insidious persecution of homosexual activities, publishers of pornography were inadvertently made aware of another potential reading audience, that of the mollies themselves. None the less, this material had to be cloaked in ambiguous language so as not to alienate other readers. Only towards the end of the nineteenth century would homosexual fiction be more fully explored.

CHAPTER EIGHT

Tribadism: 'A New Sort of Sin'

Woman with Woman act the Manly Part,
And kiss and press each other to the heart.
Unnat'ral Crimes like these my Satire vex;
I know a thousand *Tommies* 'mongst the Sex

The Adulteress (London, 1773)[1]

The cadaver lay on the mortuary slab. The surgeon called to examine the body of Catherine Vizzani was surprised at what he found. He had suspected a case of hermaphrodism and had expected to find an enlarged clitoris on the corpse – this would explain the lascivious nature and 'unnatural' desires that had been observed in her behaviour. Everyone knew that women who indulged in same-sex activities were hermaphrodites and Vizzani had been known to have dressed and acted like a man. The servants had first suspected the true sexual identity of the corpse when they came to remove the body from the bed and had noticed the prominent breasts. They had also discovered a dildo, 'the leathern Machine' as it was named, under her pillow which they had ripped open in the vain hope of finding money or something else of value, but found it stuffed only with old rags. To his mystification, on dissection, the surgeon found Vizzani's body to be that of a normally formed woman. 'The Clitoris of this young Woman was not Pendulous, nor of any extraordinary Size,' he assessed; 'on the contrary, hers was so far from any unusual magnitude, that it was not to be ranked among the middle-sized, but the smaller.' Furthermore, he found her to be still a virgin: 'I found . . . the Hymen to be entire, and of a circular Figure, like the Valves of the Intestines, to those Rings, called Diaphragms, placed within telescopes to reverberate the Rays of Light.' In this and other cases throughout Europe, the authorities would unite in agreement – that a woman taking the role of a male was usurping a man's place and putting masculinity under threat. Upon physical examination though, few such women were found to be hermaphrodites.

The case had come to public attention through a pamphlet translated by John Cleland, *The True History and Adventures of Catherine Vizzani* (1755), a story about a girl 'who, so far from being inferior to *Sappho*, or any of the *Lesbian* nymphs, in an Attachment for those of her own sex, has greatly surpassed them in Fatigues, Dangers, and Distress, which terminates in a violent Death'.[2] In the 1740s, Catherine Vizzani, an Italian woman (**FIG. 32**), met and became infatuated with a young women called Margaret, while keeping her company pretending to learn embroidery. Still

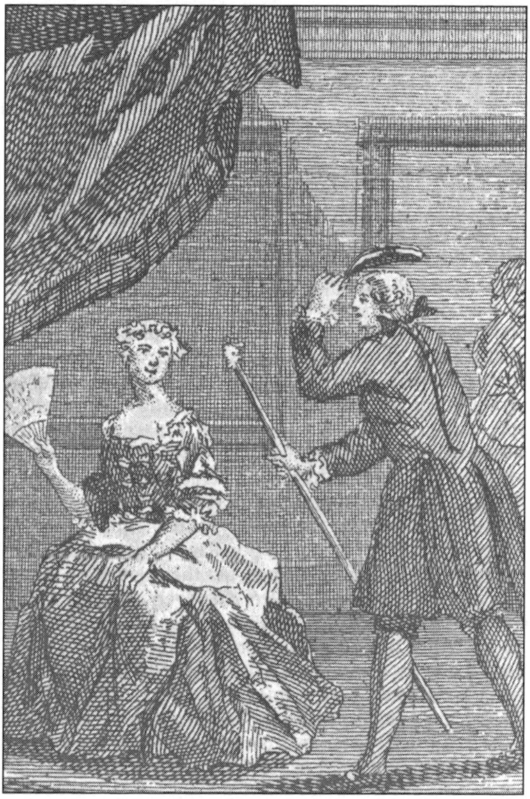

FIG. 32 Catherine Vizzani as Giovanni Bianchi, 1755

only fourteen, Vizzani began to appear beneath Margaret's window dressed in men's clothes in an attempt to woo her. She kept up this courtship for two years, by which time her paramour's father had become so incensed that he threatened to involve the governor of the City. Fearing trouble, Vizzani hastily left town, taking on a masculine persona and assuming the name Giovanni Bordoni.

Some time later, she returned in order to be near the woman she admired, and sought employment as a domestic servant at the church of Santa Maria, still in the guise of a man. She quickly tired of this type of work and, in an attempt to free herself from domestic drudgery, wrote to her mother asking her to help obtain employment with a certain captain at Arezzo. Although her mother supported this enterprise and did her best to recommend her daughter, a job with the captain did not materialize. Despite remaining in domestic service, Vizzani could at least find comfort in the attractions of the young women around her – so much so, that she was accused of 'incessantly following the Wenches, and being so barefaced and insatiable in her Amours'.

As Giovanni, she wooed the niece of the minister of the village and they both grew passionately fond of each other. She suggested that they run off to Rome together where they could marry. After acquiring two horses, they made good their escape, taking with them the younger sister of Vizzani's lover. Since she had discovered their plan and she, too, was eager to escape from her family's clutches, they had little option but to allow her to join them. The three were stopped at Staggia by the chaplain, a young blade sent after them by the girls' enraged uncle. All drew their pistols and there was a stand-off between Vizzani and the chaplain. She decided to be sensible and gave herself up, judging 'that one girl's running away with two others might, in a Court of Justice, if it should go that Length, be slightly passed over as a Frolick, rather than severely animadverted upon as a Crime'. After she relinquished her gun, the chaplain then proceeded to shoot anyway, hitting her in the thighs. The girls were sent away to a conservatory and Vizzani ended up in hospital where she contracted a fever and died.

Anxieties and 'Irregularities'

Hermaphrodism was thought to be connected to lesbian tendencies and the surgeon's suspicions in the case of Vizzani serve as an example of eighteenth-century medical thought. The Hippocratic model of the body (dating from the fifth century BC) was still circulating in the eighteenth century: it described sex as a continuum, with manly men at one end of the spectrum and feminine women at the other end, with hermaphrodites in the middle. As a result of concerns about cross-dressing, sodomy and shifting gender roles, there was an increasing interest in hermaphrodism, with a wide variety of differing interpretations and descriptions.[3] *Rare Verities*, a seventeenth-century medical advice book that was still popular, provided a chapter entitled 'Whether females may change their sex?' The author believed that 'Histories are full of such accidents', giving an example:

> a maid by a violent jump was changed into a man, her Clytoris issuing forth. *Fulgosius* writes of a maid of fifteen years of age, being married, the first night her husband lay with her, was thus changed: whether it was by reason of her too much motion in the venereal act, of the fervent heat of those parts, I cannot tell; but probably it might happen by an extraordinary dilation of the Clytoris, by much heat, and thereby being provok'd, and by reasons of its swelling on every side, not able to contain it self within any longer, issued out. This Clytoris lies latent within a woman's pudenda, which answers to a man's virility; this if it chance to grow over-much, may stand, instead of a man's members, yet without effusion of seed.[4]

The possibility of a woman changing into a man therefore sprang from the belief in a one-sex medical model of the body. Women were essentially seen as imperfect men with their genital organs kept within their body; the uterus was the female scrotum; the ovaries were the testicles; the vulva was the foreskin and the vagina was the penis. Heat was necessary for a body to develop fully. According to the humoral theory, women's humours were cold and wet, which meant they never fully developed. In contrast, a man's body was hot and dry, heating him sufficiently to allow his sexual organs to come out of his body. Although an over-simplification, based on this theory a woman, if she was heated up properly, could theoretically turn into a man.

Women could also take on masculine qualities if they masturbated. This activity was seen as threatening to women's health, as it enlarged the clitoris into the semblance of a penis and so would increase their sexual inclinations towards their own sex. Thus, physiological differences were often blamed for a woman's behaviour, an extended or elongated clitoris thought to be responsible for inciting women to make use of it as a penis. Any woman might be seen to be a hermaphrodite if she was attracted to other women – it was believed she would use her female 'yard' (the common word for penis) through rubbing or even penetrating her lover. In his diary entry for 3 March 1717, John Tomlinson wrote about 'Sir John Brownlow's Lady [who] abused other women with her clitoris'.[5]

Various debates circulated about hermaphrodites and questions arose as to whether in fact they existed. In one such confusing case, a person declared a female at birth did indeed turn out to be a man. Cornelius Wijingraef told the court in 1732 that he had been ascribed to the female sex at birth and christened Lizbeth but, on marrying and finding that he could not have sex, his parents shut him up in a lunatic asylum. After six months he was examined and deemed to be a man, discharged and told to wear men's clothing. Later doctors found him to be 'constituted as any other female . . . no parts or members have been found contrary to this.' By 1741, James Parsons in his *Medical and Critical Enquiry into the Nature of Hermaphrodites* had iterated his disbelief in their existence, blaming midwives for mistaking a baby's large clitoris at birth for a penis.[6] Yet in 1771, society doctor William Cadogan declared he had seen many such cases.

Women who were attracted to, or had sex with, other women were usually described as 'Tribades' or 'Sapphists'. 'Lesbian' was not as yet a common term but it was in use and writers and commentators of the day were aware that such activities existed. William King's *The Toast* (1732) refers to 'Lesbian Loves'; and Dr Johnson's friend the writer Hester Thrale and her circle debated 'Sapphic passion'. However, sex between women was generally more frequently spoken about in disparaging terms, reflecting the concerns of an overtly heterosexual society. Delariviere Manley wrote of 'unaccountable intimacies' in *The New Atlantis* (1709); Henry Fielding in his case study *The Female Husband* (1746) pointed to 'unnatural affections';[7] Cleland, in his account of the female cross-dresser Catherine Vizzani pointed to 'vicious Irregularities', the activities of Vizzani and her mate referred to as 'so odious and so unnatural a Vice', that one woman even described her as 'the Monster'. Women were sometimes referred to as 'tommies' although there were two different meanings in circulation: in the homosexual molly-houses, men called their wives tommies as a derogatory term but, by the mid-nineteenth century, this would be applied to masculine women-about-town, or a male prostitute.

Certain women who worked in the brothels were seen as particularly fond of passionate displays of affection towards each other. The author of *Plain Reasons for the Growth of Sodomy* (1728) noted that some of these women were 'criminally *amorous* of each other, in a *Method* too gross for Expression. I must be so partial to my own *Country-Woman* to affirm, or at least hope they claim no Share of this Charge; but must confess, when I see two Ladies *Kissing* and *Slopping* each other in a *lascivious Manner* and frequently repeating it, I am shocked to the last Degree.'[8] One tract, *Satan's Harvest Home* (1749), issued warnings about the spread of lesbian activities; the Turkish all-female bagnios were regarded as places where women, because they bathed together, sometimes became attracted towards one another. There was particular concern that this sort of activity was spreading to the ladies of England; the author pronounced that a 'most abominable Vice has got footing among the Women of *Quality*, by some call'd the Game of Flats'. The ancient influence of Sappho was cited as the source of such behaviour, teaching women 'a new Sort of Sin, call'd the *Flats*, that was practis'd frequently in *Turkey*, as well as *Twickenham* at this Day'.

The diarist Hester Thrale was most disapproving of these activities. Although she accepted some women who lived together in domestic bliss, such as the celebrated Ladies of Llangollen, she condemned other lesbian behaviour. She despised the aristocratic Marie Antoinette, declaring in 1789 that 'The queen of France is at the head of a Set of Monsters call'd by each other *Sapphists*, who boast her example and deserve to be thrown with the *he* Demons that haunt each other likewise, into Mount Versuvius.' During the French Revolution, when attacks were being made on the royal family, Marie Antoinette was accused of having lesbian sex with her maidservants; these stories were published in scandal sheets and pornography depicted her in various promiscuous lesbian scenarios. Mrs Thrale also declared that the town of Bath had become 'a cage of these unclean Birds'. Furthermore, she noted that the actress Mrs Sarah Siddons, commenting on her sister, believed her to be 'in personal Danger once from a Fiend of this Sort'.[9] Meanwhile, Mrs Anne Damer, the daughter of a general, Seymour Conway, and both friend and second cousin of Horace Walpole, was also suspected of 'liking her own sex in a Criminal Way'. She had married at eighteen, but nine years later, after her husband had shot himself when he fell into debt, she adopted men's garb and became known for her preference for women, most notably the thirty-five-year-old Mary Berry.

Anxieties about lesbian activities were being voiced in anonymous pamphlets, diaries and plays. Yet although they made society nervous, tribades were not sufficiently prominent as to be completely ostracized. To some extent, there was still a curiosity about women who desired other women, as many people did not fully understand what these women were doing. On the other hand, tribadism was transgressing the rules of a heterosexual society and action would be taken against it, particularly against those women who dressed as men.

Women in Masculine Guise

The most threatening of female behaviour was that where a woman passed herself off as a man in order to live with another woman as her husband. Although this butch archetype of the 'female husband' fits one category, not all women who married as men were necessarily 'butch'. Some dressed as men for economic reasons: living as a man would not only help the woman to conduct her daily business and earn an income for the household but also would enable the couple to live and have sex together without being subject to ridicule or specious gossip. Within these relationships, the women who lived the male role appear to have been persecuted more than the partners who continued to live as women. Women who disguised themselves as men were perceived to be imitating men, their 'superior' sex – it was felt they were trying to attain a higher status that should not be afforded to them.[10]

Splendidiello, the Lesbian Angel

One early case discovered in the archives of the records of the Inquisition in Florence describes the case of two lesbian nuns, Bernedetta Carlini and Bartolomea Crivelli. Their affair was the subject of an investigation between 1619 and 1623: Carlini had been taken to the Convent of the Mother of God at the age of nine to fulfil a vow made at her birth by her parents, a well-to-do family from a small mountain village called Pescia. She was an intelligent girl and rose in the ranks to become abbess. During this time, she asserted that she had mystical visions in which she saw angels and received the stigmata. Because of her claims, Carlini was brought to the attention of the Church authorities who, after an investigation, also uncovered her more carnal activities. They were shocked to discover that she was having sex with another nun: 'A crime so horrible and against nature is so detestable and because of the horror of it, it cannot be named.' They did, however, note the details:

> For two continuous years, two or three times a week, in the evening after disrobing and going to bed and waiting for her companion, who serves her, to disrobe also, she would force her into bed, and kissing her as if she were a man she would stir herself on top of her so much that both of them corrupted themselves because she held her by force sometimes for one, sometimes for two, sometimes for three hours . . . Benedetta, in order to have greater pleasure, put her face between the other's breasts and kissed them, and wanted always to be thus on her.[11]

Carlini, the instigator of the relationship, sometimes obtained her pleasure by force. She would also resort to subterfuge: she first pretended to be sick, then 'she grabbed her companion's hand by force, and putting it under herself, she would have her put her fingers in her genitals and holding it there she stirred herself so much that she corrupted herself.' Carlini would also fall to kissing Crivelli while masturbating her.

The most puzzling fact of the case was that Carlini envisioned herself as a male angel, Splendidiello, when she made love to Crivelli. Even stranger, the angel was only about eight or nine years old. 'This Angel Splendidiello, through the mouth and hands of Bernedetta, taught her companion to read and write, making her be near her on her knees and kissing her and putting her hands on her breasts . . . This Splendidiello called her his beloved: he asked her to swear to be his beloved always and promised that after Bernedetta's death he would always be with her and would make himself visible.'

It would be easy to assume that Carlini could not imagine a sexual relationship with another women except in the guise of a male and, at that, a childlike, non-mortal one. By this method she might absolve herself from any possible wrongdoing as it was not she who was involved. However, one of the most important features of this case is not merely the sexual acts involved but the very strong emotional attachments which were evident in the depositions. Carlini obviously had great affection towards her lover, not merely sexual stirrings. The fact that she had to engage in bodily contact through the intermediary of an angel was connected to her religious immersion and would perhaps have contributed to the spiritual intensity of her emotional commitment, while simultaneously distancing herself from any possible sin. Her religion enabled her to believe that these acts occurred through a divine interpreter.

The all-male team of examiners, having restored a semblance of order through their investigation, did not take any further immediate action. This indicated either that the Church wanted the scandal covered up, or that the incident was not taken too seriously. The nuns were sent to live in different convents.

The Case of Catherina Linck

A case that took place in the 1720s, found in the Prussian Secret Archives, was taken much more seriously. Catherina Margaretha Linck had originally begun to dress in men's attire in order to lead a life of chastity. She had joined a religious group called the Inspirants, later converting to Catholicism and then to Lutheranism. Afterwards, she continued to dress as a man to serve in the Prussian volunteer corps but later deserted to work as a spinner, reverting to female dress. At some stage, she had undertaken a marriage ceremony with another woman, Catherina Margaretha Mühlhahn. Her sexual activities only came to light when it was alleged that she had beaten up her 'wife' and stolen linen, clothes and sheets. After hearing complaints from her daughter, the mother 'took her sword, ripped open Linck's pants, examined her, and discovered that she was indeed not a man but a woman'.[12] According to Linck, this was not at all true; both the bride and her mother knew full well that she was not a man before the wedding.

Linck's defence was that she had been deluded by Satan, adding that, in any case, it was not a sin for a maid to dress as a man. Such was the confusion about her real sex that she was inspected at the town hall to confirm her gender. It was disclosed that she had fashioned herself a dildo to use as a penis in order to penetrate her wife, the device made up of a leather-covered horn through which she urinated and which she kept fastened to her body; attached to this was a pig's bladder and two stuffed testicles. After some contemplation, the municipal government reasoned that, since the instrument could not emit semen, the crime of sodomy could not apply. The court considered that 'it might appear that no genuine case of sodomy could be committed with a lifeless leather device, in which case capital punishment would not apply'. Fatally for Linck, however, they decided that the fact that she had practised oral intercourse on Mühlhahn was enough to warrant capital punishment.

The case led to much discussion in the Church courts, mainly because these events were rare and little experience had been built up in addressing such situations. The problem for the male authorities in considering Linck's 'crime' was the deficiency of biblical references to lesbianism, and thus a lack of guidance on what should be done with a woman who had sex with another woman. The court advocated that she be 'put to death by the sword' in accordance with the gravity of her crime. But, at the same time, they added,

> Should your Royal Majesty be of the opinion that the Holy Scriptures nowhere expressly recommends the death penalty for women as well as for men who had committed lewd acts; and if furthermore, in cases of different types of sodomy, when it was not committed for the purpose of emission of semen, which, for natural causes, could not be achieved in this case; then according to the opinion of many jurists, the death penalty should not be applied but only flogging.

None the less, Linck was beheaded in 1721 while her lover, Mühlhahn, was sentenced to three years in a penitentiary and afterwards banished from the town. The major accusation against Linck was that she had made up a dildo, or substitute penis, while passing as a man – a sin felt to be much more heinous than that of Mühlhahn who was seen as the 'passive' partner. Eighteenth-century Germany seems to have taken a much harder line on sex between women than seventeenth-century Italy. This could be connected to the disparity in religious and social conditions in the two countries. More likely it was because of the difference in the cases themselves: a self-fashioned dildo was involved in the German case; penetration of some kind had taken place and this was considered a grosser violation than the mere mutual masturbation between the two nuns. This, together with the fact that Linck had tried to pass as a man in the secular world, ensured a heavier retribution from the courts.

The Female Husband

According to at least one pamphlet circulating in London, Mary Hamilton had allegedly married fourteen women, deserting each of them shortly after the wedding. This was a gross exaggeration and she probably had only three wives. She was arrested in Glastonbury for posing as a doctor and for tricking Mary Price into marrying her a couple of months previously. Her last 'wife' confessed that she was unaware that her 'husband' was not a man, as Hamilton had used a dildo to penetrate her. Hamilton was sentenced to be publicly whipped through four market towns during the winter of 1746 and imprisoned for six months.[13]

Born in Bristol, by the age of fourteen, Hamilton had been seduced by her Methodist neighbour, Anne Johnstone. After the affair had ended, Johnstone opted for the conventional life and married a man but Hamilton took to travelling around Ireland preaching as a male Methodist minister. She made various attempts at wooing other women, seemingly with a view to defrauding them: one widow rejected her for an Irish cadet but another, a sixty-seven-year-old wealthy widow, did in fact go through with the marriage before discovering Hamilton's female identity. Back in England, now disguised as Dr Charles George or William Hamilton, she took up practising quack medicine, eventually eloping with a 'Miss Ivythorn'.[14] Upon discovering that her husband was in fact a woman, Miss Ivythorn could not be persuaded to continue living with her. Finally, Hamilton met up with Mary Price which eventually led to the court case.

The novelist Henry Fielding reported the story of Mary Hamilton in *The Female Husband*, adding his own variations to the real court depositions. In his version, it was the mother who exposed Hamilton's real identity after finding her dildo in a trunk, but in real life it was Mary Price herself who reported Hamilton. Fielding dished out salacious tit-bits, reporting that, on the very evening she had suffered her first whipping, Hamilton offered the gaoler money to procure her a young girl to satisfy her 'most monstrous and unnatural desires'. Even in court, she appeared bold and impudently dressed in periwig, ruffles and breeches. Fielding cited Hamilton's case as an example of unfettered female sexuality, warning his audience to keep their desires under control: 'But if once our carnal appetites are let loose, without those prudent and secure guides, there is no excess and disorder which they are not liable to commit even while they pursue their natural satisfaction.'[15] It is obvious from the pamphlets of the case that lesbianism elicited much gossip.

Mary Hamilton was not arrested for sodomy or for having sex with another woman but for fraud and posing as a doctor. It was this flouting of the law which had led to the harsh punishment meted out to her. Her crime was to have lived above her real station in life in terms of class and gender, pretending to be both middle-class and male.

'Female Friendships'

Declarations of love between women in the early modern period have frequently been compartmentalized into heterosexual fashions of the time. Passionate friendships were often thought to be a natural outlet for young women prior to marriage. Strong displays of affection between the same sexes were therefore permissible and touching, kissing and sharing beds were all acceptable customs. By this means, women would have had the opportunity to explore a physical relationship together without the knowledge of others. It would have been easy for a woman to carry out, or even to fall into, a sexual relationship with another woman in eighteenth-century England – at least on a temporary basis – under the guise of a female friendship, without any queries from others as to its true nature.[16]

It would, however, have been difficult to continue the relationship on a long-term basis. Firstly, a women's proper place was seen to be either living under the protection of her father, her husband or another male family member. Two women living together would invariably, at some point, attract unwanted public attention. Secondly, women living alone did not carry the status of married women, so two women sharing a house would have been presented with problems in trying to contract their daily business. But the biggest concern would have been financial. In view of the lack of employment opportunities for women, and the fact that women's wages amounted to less than half those of men, two women would have found it difficult to afford to set up house together.

The Ladies of Llangollen

In 1768 Eleanor Butler, a handsome women of twenty-nine, met Sarah Ponsonby, a feminine, retiring young thirteen-year-old. Some years later, they were to elope, outraging both their families (**FIG. 33**). Much as their relationship elicited gossip, these women did not project any overt sexual images and were sometimes considered purely female friends.

Eleanor came from an ancient Roman Catholic family who had inherited Kilkenny Castle in Ireland and had had an easy life, brought up

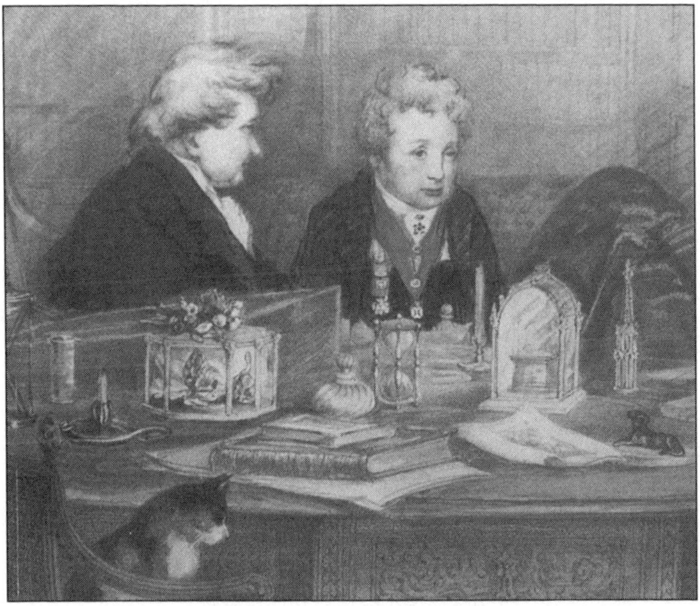

FIG. 33 Ladies of Llangollen

by her wealthy parents. For Sarah, life had been tougher. Both parents died when she was young and she was shunted between various step-relatives and half-cousins. The two girls were educated in the usual fashion for women of their class and sent off to boarding schools, Eleanor in Cambrai, France, and Sarah locally. After leaving school, Sarah went to live with a kindly but distant cousin, Lady Betty Fownes at Woodstock, whose husband, Sir William, made various unsuccessful attempts to force himself upon her.

Eleanor and Sarah had met some years earlier and despite the age difference their relationship had grown strong – they now loved one another and no longer wanted to live apart. They made a pact to run away together and waited to put their plan into action. One night, when the rest of the family was in bed, Sarah got up, dressed herself in men's clothes and packed some things into her bag. She armed herself with a pistol, picked up her small dog, Frisk, and crept downstairs. Pulling up the sash window, she climbed out into the fresh night air, looking for the friendly labourer whom she knew would take her to the eagerly waiting Eleanor. Eleanor and Sarah met up and made off to Waterford together, twenty-three miles away, with the intention of boarding a packet boat to England. However, before they could reach the boat, they were caught and brought home.

The initial relief on discovering that the girls had not run off with men gave way to distress as the extent of the passion between the two women became known. The families did not know what to make of the situation; initially at least, Mrs Tighe, daughter of Lady Betty, wrote to Mrs Goddard, her friend, that she thought the relationship 'void of serious impropriety' since there were no gentlemen involved and that it was nothing more than a 'romantic friendship'. However, Mrs Goddard took a sterner view, telling Sarah that she had a 'debauched mind, no ingredient for friendship, that ought to be founded on virtue'. Despite such opposition, Sarah resolved to 'live and die with Miss Butler' and threatened that, if she was prevented in any way, 'it would provoke her to an act that would give her friends more trouble than anything she had done yet.' Equally determined, Eleanor declared that she would not live without her friend. Thus resolved, the women took off to tour Wales, eventually settling in Llangollen.

By 1790, the ladies had become well known and gossip began to circulate about their relationship. One newspaper, the *General Evening Post*, ran an article on 'Extraordinary Female Affection' which contained revelations about their elopement and described their domestic arrangements. Even worse, it inferred that the women had Sapphist leanings. 'Miss Butler is tall and masculine, she wears always a riding habit, hangs her hat with the air of a sportsman in the hall,' the article ran, 'and appears in all respects as a young man, if we except the petticoats which she still retains. Miss Ponsonby, on the contrary, is polite and effeminate. Fair and beautiful.'[17] Eleanor, insulted at the newspaper's implication of lesbianism, wrote to their friend, the Whig politician Edmund Burke, for advice as he had had experience of suing for libel. Unfortunately, having failed in his own attempts, he could only advise them not to pursue the matter, believing that it would elicit more trouble than it was worth and, in the end, cause even more gossip. Although he sympathized with them, he doubted that they would be successful and recommended them to leave well alone.

Despite the unwelcome publicity, Eleanor Butler and Sarah Ponsonby attracted many visitors to their Welsh cottage. Their own accounts of their daily lives conveyed a domestic bliss, although their path was not entirely without ups and downs. Finances were tight as they waited on handouts from relatives, small annuities and unforthcoming pensions. They frequently ran up debts to local salespeople and were unable to find the cash for their living expenses. But the strength of their feelings for each other is revealed in their descriptions of the happiness they felt at sharing their lives. Eleanor wrote about Sarah's attention during one bout of illness: 'I kept to my bed all day with one of my dreadful Headaches. My Sally, My Tender, My Sweet Love, lay beside me holding and supporting My Head till one o'clock when I by Much entreaty prevailed her to rise and get my breakfast.' She kept watch over Eleanor all that day and Eleanor expressed her gratitude and appreciation of Sally's kindness: 'My Sally, How can I acknowledge the grateful Sense My Heart labours under, Your Tenderness, anxiety and incessant attention to your B.'[18] They expressed their love by giving each other various tokens of affection and commitment; they bound their books together with their golden embedded entwined initials, E.B. and S.P.; they signed all their letters jointly; they called each other 'Beloved', and shared a four-poster goose-feather bed with posts of carved oak. After an intimate relationship which had lasted over fifty years, Eleanor peacefully passed away in 1829, followed by her 'beloved' only two years later.

Although neither of them mentioned sexual activities in their writings, it is obvious that these two women shared a strong emotional and physical bond. Unfortunately, their life was blighted by financial problems; they were left to rely on meagre pensions and gifts from friends. Only as a result of this generosity, by frugal housekeeping and constant financial vigilance were they able to live out the rest of their lives as two women sharing a household.

Anne Lister's 'Manly Feelings'

Unlike the Llangollen ladies, Anne Lister wrote down all her sexual activities in code in her diary. Born in Yorkshire in 1791 into a family of minor gentry, she came to inherit Shibden Hall in Halifax in her mid-thirties. She spent much of her time managing the estate, studying languages and literature and travelling. She had a self-confessed lust for young women and described her exclusive desire for women in her own words: 'I love, and only love, the fairer sex . . . my heart revolts from Any other love than this.'[19] Although she had long-term relationships, she was always in danger of getting into 'scrapes', as she called her sexual flings with other women. Her attraction to them was often purely sexual, sensations she described as 'manly feelings', admitting ''Tis well I have not a penis. I could never have been continent.'

One of Anne's longest sexual relationships was with Isabella Northcliffe, whom she called 'Tib'. Six years older, like Anne, she never married. She was, however, a heavy drinker and arguments erupted because of the amount she imbibed. Anne's diary entry for Friday, 17 November 1820 announced, 'Tib and I . . . had a rowe [*sic*] . . . about drinking so much wine. Tib was very violent after she came into bed at night. We renewed the conversation & she was a good deal more violent than before . . . I stood by the fire, talking very calmly . . . Still she swore by all that is sacred she never took more than five glasses a day . . .' The conversation continued next morning, with Anne rather meanly pointing out how much drinking had aged Tib. This had the intended effect. Anne wrote, 'She was afraid I must be tired of her & could never like to be with her. She had rather do anything than cease to be loveable and desirable to me.' During this affair, Anne did not stop making advances to other women; Tib was well aware of Anne's flirtations and was concerned that there might be a problem if people began to notice. Anne recalled in her diary, 'Just before dinner, Tib very kindly told me I was beginning to be too pointed in my attention to Miss Vallance; that observations might be made & I had better take care.'[20] Both women were aware that any overt displays of sexual attraction to another woman could create gossip and provoke adverse public reaction.

Anne fell deeply in love with Marianne Belcombe, to whom she was introduced by Tib in York in 1812. After visiting the Ladies of Llangollen, Marianne wrote to Anne declaring that she wished they could have such a relationship.[21] They were obviously aware that the Llangollen ladies had a loving lesbian relationship and it was evident that Anne would have liked to live in a similar set-up with Marianne. Although she loved Anne, Marianne none the less preferred to adhere to convention and married Charles Lawton. While staying with friends, Anne lamented, 'the last time I slept in this room & in this bed, it was with Marianne, in 1815, the summer of. Surely, no one ever doted on another as I did then on her. I fondly thought my love and happiness would last forever. Alas, how changed. She has married a blackguard for the sake of his money. We are debarred all intercourse.'[22] Charles had become suspicious of their relationship after finding one of Anne's coded letters to his wife. In order to avoid his constant vigilance, rather than meet at the marital home, they contrived to meet at Marianne's family home in York where they could share a bed together unhindered.

Anne continued to have sexual relationships with both Marianne and Tib whenever she had the opportunity. After Marianne's marriage, when they were together again, Anne remarked to Marianne, '"Well, come, whatever C [Charles, Marianne's husband] has done to me, I am even with him. However, he little thinks what we are about. What would he do if he knew?' Marianne answered, 'Do? He would divorce me.' She then proceeded to kiss and fondle Anne. 'From the kiss she gave me', Anne wrote, 'it seems as if she loved me as fondly as ever. By & by, we seemed to drop asleep but, by & by, I perceived she would like another kiss & she whispered, "Come again a bit, Freddy" [her nickname for Anne] . . . so, I got up a second time, again took off, went to her a second time &, in spite of all, she really gave me pleasure, & I told her no one had ever given me kisses like hers.'[23]

Anne pursued various lovers and became infatuated with one of the local girls, a Miss Elizabeth Browne. 'I wonder what she thinks of me?' Anne mused. 'My attention to her is certainly sufficiently marked to attract her notice. Is she flattered?'; and again, 'Thinking of Miss Browne all the way home & while I was getting into bed'; and yet again, 'I either am, or fancy I am, in love with the girl. At least I think more of her than ever & felt quite low & vapourish at not seeing her.' They began to meet regularly and soon became the target of neighbourhood gossip.

Although Anne continued to wear petticoats, her short hair and masculine manners caused malicious speculation about her sexual identity in Halifax society. The locals nicknamed her 'Gentleman Jack' and she eventually became the victim of harassment. In her journal, she wrote, 'The people generally remark, as I pass along, how much I am like a man.' In one incident she was jibed at by three young men who shouted after her, 'That's a man', and one asked, 'Does your cock stand?' Nevertheless, she was obsessed with Miss Browne and carried out her business as usual, refusing to be demoralized by the locals' spiteful comments. A more frightening episode occurred one night when two men were hanging around outside her house. Anne, refusing to be subdued, charged her pistol and declared that she would 'blast their brains out if they did not immediately go about their business'. In another incident, when travelling with the mail coach, she was subjected to an assault: 'There were several bad women standing about the mail. They would have it I was a man & one of them gave me a familiar knock on the left breast & would have persisted in following me but for James.'[24]

In 1820, Anne began to receive anonymous letters. None the less, she was determined to carry on with her preferred lifestyle, a choice made easier by her wealthy background. She had money and her wealth brought her status. Anne could also be a snob and thought that many of the friends she visited were beneath her, so she could easily dismiss the reactions of the lower-class local villagers. Her family's position in the area must have alleviated pressures to some degree, allowing her to continue on her chosen path without serious trouble.

In August 1820, she noticed that she had contracted a sexually transmitted disease, probably from Marianne who had received it via Charles. 'I have felt the discharge a good deal today,' she complained, 'as if my linen, rubbing against my thighs, made them feel hot & irritated. There can be no doubt, surely, of its being venereal.' She obtained a prescription, 'a scruple of calomel gradually mixed in a marble mortar with an ounce of sweet oil . . . Two or three drops a day after making water generally cure in two or three days.' She injected the liquid at bedtime, using two borrowed ivory uterine syringes. Her medication also included powders, pills and lotions: 'The liniment for the injection, according to Mr

Duffin; fifteen of his pills, Steph's cubeb powders & lotions. That is an ounce of cubebs – pulvis cubebs – in twelve equal powders, one to be taken three times a day, & for the lotion, ten grains of hyd. oximur, that is, corrosive [*sic*] sublimate, with two drams of tincture of opium mixed with a quart of water.' The treatment failed and she and Marianne suffered the disease on and off for years. She eventually passed it on to Tib, sleeping with her once, having 'forgot' she had it.[25]

It is obvious from her diaries that Anne Lister saw herself as part of a group of women who were mutually attracted to other women. She did not view herself as a female husband, nor did she see her relationships merely as romantic friendships. Although she loved a number of women, she did not hesitate to chat up a pretty neighbour and to make her feelings known. Courageous enough to spend her life pursuing her own needs regardless of convention, she had a reputation as a loner and a bluestocking. Notwithstanding, however, it was her financial independence and superior social status which largely afforded her protection within the village, despite some gossip and harassment, and allowed her a greater freedom to pursue her own private life.

Trials and Tribadism

Sex between women did not pose the same threat to social order as did sodomy, and consequently it was never made illegal in England. Thus, technically speaking, women who had sex with other women might do so with legal impunity. However, although women who had sex together were not accused of sodomy, same-sex activities could lead to trouble and they would rarely escape malicious gossip if the matter became public. In fact, in many of the cases which came to light, the women had already been accused of a crime, usually fraud. Most often these were cases of cross-dressing where a woman disguised herself as a man in order to marry a richer woman. The *Annual Register* of 19 June 1773 recorded the case of a young woman who was brought before the Lord Mayor for dressing as a man in order to marry an old woman who possessed £100. Five years later, a woman was convicted at the Westminster law courts for dressing as a man, having married three different women under a fictitious name and defrauded them of their money and clothes. Likewise, in July 1777, Ann Marrow was sentenced to six months' imprisonment 'for going in a man's cloaths, and being married to three different women by a fictitious name, and for defrauding them of money and effects'.[26] Marrow was sentenced to the pillory where she was pelted by the crowd so violently that she lost both her eyes. However, these women were not punished for being lesbians or for having sex with another woman but for non-sex-related crimes.

In contrast, women in Holland and Germany were punished for having sex with other women. In 1792, Bets Wiebes was exiled from Amsterdam for six years because she had slept with another woman 'in the way a man used to do when he has carnal conversation with his wife'.[27] Prior to this, although male sodomy trials had swept through Holland, there had been no equivalent trials of females. This case was significant as it marked the start of a focused persecution of lesbians which failed to take place in England. A series of further trials took place in Amsterdam between 1795 and 1798 of women accused of engaging in 'caresses and filthy things'. Such cases also often came to court as a result of some other incident; in the case of Bets Wiebes, she was accused of killing her friend Catherina De Haan. It turned out, however, that Bartha Schuurman, Wiebes's lover, had committed the murder in a fit of jealousy after all three women had been drinking heavily together. Schuurman was garrotted and hanged at the gallows field. Although sodomy trials and the persecution of male sodomites were evident in England in the 1720s, women were never targeted *en masse* for sexual deviance. Lesbian activities in themselves simply did not pose the same threat in England as they did in many other countries, nor did lesbians suffer the same level of persecution as in Amsterdam.

Lesbian history has so far concerned itself with when, and under what circumstances, lesbianism evolved. Investigations have tended to focus on one of two categories: either that of the 'female husband' (the 'butch' in the femme/butch relationships roles); or that of female friendships. However, this is a very narrowly defined set of relationships and, clearly, women of the eighteenth century lived their lives in a varied way, with sexual boundaries less rigidly defined. Historians are now branching out to uncover a greater variety of lesbian identities and relationships within lesbian history. Neither the women placed on trial in Amsterdam in the last decades of the eighteenth century, nor certain relationships involving sexual attraction between women in England, fit the transvestite tradition of the 'female husband' or 'romantic friendship'.

Sapphic Sex in Erotica

The fantasy world of erotica often depicted women in a different light from the images established in the real world. In eighteenth-century erotic fiction, sex between women was portrayed as a natural phenomenon, an exploration of natural sexual desires. Women were described as both lascivious and inquisitive and, therefore, investigating another woman's body was a good introduction to sex. Although the female characters had sex together, they were none the less depicted as heterosexual women – sex with another woman was seen merely as a substitute for sex with a man and, as such, was thought to be an inferior sexual activity. The heroines would invariably go on to have full-blown penetrative intercourse with men. Thus, in erotica, the reader is guided through the rules of sexual initiation in a three-stage process: masturbation, lesbian sex and, finally, heterosexual intercourse.

French erotica was the first to introduce the British audience to scenes involving sex between women in books such as *L'Escole des Filles* (1655), *L'Académie des Dames* (1680) and *Venus dans la Cloître* (1683), translated respectively as *The School of Venus, The School of Women* and *Venus in the Cloister*.[28] This type of pornography came in the form of dialogues about sex between two women. Usually a slightly older and more experienced woman would be introducing the younger, more naive one to the joys of sex through conversation followed by experimentation. In both *The School of Venus* and *The School of Women*, tales of love and sex are related by the two female characters in the form of verbal foreplay, the older instructing the younger in anatomical details and then proceeding to show her how it works. Jean Barrin's *Venus in the Cloister* introduced the nunnery as a setting for lesbian love, a backdrop to appear in other French pornography: *Thérèse Philosophe* (1748) and *Dom Bougre, ou*

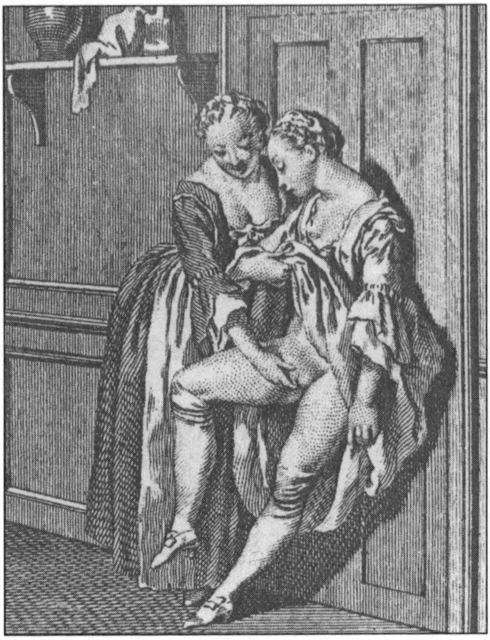

FIG. 34 Phoebe and Fanny in *Memoirs of a Woman of Pleasure*, 1766

Le portier des Chartreux (1741). Although French pornography experimented with woman-on-woman sex in the seventeenth century, this was yet to emerge in British pornography.

One of the first scenes of tribadism in British pornography can be seen in John Cleland's *Memoirs of a Woman of Pleasure* (1749) in which Fanny Hill is introduced to sex by Phoebe, her brothel-mate (**FIG. 34**). Fanny described her induction:

> I lay then all tame and passive as she could wish, whilst her freedom raised no other emotions but those of a strange, and, until then, unfelt pleasure. Every part of me was open and exposed to the licentious courses of her hands, which, like a lambent fire, ran over my whole body . . .[29]

Fanny and Phoebe were portrayed as essentially heterosexual, sex between women again presented as a first introduction to sex.

Women having sex with other women in erotica generally started with mutual masturbation. On occasions, a dildo might be introduced into the scene. In *A New Atlantis for the Year 1758*, the heroine, Tonzenie, abandons herself to pleasures of the flesh, assisted by her female servant: 'One of the middle-sized dildo-tribe was procured for her private amusement; through it her French maid, well skilled in such practices, would in the moment of rapture, dart a warm-injection; nay, sometimes artfully gird it to her loins, and act the man with her young mistress, who grown too sensible of the inefficacy of all such weak representations, was determined to enjoy the essence ere long.'[30] She is resolved to have a sexual experience with a man as soon as she can, thus confirming that basically she is heterosexual.

Dildos were regarded as an essentially female toy, a substitute penis for use by women characters in British erotica – they were never used on men, and only rarely used by men on women. They came in all shapes and sizes but there were two main designs: those to be used by hand, and those which could be strapped on. The first sort was made of ivory, or an ivory substitute, such as whalebone. Some were made of glass and filled with warm milky liquid so that, at a particular point in the activities, a bulb could be pressed to emit the fluid. The second sort, the 'strap-on' dildo, was made with what was called a 'stomacher and bands' in order that a woman might strap it around her waist so that she could have sex with another women. These might be made out of animal membrane or leather, and were filled with rags.

One early piece of erotica mentioned dildos made of indiarubber which 'cause them to perform as well, if not better than the real thing'. Although female mutual masturbation using hand-held dildos for manual stimulation was mentioned in fictional erotica, passages involving strap-on dildos were less frequent. This suggests that a woman using such equipment was perceived as more threatening by the male reader. Where strap-on dildos were used in erotic fiction, they tended to be in a convent or monastery setting, thus reinforcing the idea of just how debauched Catholics really were to the anti-Catholic readership. Real-life cases which came to trial in this period confirm that lesbian activities involving penetration with a dildo were seen as much more menacing than the passionate 'friendship' type of love between women.

*

As we have seen, lesbian relationships of the eighteenth century have been divided into either 'female friendships' or 'female husbands'. Within these models, middle-class lesbians have often been categorized as 'female friends' and working-class ones as 'female husbands'. Yet the division has bisected the world of eighteenth-century lesbians in a way that just did not exist. This has largely come about because literate, upper- and middle-class women recorded their experiences in their diaries and letters, and we are left with fewer personal opinions from uneducated working-class women. Most cases of lesbianism from the lower class come to our attention through trial reports, which biases the larger picture because the women concerned had already been classified as criminal.

Lesbian culture was diverse: there were several types of lesbian and they employed a wide range of strategies to allow them to follow their preferences: penetrative delight with one's 'wife'; passionate friendships with (or without) sex; mutual masturbation for fun; and sex without love. Some women lived their lives as 'feminine' women and managed to conduct love affairs and have sex with other women without becoming entangled with the law, sometimes hiding behind heterosexual marriage, as did Marianne, Anne Lister's lover. Others, as with Lister herself, wore 'manly' attire and cropped their hair short but retained their petticoats, provoking public attention and usually ending up in trouble. Lister fitted neither the archetype of the 'female husband' nor that of the 'female friend'. Among her group there existed a consciously shared subculture – these women knew exactly what they wanted and enjoyed initiating other women into lesbian relationships. Yet others might well not have even understood themselves to be lesbians, as Miss Browne's initial feelings for Anne Lister suggest. Some women presented themselves as close friends who shared a home together, as did Sarah Ponsonby and Eleanor Butler. But it is evident that these 'female friends' went further than mere friendship – they shared beds and called each other by lover's endearments. Those who underwent the full transition, and pretended they were men, the 'female husbands', were mainly detected after being brought to court, but they might also love their spouses and did not necessarily only want to obtain sex or defraud. The categories are therefore not always applicable or even useful. In these situations, male guise was generally adopted to make it easier for a woman to earn a living and enable a couple to share a comfortable life together, not because of any innate sexual desire to dress up in men's clothes. None the less, where dress violation did occur, society's reaction was punitive, the woman usually given a whipping or a prison sentence. Women in England, unlike in Holland and Germany, were not punished for the crime of having sex with another woman or for sodomy (using a dildo). They were, however, punished for crimes such as extortion and fraud conducted in the guise of a man.

In England, the different punishments meted out to male sodomites and certain lesbians were connected to the way in which men and women were perceived in a social, sexual and medical way. Firstly, some people in the eighteenth century could not conceive of the notion of women having sex with other women (although, as we have seen, plenty of others were well aware of it). It may be that lesbians managed to keep their activities hidden. If women merely presented themselves as having passionate 'friendships' rather than overt sexual relationships, the real nature of their relationship would remain secret. Secondly, if penetration with a dildo had not occurred, the women would technically still be virgins and therefore their sexuality was seen to be contained. Once dildos were involved, the activity was deemed more significant, even criminal. Finally, in erotica at least, sexual activity between women, unlike that between men, was seen as part of their heterosexuality and, as such, caused no threat at all. It was merely an initiation into sex whereby women would go on to have the 'normal' heterosexual sex with men. Sex between women was viewed merely as a substitute for the 'real' thing and, as such, was merely titillating.

There can be no doubt that in England lesbianism was much less of a threat than male homosexuality. Male-on-male sex was seen as a blatant offence against nature and an affront to civilized society. Sodomy between men was still a capital offence, whereas such sentencing for women, at least in Britain, was rare. By the early nineteenth century, however, it is possible to detect a change in attitude towards certain female sexual activities. Malicious gossip was emerging about women who wore 'mannish' dress and who lived with other women. Middle-class women, such as George Sand, began to wear masculine clothes and flaunt their sexuality. Scandal had moved from the bedroom politics of Marie Antoinette to attacks on overtly Bohemian women.[31]

CHAPTER NINE

'Strength to Wear a Dress'

'You are destined to be female; accept it. Since you had the weakness to wear a uniform into war, you have the strength to wear a dress during peacetime.'

Chevalier D'Eon's mother to her son

'Madame D'Eon is a man', declared the astonished physician on examining the body of the swordswoman, spy and courtier who lay before him. This was the conclusive end to what had become one of the strangest stories of eighteenth-century cross-dressing. It was surprising, perhaps, but not unique: D'Eon (**FIG. 35**) was following in the footsteps of the lesser-known

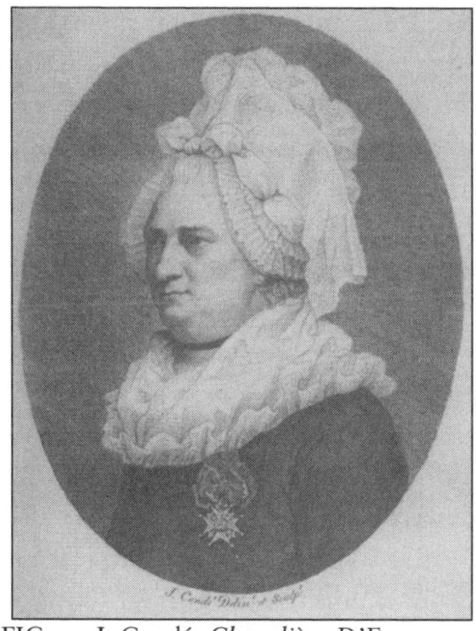

FIG. 35 J. Condé, *Chevalière D'Eon*, 1791

Chevalier De Choisy who had already created a stir with his feminine guise in France in the previous century.

Both De Choisy and D'Eon were from noble backgrounds; they had both been involved in life at the French court and left insightful memoirs as to their reason for cross-dressing and its effect on their daily lives. Abbé De Choisy wrote about his experiences in *Mémoires Pour Servir á L'histoire de Louis XIV*,[2] Chevalier D'Eon in *Lettres, Mémoires et Négociations*. Although they both visited England, only D'Eon left an account of what he did there.

Neither De Choisy nor D'Eon were homosexual in the modern sense of the word: neither were attracted to men. The fact that De Choisy was sexually attracted to young women, and that D'Eon was notably, by his own admission, not interested in sex with either men or women, probably saved them from greater persecution. These men chose to live part of their lives dressed as women and were encouraged to do so by their mothers. They obviously liked themselves in women's clothes as they had their portraits painted in full female garb. Neither were accused of sodomy or legally pursued for it.

During the eighteenth century, there was no terminology to define the behaviour of men like De Choisy and D'Eon. Transvestism, as a term, was only introduced in 1910 by the sexologist Magnus Hirschfeld in his book *Die Transvestiten*. He described it as the desire of men and women to dress up in clothes of the opposite sex. Havelock Ellis would later identify the desire to live as a woman as a 'pathological' condition and connected it to Chevalier D'Eon, labelling it D'Eonism. Cross-dressing might occur where there was no intention of having sex, either with a member of the same or the opposite sex.

Men dressing as women was seen to be an intentional desire for loss of status, an aspiration to be less than a man. It was therefore a non-rational achievement and, as such, perceived as a threat to the existing hierarchy of the sexes.[3] In his book *Sexual Dissidence*, John Dollimore believes that 'street transvestites transgress the natural and fixed order of things by wilfully confusing distinctions which it was thought imperative should be kept distinct, especially within the categories of rank, class, and gender.'[4] This was certainly the case with homosexual cross-dressing mollies who caused so much antagonism in London. However, in both France and England there appears to have been a greater tolerance of aristocratic cross-dressing men than of their homosexual working-class counterparts. Lords Stanhope, Hervey and Germain all had reputations as flamboyant sodomites yet none were ever arrested or tried for sodomy.[5] The English aristocrat Beau Wilson was accused of sodomy and dressing as a woman some time after he was killed in a duel in 1694. A description of the affair was aired in *Love-Letters between a Certain Late Nobleman and the Famous Mr Wilson* (1723), showing Stanhope as a villain. The writer Mrs Delariviere Manley had earlier described the surrounding events at some considerable length in her 'Lady's Pacquet of Letters' in Marie Catherine D'Aulnoy's *Memoirs of the Court of England in the Reign of Charles* (1707). British accounts of male cross-dressing, particularly in cases where no sexual activity with other men was involved, are none the less rare. So far, little has been uncovered on eighteenth-century heterosexual male cross-dressers. *Hell upon Earth* (1729) related the tale of an Irishman who, after bragging that he had spent a night with two lovely young women, was left baffled and ashamed on discovering that they were actually young men who, 'to pass the Time away, had purposely put on the Disguise to conceal their Sex'. The work is, however, of doubtful authenticity and probably a fabricated joke.[6]

Abbé De Choisy: Cross-dressing Seducer

François Timoléon De Choisy, whose uncle was the King's Chancellor, was dressed in girl's clothes from an early age by his mother. As he described in his memoirs, 'my mother almost from my birth, accustomed me to women's garments and I continued to wear them in my youth.'[7] She had his ears pierced and applied a depilatory cream from the age of five or six in an attempt to avoid the development of facial hair. Some say De Choisy's mother wanted a girl (he was the youngest of three boys); others say that the unconventional dress was adopted for political reasons, so that he could act as a companion to Louis XIV's younger brother, Philippe de Orléans, who had also been forced to dress as a girl to dampen any possible attempts to assert power over his older brother. Yet De Choisy so enjoyed the experience that he continued it into adulthood, living, on and off, dressed as a woman.

De Choisy's mother had instructed him on the type of people with whom he should mix, advising him to choose only those of quality, and never to socialize with administrators or officials. After attending the Sorbonne, he left Paris for about five months, appearing on the stage in Bordeaux, masquerading as a woman while entertaining male suitors. Following his mother's death, he donned male attire again, but soon reverted back to women's clothes to assume the role of a countess in the country at Bourges. With agreement from their families, he took in young girls and acted as their patron in the guise of an experienced woman of the world. Although the parents were not always aware of his true sex, some of them knew and chose to ignore the fact for the sake of his money. He taught the girls how to style their hair and how to dress properly. And he always took them to his bed. This in itself would not have been unusual or necessarily have raised superstitions as older hostesses often had their young companions sleep with them. In De Choisy's case, however, he was seducing his charges.

When he first started his affairs with the young women he was nurturing, he was fully penetrating the girls he bedded. Dressed as a woman, he met and fell in love with the eager Mademoiselle de la Grise: 'As soon as we were in bed there was no need to tell her to come near me, she wanted to devour me with caresses. I was bursting with desire and I set myself to give her real pleasure. She began to say that I was hurting her, then she gave such a cry that it raised Madame Bouju [her mother] from her bed to see what was happening.' Despite this experience, the young woman seemed quite innocent of his real sexual identity. Neither did her family seem to know or care about the true situation. De Choisy called her 'his little wife', while she referred to him as 'my little husband'. He was, however, more careful with girls who were more worldly wise. About another girl he seduced, he declared, 'I risked nothing with her,'[8] purposely avoiding penetration and the possibility of his true sex being discovered. When Mademoiselle de la Grise fell pregnant, she was married off to a wealthy nobleman, Comte des Goutes. This was to become a regular occurrence in De Choisy's life. He avoided pregnancy as far as he could but, when his paramours did succumb, he married them to rich suitors. Once they were married, De Choisy lost interest in them and never saw them again. He then fell in love with an actress, Rosalie, who he dressed as a cavalier, introducing a role reversal and this time calling her 'my little husband'. When she fell pregnant, he treated it as a malady and employed a midwife 'until the girl was cured'.[9]

De Choisy's cross-dressing so angered his relatives that he was eventually forced into exile in Italy where he proceeded to gamble away his money. He had an addictive personality; if he could not fulfil one passion, he needed the crutch of another – when he could not dress as a woman, he fell to gambling. He admitted, 'Gambling, which had always been my downfall, cured me of these minor frivolities for several years, but every time that I was ruined and wanted to cease gambling, I fell, yielded to my old weaknesses and became a woman again.' Cross-dressing and gambling were passions he pursued throughout his life, to the extent that he had to sell the family château in order to pay off his gambling debts.

In order to continue to dress as he pleased, De Choisy bought a house in the country at Saint-Marceau, assuming the name Madame de Sancy. 'I began by having my ears pierced again, the holes from earlier piercing having closed up. I wore embroidered corsets and gold and black *robes de chambre** with sleeves lined with white satin, a girdle with a busk and a large knot of ribbons behind to mark the waist, a wide trailing train, a well-powdered peruke, ear pendants, patches and a cap with a *fontage*.'[10] Gradually his dress became increasingly elaborate and more feminine; an intentional ruse, as he explained:

> . . . at the end of the month, I undid three or four silver buttons at the top of my robe so that my bodice of silver moiré, which I wore underneath, could be seen. I put on my diamond earrings, which I had bought five or six years beforehand from Monsieur Lambert, the jeweller. My peruke became a little longer and more powdered, cut in such a way that my earrings were in full view, and I put on three or four little patches around my mouth

* A long loose housecoat with a short train made from luxurious materials, generally intended for indoor wear but which De Choisy chose to wear outdoors.

> or on my forehead. I remained like this for a month, so that people would, without knowing it, become accustomed to my apparel, and would believe that I had always been the same; and that is what happened. As soon as I saw my plan had succeeded, I opened five or six buttonholes at the bottom of my gown, in order to reveal a robe of speckled black satin, the train of which was not as long as the gown. I also wore a white damask underskirt, which could be seen only when the train was carried. I ceased to wear trunk-hose . . .

De Choisy also took great care of his skin: 'every evening I laved my neck with veal water and sheep's-foot grease which made the skin soft and white.'[11] The villagers must have known he was a man but they became used to seeing him in female garb. Eventually his friends and neighbours took to calling him 'madame'.

De Choisy was an intelligent man and sought reasons for his penchant for female dress: 'I have considered carefully whence came such a bizarre taste and here is my explanation: the attribute of God is to be loved, adored; Man, as far as the weakness of his nature allows, wishes for the same but, as it is beauty that kindles love and since that is usually the lot of women, when it happens that men have, or believe themselves to have, certain traits of beauty, they try to enhance them by the same methods that women use, which are most becoming.' He concluded it was his desire to be admired that motivated him.

He enjoyed the company of women, hosting suppers for his lady friends and taking them to the opera and comedies. His private chaplain held Mass every day, an event which attracted all the 'idle women in the neighbourhood'. But he knew that being too blatant in his behaviour would attract adverse comments from other sections of the community. On reading in a newspaper about a man of quality who dressed as a woman, he recognized the description of himself. He admitted to a friend that he would only ever dress like that in close company as he knew that society was fickle and liable to condemn him for cross-dressing: 'The world is so wicked, and it is so uncommon to see a man wishing to be a woman that one is often exposed to distasteful pleasantries.'[12] Despite society's disapproval of such behaviour, the Church astonishingly accepted his position without question, although, like the parishioners, they must have suspected his true sex. The churchwardens always sent a lighted candle for De Choisy to join them in the procession; then they bestowed further honours on him, accepting him as a woman:

> After five or six months I was given the *chanteau** to provide the bread for consecration. I played my part wonderfully well, but I had no wish for acclaim. The churchwardens told me that the consecrated bread had to be presented by a woman and the collection taken by her, and they flattered themselves that I should be willing to accept this honour.[13]

De Choisy grabbed the opportunity to flaunt himself in elaborate, extravagant dress. 'I needed no more pressing, but prepared myself as if for a grand occasion which would show me off magnificently to the whole populace. I had a *robe de chambre* of white damask from China, lined with black taffeta: I had an *échelle* of black ribbons, ribbons on the sleeves and, behind, a large bunch of ribbons to mark the waist.' His attention to the details of his attire was obsessive. It obviously had the desired effect on his audience, as he declared immodestly: 'I do not wish to boast, but they had never taken so much money at Saint-Médard.' Such was the eagerness to see him that people turned out from other parishes. He revelled in this display, placing himself on exhibition to be admired. Curious spectators declared, 'But is it really true that that is a man? He is quite right to pass himself off as a woman.' So he would come up with further excuses to give them the pleasure of seeing him again, this time closer up. He was delighted to be treated as a woman.

De Choisy was strongly attracted to women and, surprisingly, girls in the village were attracted to him, despite his female attire. Two young women in the parish were not at all deterred by the fact that he dressed as a woman, and vied for his attentions. They kissed him on his lips, and 'it became clear that this was a demonstration of more than simply good

* The term used for the blessed bread sent to a woman who would offer it to the church the following Sunday; not to be confused with the Host.

friendship.'[14] He and one of the girls, Mademoiselle Charlotte, wrote to each other every day despite being constantly in each other's company. At first she called him 'Madame' but, after the affair had been initiated, in her letters she addressed him as 'Monsieur'. Despite his cross-dressing she became emotionally attached to him, declaring, 'I am in truth, monsieur, quite wretched in my love for you.' In her eyes at least, De Choisy was a man.

For a masquerade, he dressed Charlotte as a man, complete with periwig. She acted as his escort for the evening, thus beginning a relationship in which there was a complete reversal of gender roles. Not only were they unabashed at this inverted status but they blatantly showed off. Charlotte took off her mask at the ball and De Choisy enquired to his hostess, 'There, madame, this is my little lover; is he not pretty?' From then on, whenever they met, Charlotte was 'en garçon' and De Choisy dressed as a woman. Charlotte's aunt, her parents being dead, made a slight fuss but quickly relented, even allowing De Choisy have her niece's portrait painted dressed as a cavalier. At the same time, he commissioned a picture of himself dressed as a woman. He proudly hung both pictures in his summerhouse much to the glee of his neighbours who declared, laughing, 'There's a fine couple; they should marry, they would love each other so.'

Although Charlotte's aunt was perturbed by the relationship, she even agreed to a ceremony of 'marriage' between the pair. All Charlotte's other relatives attended and wished the couple well;

> The ceremony took place before supper, so that the evening would be more festive. Wearing a robe of silver moiré and a small bunch of orange-blossoms behind my head, like a bride, I said in a clear voice, before all the relations, that I took Monsieur de Maulny [Charlotte] for my husband, and he said that he took Madame de Sancy for his wife. We touched hands, he put a small silver ring on my finger, and we kissed each other . . .

All the relations came to kiss them goodnight and to give them their blessing on the wedding night, and the aunt even drew the wedding curtain around the marriage bed. They all knew the real nature of the relationship but were obviously persuaded by De Choisy's status and his money not to make a fuss. After the 'wedding' ceremony, the couple slept together. The relationship involved sex but, by this time, De Choisy was avoiding intercourse because of his abhorrence of pregnancy. De Choisy remarked, 'It was then that we gave ourselves to joy, but without overstepping the limits of propriety. That may be difficult to believe but it is none the less true.'[15] He did not want to upset their current relationship with the burden of children and had learned from his previous experiences to avoid intercourse. It was impossible to continue his role-playing fantasy once his girlfriends fell pregnant.

De Choisy and Charlotte, of course, could have married legally, but this was not what De Choisy was seeking. Rather he wanted confirmation of his inverse relationship with Charlotte in the eyes of others. He wanted people to accept him as a woman and her as his husband. The monetary gains for Charlotte and her family were great and, because of his wealth, they were wily enough to accept his cross-dressing as a minor eccentricity. He took on the responsibility for both her and her aunt, allowing them to live with him.

From then on, Charlotte always dressed as a man in his house. Part of the enjoyment for De Choisy was exhibitionism and he often called in tradesmen to see them breakfasting in bed together. He was respected and accepted in his local neighbourhood, carrying out good works for the poor, but only ventured twice into wider society. At the Opéra, the audience was discreet and did not comment but when he took Charlotte and her aunt to the Comédie Française, people stared and whispered. Fearing scandal, from then on he decided to remain in his own neighbourhood.

Gossip was circulating about De Choisy and scandal was imminent. His nephew rebuked him for making an exhibition of himself, a fact of which De Choisy was well aware since showing off was part of his pleasure. Worse still, songs were being written about him and he began to receive anonymous letters. One of these letters criticized him for living with a young girl, yet surprisingly did not mention his cross-dressing. Nonetheless, because of the vindictiveness of others, he began to stay in during the day. He loved Charlotte dearly but admitted that he only 'caressed and kissed her' and lamented the fact that he did not satisfy her like a 'genuine husband'. Because of this, when the time came, and she was proposed to by a very wealthy man, he did not stand in her way, but wished her well. As with his other lovers, he was never to see her again.

De Choisy liked to pick up poor young girls and train them for ladyhood. His next protégé, fifteen-year-old Babet, was an orphan whom he found in a draper's shop. Although attracted to her, before he bought her out of her apprenticeship, he inspected her like a horse. 'I called her to me, I looked at her teeth and her bosom which had begun to form; her arms were a little thin.'[16] He even had his old maidservant inspect the girl to ensure she 'is clean'. Stripped naked, her body had an obvious effect on De Choisy who admitted, 'I was dying to embrace the little wisp.'[17] Rather than dress Babet as a man, this time he dressed her elaborately as a lady: 'I could not refrain from dressing her in the most lovely clothes and the finest linen in Paris; I bought for her from Monsieur Lambert, the jeweller, earrings of brilliants, which cost me eight hundred and fifty livres; I had her hair dressed with silver and blue ribbons; I always put seven or eight little patches on her.' Finally, to complete the transformation, he renamed her Mademoiselle Dany.

Part of De Choisy's pleasure lay in the reinvention of these girls, transforming them into new people. Yet this process involved much kissing and fondling, usually while others looked on, thus satisfying De Choisy's exhibitionist streak. The attraction he felt for his girlfriends was not merely sexual – he was obviously very fond of them and enjoyed providing them with the best clothes and most opulent lifestyle that money could buy.

In later life, De Choisy enjoyed socializing and even formed a club, with many academics convening at his living quarters in the Palais du Luxembourg. At another club in which he was involved, Le Club de l'Entresil, formed in 1724, they discussed his *Imitation of Jésus-Christ*, a scandalous bestseller containing shocking engravings of the erstwhile King's mistress, Madame de Maintenon, kneeling before a crucifix. De Choisy never lost his love of donning women's clothes and, although he could no longer afford the extravagant dresses and jewels he had adorned himself with in his earlier days, this passion continued for the rest of his life. He wrote his memoirs when in his late sixties or early seventies, and died at the age of eighty on 2 October 1724.

Chevalier D'Eon: the 'Female' Spy

Charles-Geneviève-Louise-Auguste-André-Thimothée D'Eon de Beaumont was born in the picturesque Burgundian town of Tonnerre on 5 October 1728. Throughout his life D'Eon displayed no sign of the sexual passions of De Choisy. He admitted to the Comte de Broglie in 1771: 'I have never wished for wife or mistress . . . I am somewhat mortified to be still as Nature made me and that, since the calm of my natural temperament has never made me addicted to sensual indulgence, this has given my friends in France, as well as in Russia and England, grounds for imagining in their innocence that I was of the female sex.'[18]

D'Eon first served as a diplomat under Louis XIV, then spent some years acting as an agent of the Secret du Roi, the royal secret service, on behalf of Louis XV. He had been given a commission as lieutenant of the Dragoons as a reward for his diplomatic work in Russia, followed by the command of a company on the Rhine. His military career only lasted a few months but he fought bravely against Scots and Prussians. He helped to negotiate terms for ending the Seven Years War where his secret service work earned him the Order of Saint-Louis.

D'Eon first came to London in 1762. Full of charm and witty conversation, he worked wonders in diplomatic circles, assisted by the cache of fine wine he had brought from his home town, which he liberally dispersed among his friends. D'Eon had been appointed secretary to the ambassador Comte de Guerchy, but their working relationship was far from easy. For some time, Guerchy had been jealous of D'Eon's successes on the Rhine, a campaign in which the Comte himself had shirked his duties. Resentful of D'Eon's accomplishments, he wanted to make life difficult for his rival. A bitter enmity broke out between the two men and the antagonism eventually came to a head when Guerchy accused D'Eon of being a hermaphrodite, a charge usually laid at the door of women with masculine tendencies. Although D'Eon was to emerge victorious from the scrap, it was a hollow victory as Guerchy's plotting and scandalmongering resulted in the loss of D'Eon's reputation. Louis XV now distrusted him to the extent that he became convinced that D'Eon was mad. His greatest concern was that D'Eon might divulge incriminating evidence about the

King's secret service. Growing hostilities between the foreign ministry and D'Eon eventually led to his being recalled to France. As a member of the secret service, D'Eon was in the precarious position of having to rely on the King just as he was withdrawing his support. As a consequence, the French government failed to pay his debts, his financial problems grew worse and the threat of extradition hung over him. In retaliation, D'Eon dug in his heels and refused to return to France, remaining in London. It was around this time that the furore about issue No. 45 of *The North Briton* exploded, and Wilkes and D'Eon became good friends, the similarity of their cases not escaping the British political establishment.

Concern mounted as to exactly how much incriminating evidence D'Eon actually possessed, the French government now furious that he was using the threat of exposure to blackmail them. D'Eon published his *Lettres, Mémoires et Négociations* in March 1764 and was fast becoming a household name, adding to the anxieties of the King. Finally, in 1775, an agent, Beaumarchais, was sent by the new King, Louis XVI, to negotiate with D'Eon and attempt to settle the affair without undermining the French secret service. It was at this point that D'Eon and the French government came to an agreement whereby D'Eon would surrender all the French documents in his possession in return for the payment of all his debts and the provision of a royal pension. A further stipulation was added: that D'Eon must dress as a woman for the rest of his life. Strange as it might seem, the French court believed that D'Eon was, in fact, female and had fought in the army as a brave woman impersonating a man – it was now felt to be an appropriate time for him to resume the role of a woman. Despite these deliberations, the overriding intention of the government was to disable him politically since, as a woman, he would have less power.

During the 1770s, gossip about D'Eon's true sexual identity started to flourish and the confusion about his real gender saw all of London making and taking bets. Public curiosity was fuelled by British newspaper reports and French pamphlets about him. The *Public Advertiser* of 12 March 1771 noted, 'The discovery of her sex was occasioned by her lately discharging a favourite footman, to whom she had entrusted the secret'; the *London Evening Post* for 11–14 May 1771 went as far as to declare 'that a

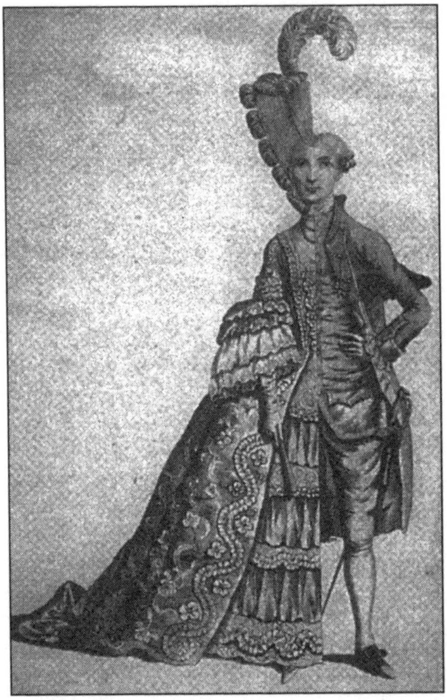

FIG. 36 D'Eon, *The London Magazine*, September 1777

celebrated Chevalier [D'Eon] has within a few weeks past, been discovered to be of a different sex'. A picture of the chevalier was even circulated in the *London Magazine* for September 1777 to inform people what D'Eon really looked like (**FIG. 36**). By 1778, the interest was so intense that the journalist for *L'Espion Anglais* (The English Spy) wrote: 'Since the return to France . . . of the Chevalier D'Eon, of this amphibious being, male in London, female in Paris, I have focused all my efforts on verifying the condition and adventures of this celebrity . . .'[19]

While in England, D'Eon had amassed a library of over six thousand books and five hundred rare manuscripts. Some fifty books were about women, ranging from Catholic tracts to feminist assertions such as Judith Drake's *An Essay in Defence of the Female Sex* (1696), Mary Astell's *Some Reflections upon Marriage* (1700) and the anonymous *Female Rights Vindicated* (1758). D'Eon was obviously not just a learned man, but one who was interested in the position of women in society and their rights.

On his return to France in 1777, in keeping with the King's order, D'Eon was obliged to take to dressing as a woman. Until this point, he had dressed as a man, wearing military uniform to fight while actively trying to convince everyone that he was really a woman. Now D'Eon had no option, his choice had been eradicated. The enforced gender change began to affect his behaviour and mental attitude – the order had 'killed in her the old Dragoon captain'. He wrote in a female voice in the third person, as if to exemplify the distance he felt from his female persona, complaining, 'Such a change completely transformed her mind, her heart, her conduct, her manners, her habits, and her inclinations. It forced her to come alive, move forward, and act as an entirely new creature . . . resuscitated to all the decency, wisdom and dignity of her sex.'[20] D'Eon was now pressured into completely giving up his male identity for his female one, a situation with which he was not at all happy.

For the French government, the situation was simple: they were hoping to rid themselves of D'Eon, encouraging him to enter a convent and become a nun. Indeed, D'Eon did give it some consideration and he visited two nunneries to see how he might fit in. In 1778, as France joined the American colonists against Britain in the War of Independence, D'Eon desperately wanted to rejoin the army and fight with the Dragoons. Ignoring the royal decree, he dressed up in his full military outfit and was promptly arrested for breaching his agreement with the King. He made incessant appeals to the government requesting consideration of his application to fight, and sent more than forty letters to various well-connected people in the hope of being readmitted to the Dragoons. The government took forceful action against him: his family estate was confiscated, his pension was withdrawn, and D'Eon was ordered to return to his family in Tonnerre.

Once home, D'Eon's mother pressed him to continue dressing as a woman – she wanted him to stay with her rather than go to war. 'I would like you one hundred times better wearing a dress', she told him, 'than to see you suffering and being the silent object of public scandal. A little kindness is soon passed. Put on your dress . . . and you will live happy and at peace near me.'[21] D'Eon was later to complain that his mother had encouraged his taste for finery. 'She tormented me day and night,' he moaned, 'and to encourage me, she gave me all her beautiful dresses and lacework.' Regardless of her entreaties, the quiet life was not for the chevalier; he was determined to fight the edict, despite the fact that all of France and England now believed him to be a woman.

Unconvinced by the urgings of his family and friends to comply with the government's demand, D'Eon did not want to relinquish his masculine role entirely. He therefore continued to press his claim to dress as a man via the patronage of influential politicians. Meanwhile, Queen Marie Antoinette's own dressmaker, Rose Bertin, was busy creating a female wardrobe for him in an array of exclusive silks and satins. Although the clothes were exquisite, D'Eon could take no pleasure in them. After Bertin had spent more than four hours dressing him up, he could still not bear the thought of giving up his male identity. 'I left . . . the room and locked myself in my bedroom and sobbed bitterly,' he complained. 'Despite the complete change in my clothing my heart did not feel any different.'[22] Seeing no reason why he should pay for his new clothes, he had at least ensured that the French government would foot the bill as part of the agreement.

Although D'Eon had earlier blamed his father for dressing him as a boy while being born a girl, allegedly in order to gain access to an inheritance, it had been his own autobiographical account of his early escapade in Russia which had been responsible for spreading the rumours about his gender. In his own writings, he had related how the King's cousin, Prince de Conti, was let in on the 'secret' of his identity and that he and the King thought that the country's interest would best be served with D'Eon dressing as a woman in order to become closer to the Empress Elizabeth of Russia. Historians argue about the veracity of D'Eon's tale.[23]

For all his prevarication, it seems that D'Eon felt more comfortable dressed as a man while pretending to be a woman. His cultural background must have had an influence on him; he grew up at a time of political flux when the uneasy climate of France during the last decades of the Old Regime was challenging both social and gender roles. A month after his return, he was presented, dressed as a woman, to the King and Queen and warmly welcomed back into the court at Versailles. To some extent, this smoothed his passage back into French life; after all, he had been increasingly convinced that his political career was over. He had feared, not without some justification, that he would be unable to continue serving the court and government as a woman. A woman's position was inferior, political power less accessible, and he was also worried that his liberty would be curtailed. The fact that the monarchy had approved the feminization of his title to *chevalière* meant that D'Eon would at least retain his honours for his military record.

In 1785, as a result of continued harassment from D'Eon, the French government awarded him 6,000 livres in order to pay off his debts in England, and he left France for good. Once back in London, his financial situation had so deteriorated that he was obliged to sell off his belongings at auction at Christie's, including his favourite jewellery and his substantial collection of books. Still in the guise of a woman, he moved to 38 Brewer Street in Soho, where he lived modestly. In order to finance himself, he teamed up with a former servant of his, Jacob de Launay, and a Mrs Bateman and gave fencing lessons, teaching as a woman. They toured the South of England, putting on shows, giving demonstrations and inviting challenges from the audiences. Unfortunately, a fencing accident was to have serious consequences for the chevalier. During one demonstration, De Launay's foil broke and injured D'Eon enough to prevent him from continuing in this line of work. As a result of an infection in the wound, he suffered blood poisoning and had to return to London where he set up home with a Frenchwoman, Mrs Marie Cole, widow of a British naval engineer, at 33 Westminster Bridge. It was a purely domestic arrangement with no physical aspect to the relationship. His financial situation remained dire, despite sympathetic friends helping him out with small gifts of money. Queen Charlotte was good enough to provide an annual pension of £50 but it was not enough to keep him afloat.

In 1804, at the age of seventy-five, D'Eon ended up in debtors' prison. Mrs Cole managed to raise enough money to secure his release and they both moved to 26 Milman Street in Holborn, where they continued living as platonic companions, now in even more straitened circumstances. Only on his death did Mrs Cole discover that the person she had been sharing her life with for the last fifteen years was in fact a man. The doctor-priest who had looked after D'Eon throughout his last years was also unaware of his real sexual identity until he examined him after his death. Because of the curiosity about his gender, D'Eon's corpse was subjected to dissection and countless physical inspections before the surgeon, Thomas Copeland, signed the following document:

> I hereby certify that I have examined and dissected the body of Chevalier D'Eon in the presence of Mr Adair, Mr Wilson and Pére Elysée and that I found the male genital organs perfectly formed in every respect.[24]

Even Casanova, the Italian lover and alleged expert on women, had mistakenly described D'Eon as 'a beautiful woman, who, before adopting the career of diplomacy, had been a barrister, and then a captain of the Dragoons'. He added, 'I had not been a quarter of an hour in her company before I knew her for a woman. Her shape was too rounded for that of a man, and her voice was too clear.'[25] Thus, D'Eon fooled even the most sexually experienced of men about his real gender. He died in Bloomsbury in 21 May 1810 after having lived for eighty-two years, and was buried in the graveyard of St Pancras Church as he had requested.

*

For De Choisy, who wanted to lead the life of a man while dressing as a woman, part of the enjoyment involved publicly exhibiting himself as a female. He adored women and revelled in dressing them up as men. To some extent this usurping of roles was undertaken to test the extent of public reaction. He continually provoked those around him to pass comment on his relationships, and was happiest when he was the centre of attention. D'Eon, on the other hand, projected a more complicated image. He wanted people to believe he was a woman dressed in men's clothing. His sexual persona was muted and he was happy to keep it that way. He was disgusted that a person's body could become the subject of so much gossip and the wagers on his gender revolted him. To some extent, he fought for women's right to be involved in the public world, particularly the right to bear arms. His collection of feminist tracts written by women conveys a keen interest in their social and political position. He was less happy, however, to give up his men's clothes entirely and recognized that, forced to live as a woman, his standing with the government would be lost. Yet, interestingly enough, he continued to dress in women's clothing even after moving to London. The French government's persecution of D'Eon was less to do with his manner of dressing than with his secret service work; also, it was presumed that he was in fact a woman dressing as a man. In England, D'Eon was made into a *cause célèbre*, in the time-honoured tradition of women who dress as men to take up arms.

Although both De Choisy and D'Eon were harassed at various times in their lives, they avoided prosecution for crimes connected to any sexual transgression, which suggests that wealthier men could indulge in cross-dressing with less persecution than working-class men. The fact that neither was seen to be a sodomite also meant that they posed less of a problem: De Choisy was essentially heterosexual, and D'Eon was considered a woman without any apparent sexual element to his life. Yet cross-dressing for these two men had been important to the extent that they had continued to dress up even when endangering their elite positions in society and, despite the threats, battled throughout their lives for acceptance as women.

CHAPTER TEN

Women in Breeches

> In the moral system, there seems at present to be going on a kind of Country-Dance between the Male and Female Follies and Vices in which they have severally crossed over, and taken each other's places. The Men are growing delicate and refined, and the Women free and easy.
>
> George Colman, English playwright, 1762–1836[1]

Chapbooks, ballads and poems rejoiced in the tale of brave Long Meg who kept an infamous tavern at Islington and killed men while dressed as a man. She had gained her reputation fighting against the French. 'On the day the Frenchman came, Meg met him and without any salute, fell to blows; after a long combat, she overcame him, and cut off his head. Then pulling off her hat her hair fell about her ears. By this the Frenchmen knew it was a woman . . .'[2] *The Life and Pranks of Long Meg of Westminster* (1590), found among Samuel Pepys's collection of 'Penny Merriments', provided a jocular anecdote: 'It chanced one Evening that Meg in a frolick humour did put on a Suit of Man's Apparel, and with her Sword and Buckler walked the Streets.' That night, a merry young nobleman, strolling down the Strand, came upon Meg. He joked and teased her, 'putting his Thumb to Megs Mouth, said, there's a Tester'. Meg retaliated by giving him 'a good Box on the Ear', declaring, 'There (Sir Knave) there's a Groat again, and now I owe you but two pence.'[3]

Similar tales of female daring related the adventures of pirates and soldiers and even of a woman highway robber. Joan Philips, the daughter of a wealthy farmer, was born in Towcester, Northamptonshire, in 1656. Her father hoped to find her a husband but she was hard to please and quite ungovernable; the ballad she inspired was a warning that, for such women of spirit, there would be dire consequences: 'Being of a wild disposition, she could settle her affection upon none of them, being reserved for a worse End.' The tale related how Joan had become acquainted with Bracy, a Highway-Man, who, after seducing her, persuaded her to steal from her own father, and go along with him 'on the Pad', robbing as they went. They passed as man and wife, thieving from coaches on the highways. Sometimes Joan would dress in men's clothing, at others, she practised what was called the 'Crocodile Cheat'. First, she cut her finger, smearing her face with blood; then, she pulled off her cap and ordered her husband to tie up her hands and legs and put her in a ditch. She would then lie in wait, crying and sobbing for the first good man to come along and rescue her from her feigned plight, whereupon her husband would jump out from his hiding-place, taking his victim unawares. Fearing that the law would catch up with them, they ended their careers as highway robbers and set up an inn in the Bristol suburbs. Philips, however, continued to steal, only now it was from her own customers. Under the pretence of accepting their flattery, she would entice them into her bed, then, with her maidservant, would rob them and throw them down the stairs. The inn achieved such a scandalous reputation that Philips and Bracy were forced to close it and return to their old ways. She was eventually caught robbing some wealthy travellers in their coach on the way to Nottingham, condemned and executed in April 1685 at the age of twenty-nine. Although her husband had been apprehended at the same time, he escaped sentence, but was eventually fatally wounded by one of his earlier victims.[4]

Roaring Girls

Eighteenth-century British society to a large extent tolerated female cross-dressing, particularly in cases where women had joined the army or gone to sea.[5] Indeed, female soldiers and pirates were frequently fêted in street literature which related their military exploits and seafaring adventures. Plays were inspired by lives of cross-dressing women: Middleton and Dekker's play *The Roaring Girl* (1608–11) was based on the life of Mary Frith, alias 'Moll Cutpurse', highway robber, and her tale recounted in a chapbook, *The Life and Death of Mary Frith* (1662). Usually, these tales were at pains to point out that the women who had fought, robbed or sailed as men were in fact 'real' women who were sexually attracted to men, and that their cross-dressing was merely a means by which to seek adventure. In the final stages of their careers, more often than not, they reverted to their female garb.

Female cross-dressing was not perceived as a problem as long as sex with another woman was not involved. When sexual activities were thought to be taking place, it was considered an affront to public order. This was particularly so when a woman impersonated a man in order to defraud another woman and marrying another woman was considered to be a serious offence. Generally, the women caught in this position had been brought to court for the prosecution of a non-sex-related crime, usually the taking of money or possessions, or attempting to defraud.

Cross-dressing was perhaps most tolerated and enjoyed in the theatre, where female 'breeches' parts, such as those played by eighteenth-century actresses like Peg Woffington and Charlotte Charke, were especially popular.[6] Woffington was praised for playing Harry Wildair in Farquhar's comedy *The Constant Couple* (1699). Charlotte Charke, in her autobiography, describes how she adopted the attire of a man, not only playing male parts as an actress (which was comprehensible to the public), but also working as a male grocer, clerk, pastrycook, hog merchant and manservant (which was not). Her disguise did not help her finances as she was imprisoned for debt on several occasions.[7] She even wrote a novel on the subject of cross-dressing, *The History of Henry Dumont* (1756).

Scenarios of female cross-dressing could also be found in a number of other racy novellas, in which it was employed as a ruse to allow women to follow their menfolk in dangerous circumstances. In *The Nun in the Cloister or, the Amours, Intrigues and Adventures of the Marchioness of Beauville* (1828), the Marchioness, prior to her marriage, goes off in search of her future husband, Don Carlos. She trips through adventures, including being captured by the Turks and being sold as a slave. Her clothes stolen, she dresses in breeches and a shirt, passing for a man. After she is bought by a twenty-year-old master, she is taken to Constantinople and instructed in the Turkish language and customs. Here, living as a man, she gains a new perspective on life as she follows her master into battle with the Germans. 'Having appeared so long as a man,' the heroine remarks, 'I was almost persuaded that I really was so, and therefore followed him with much less concern than I would have done two years before.'[8] Surprisingly, though, female cross-dressing was rarely employed as a sexual enticement in lesbian scenes in English erotica. Any women-on-women sex scenes involved heterosexual women dressed in female clothing.

By no means all women who dressed as men felt sexually attracted to other women;[9] some merely dressed as a man to obtain the financial independence that came with better job opportunities and greater individual freedom in a world largely dominated by men. That way they could shun marriage and avoid falling under the dictates of a husband. Such female cross-dressers could be seen as the first feminists. In men's garb, they could move about more easily and claim the privileges open to men of their class. Dressing and living as a man must have been a tempting fantasy for any adventurous young woman who valued her freedom.[10] Yet although female cross-dressers were regarded as less threatening than their male cross-dressing counterparts, certain anxieties were publicly voiced about their shifting gender roles.

Some of these concerns related to religious considerations. The Bible condemns cross-dressing: 'The woman shall not wear that which pertaineth unto a man, neither shall a man put on a woman's garment: for all that do so are abomination unto the Lord thy God' (Deuteronomy 22:5). Some eighteenth-century books echoed these sentiments, displaying particular concern over the increasing number of women who were cross-dressing or otherwise showing masculine behaviour. *Hic Mulier, The Man-Woman* specifically addressed the emergence of the mannish female and criticized such developments. Intended as 'a Medicine to cure the Coltish Disease of the Staggers in the Masculine-Feminines of our Times', the author railed:

> For since the daies of Adam women were never so Masculine; Masculine in their genders and whole generations, from the Mother to the youngest daughter; Masculine in Number, from

> one to multitudes; Masculine in Case, even from the head to the foot; Masculine in Moode, from bold speech, to impudent action; and Masculine in Tense; for (without redress) they were, are and will be still most Masculine, most mankinde, and most monstrous.

Women were also attacked for their masculine mode of dress:

> . . . you have taken the monstrousnesse of your deformatie in apparel, exchanging the modest attire of the comely Hood, Cawle, Coyfe, handsome Dresse or Kerchief, to the cloudy Ruffianly broad-brim'd Hat and wanton Feather, the most upper parts of the concealing straight gowne, to the loose, lascivious open embracement of a French dublet, being all unbuttoned to entice, all of one shape to hide deformitie, and extreme short wasted to give a more easie way to every luxurious action; the glory of a faire large hayre to the shame of most ruffianly short lockes.[11]

The *Gentleman's Magazine* and the *Female Tatler* complained about women who did not know their place, yet the objections appear to be facetious rather than any serious condemnation of female cross-dressers. The *Female Tatler* of September 1709 requested,

> The young lady in the parish of St Laurence, near Guildhall, that lately went to the Coffee-House in man's clothes with the two 'prentices, called for a dish of Bohee (black Indian tea), smoked her pipe, and gave herself abundance of straddling masculine airs . . . to do so no more.[12]

In an article on 'Female Extravagances', the *Gentleman's Magazine* of July 1732 described women wearing breeches, riding astride, shaking hands, ordering men to serve them, carrying pistols and even taking the initiative in love affairs.[13] There was, however, a grudging respect for such women.

The biggest stir was caused by women who dressed as men in order to marry. As well as duping their brides with intent to obtain money, there was a fear that sexual activities would take place between these women.

One tale which reiterated these concerns not only acted as a warning to both young girls and their parents to beware of tricksters but also pointed out the immorality of Eastern ways. *Travels into Turkey* (1744) relates the story of an old woman who falls in love with a young girl, the daughter of a poor man of Constantinople whom she encounters in the public baths. Determined to win her over, when neither wooing nor flattery works, she decides to dress as a man. She 'changed her Habit, hired a House near the Maid's Father, and pretended she was one of the *Chiauxes* of the *Grand Seignor*'; by this means she ingratiates herself with the father and asks to marry his daughter. The poor man agrees on the dowry and the couple are duly married. Upon pulling off her headgear, the bride discovers her husband to be a woman, whereupon she informs her parents who cart the offender off to the General of the Janissaries. Such 'factional' accounts were based on real-life female cross-dressers, conflating genuine biography with fabrication or exaggeration. It was thanks to these stories that women who dared to be dashingly different have passed into folklore.

Jolly Jill Tar

British piracy had been in existence from ancient times, with men fighting and pillaging one another's ships. In the Elizabethan period, Spanish galleons became a particularly favoured target. However, it was during the years between 1680 and 1730 that piracy was to come into its 'Golden Age', with vast amounts of pirates taking possession of ships in order to plunder them. Although not prevalent around the British Isles, piracy was rampant in North America and Africa, with as many as two thousand British private ships marauding the seas. The Caribbean, with its waters full of treasure-laden galleons, had become a prime location for these attacks.

At least two of the most famous pirates were women: Anne Bonny and Mary Read, who dressed up as men and went to sea as sailors. They first came to public attention in late 1720, with the trial of Calico Jack Rackham's crew in Jamaica. They were strong and hearty women who drank and cussed, and shot men dead. Dorothy Thomas, a witness who had been captured by Rackham's crew, told of how the women 'wore

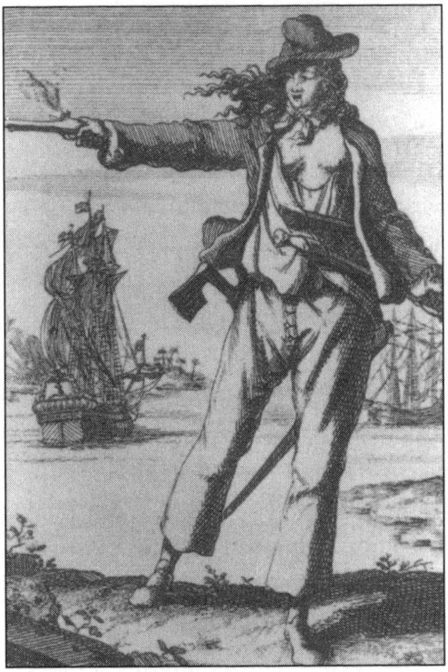

FIG. 37 Pirate Anne Bonny, 1725

Men's jackets, and long Trouzers, and Handkerchiefs tied about their Heads, and that each of them had a Machete and Pistol in their Hands'.[14] At the trial, fellow crewmen described their two female shipmates in glowing terms, as strong and bold as any of the rest of the crew. Both women had gone into piracy in their youth, the average age of pirates being around twenty-five. Both employed the 'proletarian practice of self-marriage and self-divorce'; in other words, they used a promise of marriage as proof of commitment and wife sales as a way out of their relationships. They appear to have been essentially heterosexual, neither Bonny nor Read being sexually attracted to other women.[15] Their stories appeared in various versions, including *The Tryals of John Rackham and Other Pirates* (1721), *A General History of the Pyrates* (1724) and *The Lives and Adventures of a German Princess, Mary Read, Anne Bonny, Joan Philips . . . etc.* (1755) and *The History of the Following Notorious Pirates* (1806), and proved immensely popular.

Anne Bonny, although born illegitimate, was brought up in a wealthy family in Cork in Ireland where her father was an attorney (**FIG. 37**). It was said she had a 'fierce and courageous temper', and inspired several tales, many of which proved groundless. One such anecdote described how she had killed a maidservant with a knife while in a fit of passion over a jealous affair. About to inherit a fortune from her father, she was all set to become a lady of leisure – until she met James Bonny, a man 'not worth a Groat'. It was obvious to her father that he was after Anne's inheritance. Nevertheless, she chose to marry her lover anyway, thus squandering her chances of an easy life. Her father disowned her, as he had threatened, and, with no family fortune forthcoming, James Bonny absconded.

At this stage, Captain Jack Rackham came on the scene and, obviously attracted to Bonny, courted her and persuaded her to adopt men's garb so that she could join him at sea. The problem for Bonny was that she was still officially married. In order to wed Rackham, she had to dissociate herself from her previous husband and, to this end, Bonny employed a common custom to end her marriage – she organized a wife sale. Although it was usual to have both the husband and the intended partner present to effect such an auction, the future protector bidding for the wife, this was probably not the case in Bonny's sale since her husband was absent. None the less, the new 'marriage' went ahead (such 'marriages' and 'divorces', although not legal, were considered acceptable among the plebeian classes) and Bonny joined Rackman aboard ship. After she fell pregnant, the couple decided to disembark in Cuba, in order to allow Bonny to give birth in greater comfort in the house of a friend of Rackham's. The break allowed the crew some time for leisure and enabled them to restock the ship.

Pirate crews generally organized themselves co-operatively according to the articles they had drawn up to govern behaviour, the distribution of spoils and any other eventualities which might arise on board ship. Some men on board formed same-sex unions under the common bonding of 'matelotage' which enabled them both to hold their possessions in common and to inherit each other's property after death. The captain was elected by the crew themselves, and it was he who would act as the military leader, overseeing and imposing discipline on the men. During the eighteenth century, the piracy trade was being subjected to a crackdown. Due to a concerted effort on the part of the British government, resulting in more Admiralty commissions in the colonies and the criminalization of those who had contact with pirates, wayward ships and their crews were increasingly tracked down and brought to justice. Finally, hauled in to answer for their crimes, both Rackham and Bonny were brought to trial for piracy, along with Mary Read. Rackham was allowed to see Bonny on the day of his execution. On being admitted to her cell, her final remark to her husband was that 'she was sorry to see him there, but if he had fought like a Man, he need not have been hang'd like a Dog'. Bonny, who was again pregnant, gave birth to her second child in prison and, although she appears to have escaped execution, nothing more is known about her.

Unlike her ship-mate Anne Bonny, Mary Read (**FIG. 38**) was born into a poor family. The stories about her early years are confused but it seems that Mary's mother had married and had a son. Prior to Mary's birth both husband and son had died and Mary's mother had thought it prudent to dress Mary as her deceased son in order to continue to receive money from her in-laws. One tale tells that Mary's mother married again and her husband, Mary's father, absconded; others say Mary was illegitimate. In any case they were left to fend for themselves.

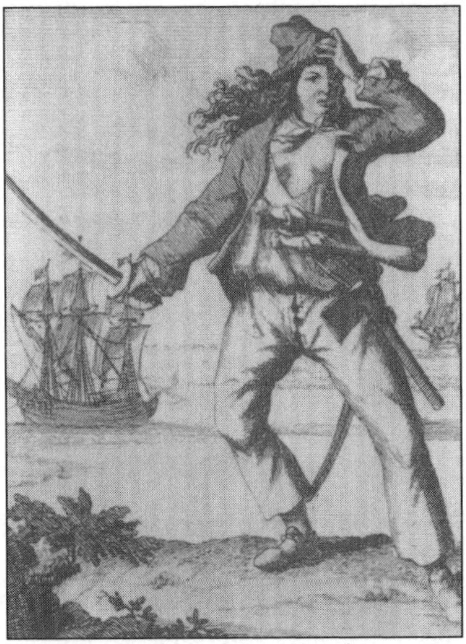

FIG. 38 Pirate Mary Read, 1725

At first, mother and child had lived quietly for three or four years until the money ran out and, in dire straits, they were forced to turn to the dead husband's relatives for support. Read's mother, thinking the grandmother would only be willing to support her son's male child, decided it best to disguise her daughter. Indeed, the ploy worked: '. . . the old Woman would have taken it [the child], bred it, but the Mother pretended it would break her Heart to part with it; so it was agreed betwixt them, that the Child should live with the Mother, and the supposed Grandmother should allow a Crown a Week for its Maintenance.'[16]

When the grandmother died, their only source of income was cut off. They were again in reduced circumstances so Read, who was by then thirteen, was put to work as a footboy to a wealthy French lady. After a succession of jobs dressed as a man, first at sea on a man-of-war, then as a cadet in the army at Flanders, Read joined the Regiment of Horse. Commissions in those days were bought and sold in what amounted to a commercial enterprise and, despite her bravery, Read was denied promotion to the rank of officer. Men from wealthier backgrounds than her would be first in line to buy such commissions, sometimes even purchasing them for their infant sons.[17]

While enrolled in the army, Read met the man who was to become her future husband, a fellow soldier to whom she revealed her secret. Her cross-dressing evidently did not lose her any friends among the other serving soldiers who presented Read with a gift of money 'in Consideration of her having been their fellow Soldier'. After having obtained a formal discharge, the money enabled the couple to set up an eating-house, the Three Horseshoes, where they worked hard to make a living. After the death of her husband, Read was unable to maintain the business and had to look elsewhere for a source of income. Donning her male garb once again, she returned to the army, this time with the Regiment of Foot in Holland. Her downfall came when she joined a ship en route to the West Indies which was seized by pirates.

So it was that Anne Bonny and Mary Read met up on board ship. According to the tales, Bonny had thought Read a fine, attractive-looking young man and intended to court her. This misunderstanding was soon cleared up when they admitted to each other that they were women and became firm friends. Unfortunately, their closeness had so enraged Captain Rackham, Bonny's lover, that they were obliged to reveal Read's true sexual identity. Meanwhile, Read had fallen in love with another man. On one occasion, he became embroiled in a duel and, concerned that he would not win, Read challenged his opponent to a duel two hours earlier. She killed him outright. In order to cement their relationship, Read and her lover entered into a marriage by promise ('look'd upon to be as Good as Marriage in Conscience') and continued as pirates on the same ship until the day they were caught. At her trial, in order to avoid execution, Read 'pleaded her belly' and declared that she and her husband (as she called him) planned to leave piracy at the first opportunity and seek an honest livelihood. Because of her pregnancy, Read's execution was stayed but she soon succumbed to a fever and died in prison.

Again Read's fellow pirates commended her bravery: 'In Times of Action, no Persons amongst them were more resolute, or ready to board, or undertake anything that was hazardous, than she and Anne Bonny; and particularly at the Time they were attacked and taken, when they came to close Quarters, none kept the Deck except Mary Read and Anne Bonny . . .' The popular tales about these two women provided examples to the public of female independence and bravery, while emphasizing the dangers which lay in wait for such adventuresses.

There is evidence in naval records of the eighteenth century of more than twenty women who went to sea with the Royal Navy or the Marines. One female sailor, Mary Lacy, told her story in *The History of the Female Shipwright*. Her parents were poor so Lacy was sent to a charity school where she could learn how to earn her own living. In childhood, she had made some money at knitting, but at the age of twelve she was put into domestic service. She quickly tired of this, escaping from the house to go dancing all night. In her twenties, she took to working at Portsmouth dockyard under the name of William Chandler, eventually running away to join the ship *Sandwich*.

Although some of the women who ran away to sea were from poor backgrounds, we know of at least one who was from the gentry. Anne Chamberlyne joined the ship of her brother, Captain Peregrine Clifford Chamberlyne, in 1690 and was commended for her fighting valour against the French. After surviving the dangers of battle, she returned to England to marry, only to die in childbirth. We also know that at least one black woman was among the crew of the *Queen Charlotte*. She was a married woman from Edinburgh who went to sea as a volunteer, disguised as William Brown, after quarrelling with her husband. She was said to be about twenty-six years of age, of great strength and a jovial character who 'takes her grog with her late messmates with the greatest gaiety'.[18] She served in the navy as an able seaman during the years 1804 to 1816 but her female name is not mentioned.

Women at Arms

Women usually became soldiers because they were poor and in need of financial security. Hannah Snell, who served under the name of James Gray (**FIG. 39**), became one of the most notorious female soldiers of her time. Her curious exploits were documented in *The Female Soldier or; The Surprising Adventures of Hannah Snell* (London, 1750) and were to result in various newspaper reports and earn a mention in the *Gentleman's Magazine* in 1750. Like many women who sought an independent existence, Snell's life was full of highs and lows. At her lowest ebb, she was to suffer the lash, a severe whipping under the auspices of a military punishment. At the end of her career, she received a pension as a reward for her services. Despite being

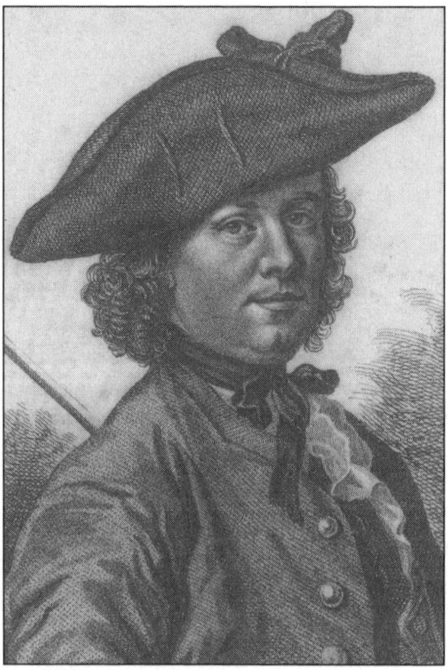

FIG. 39 Soldier Hannah Snell, 1750

partially illiterate (she could read but not write), Snell managed to carve a life for herself in the harsh male-oriented world of the military.

The daughter of a hosier and dyer, Snell was born in Fryer Street in St Helens, Worcester, on 23 April 1723. She was said to be the granddaughter of an illustrious Captain Snell who died fighting at Malplaquet, a fact which may have had some bearing on her choice of career. Little is known about her early childhood but about three years after the death of her parents, in 1740, she met and married a Dutch sailor, James Summs, who soon deserted her. Two months later, she gave birth and, having no other means of support, she travelled to London to stay with her sister Susannah and her husband, James Gray, a carpenter from Wapping. After some contemplation, she decided to go after her husband in order to seek revenge but changed her mind about going to sea at the last minute, and instead enlisted in the army under her brother-in-law's name, disguised in clothes she had borrowed from him. On 27 November 1745, Snell joined the Royal First Warwickshire regiment at Coventry.

Although women were not allowed in the army, many young men joined up as volunteers and it would have been easy for Snell to pass as one of them. Indeed, she earned the nickname 'molly' because of the smoothness of her chin. At this time recruits were not subjected to a medical inspection so she would not have been under threat of detection when enlisting. The army had a poor reputation, relying entirely on a voluntary recruitment process and so needed every hand it could muster. Those enlisting could expect little income and poor food and to mix with other soldiers who were thought to be drunk and unreliable.

At first things had gone well: while stationed in Carlisle, Snell had taken to her work, and was particularly good at the military drill, 'which she now performed with as much Skill and Dexterity as any Sergeant or Corporal in his Majesty's Service'. She fell in with a Sergeant Davis, technically her superior, but soon discovered that he was a villain, with a 'criminal inclination for a young woman in that Town'. In an attempt to seduce the unwitting young girl, Davis tried to enlist Snell as an accomplice but she refused and instead warned the intended victim of his plan. The two women struck up an intimate friendship but Davis, sick with jealousy and seeking revenge, unjustly accused Snell of neglecting her duties. Out of spite, he sentenced her to six hundred lashes. She was tied by her hands to the castle gates and allegedly 'received five hundred'.[19]

Life in the army varied from regiment to regiment but generally corruption was rife, the discipline was harsh and poor relations existed between officers and troops. In 1747, as a result of her unjust punishment, Snell deserted and went off to Portsmouth to join the Marines. From here, she sailed with the sloop of war *Swallow* bound for the East Indies, serving as assistant steward and cook for the officers of the mess under Captain Rosier. After several skirmishes, she eventually marched with the rest of the troops at Pondicherry, fighting bravely against the French. It is said that she fired off thirty-seven rounds but was eventually wounded in the groin. No doubt worried that she would be found out, she refused to be seen by the official surgeon but agreed to be treated by a black woman, who removed the bullets. She returned to Portsmouth on the *Tartar* in 1750 as a common sailor and remained there until she joined the man-of-war *Eltham*, bound for Portugal. While in Lisbon, she learned that her husband had been executed at Genoa.

The story of Snell's adventures was a huge success with the public. Indeed, her popularity was such that she eventually took to the stage, stomping up and down in uniform while carrying out her military exercises. Not all were so impressed with her accomplishments; a correspondent for the *Gentleman's Magazine* in 1750 declared, 'A more unpleasant sight can scarcely be seen than that of a woman imitating the dress of our sex; and it is infinitely worse when they go so far as to imitate that of a soldier . . . the acquiescence of the ladies in masculine vices, as it is more general, is also of worse consequence to the State.' Nevertheless, Snell was given a pension of £30 per annum in appreciation of her services to the army and the Marines.

Hints of lesbianism surfaced in one anecdote about Snell: she and a male shipmate, Jeffries, made the acquaintance of two young women who became quite attached to them. On setting sail for England, the captain ordered that no women should be allowed on board – their two female admirers would otherwise have joined Snell and her friend on the voyage.[20] Despite such stories, there is no hard evidence that Snell was a lesbian. Rather the opposite, as she married twice more: in 1759, to a carpenter called Samuel Eyles in Berkshire; and in 1779, to Richard Habgood who was found dead on a heath in Warwickshire some seven years later. In 1789, she was registered insane in Bedlam where she died on 8 February 1792 at the age of sixty-nine.[21] At her own bequest, her body was interred in the grounds of Chelsea Hospital.

Susan Cope was another woman who disguised herself as a man in order to become a soldier. Born in Ware in Hertfordshire, she was the only child of a reputable farmer, her mother having died when she was still young. As she grew up, she became very tall and acquired masculine mannerisms, her friends nicknaming her 'The Grenadier'. Despite her lack of feminine poise, Cope was pretty, had many sweethearts and received countless offers of marriage. Only too willing to put men in their place, she 'could so well take her own part that several young men in the neighbourhood who gave her offence, had felt the weight of her fist and learnt better manners'.[22] She eventually fell in love with a handsome soldier attached to the Guards and eloped with him. In order that she might stay with him, she joined his regiment dressed as a man.

In her new guise, Cope was soon being wooed by a stream of female admirers. One fifty-year-old woman who ran a tavern presented her with countless gifts, including her deceased husband's watch, and then proposed marriage, giving Cope five guineas with which to buy the wedding ring. No doubt having initially enjoyed the landlady's attentions, Cope now became worried that she was too deeply involved. She backed out at the last minute, leaving the widow standing at the church door. She wrote a poem by way of an explanation and sent it with a drummer boy to the jilted bride:

Kind loving Landlady, I find
Myself to wedlock not inclin'd
It is a thing so common,
But for your sake,
A vow I make,
To marry no other woman.

My gold I'll spend,
With my true friend,

And drink your health so free,
So don't perplex,
Or yourself vex,
Farewell, remember me!

Along with her male lover, Cope was sent with the British troops to Holland to fight the French. On receiving a wound in her breast, the surgeon discovered her true sexual identity and she was hauled in front of the commanding officer. When questioned about the motives for her disguise, Susan answered that she had become a soldier to seek her fortune and share the lot of the man she loved. After hearing this news, her lover flew to her side and married her. They were given subscriptions by way of support from their loyal commander.

Another soldier, Mrs Christian Davis, travelled from Dublin to Europe to fight with the British army but was eventually captured by the French. Davies ingeniously used a silver tube as a urinating device to prevent easy detection of her real identity. She attested that she had been given the implement by another female soldier. Davies was later awarded honours from Queen Anne for her distinctive performance in battle.

*

For the most part, women who disguised themselves as soldiers and sailors managed to earn a living, and were even admired for their strength and bravery by the men with whom they sailed and fought. It would have been easy for women to board ship since there was no physical examination prior to admission. Packed in below decks in foul-smelling cabins and with little chance to wash, the men rarely undressed and a woman might maintain her disguise. The danger of exposure would arise when a punishment was threatened, such as flogging which involved stripping the victim to the waist, or when an injury occurred. Yet women were rarely punished for going to sea or into battle disguised as men. Occasionally they would be forced to leave the ship if caught before setting sail, but they were generally treated well if their identity was uncovered, even receiving pensions and rewards.

The reasons for heterosexual women cross-dressing in order to join the army or navy ranged from financial necessity to following a lover into battle or to sea. As in other fields of work, a woman would gain a more independent lifestyle dressed as a man and she enjoyed greater freedom of choice. Consequently, many of the tales that fêted the female cross-dressing adventuress also acted as warnings about ungovernable women. The heroines could not be allowed to escape with such wanton displays of waywardness. The stories had to be morally resolved either through marriage or death: one involved the choice of a resumption of the 'natural' order of things; the other was unequivocal punishment.

While female cross-dressing might sometimes be considered acceptable (for the purpose of obtaining work), or even fun (as in the theatre), in other cases, it was unforgivable. Under normal circumstances, women and men were expected to dress according to their gender roles. Any reversal of the dress code was viewed as a threat to the status quo as it was seen to usurp male authority and invert the perceived natural order of things. On a lighter note, these tales provided jolly japes for the public and reinforced the positive characteristics of the women involved. For all the negative espousals about unruly women, their courage was applauded and their determination admired.

CHAPTER ELEVEN

Pains and Pleasures of the Birch

The arse of my love is delightful to see,
Its plumpness rejoiceth the eyes;
Her lily-white belly is heaven to me
But, ye gods! What are these to her thighs?

Theresa Berkeley, *Venus School-Mistress, Or Birchen Sports* (*c*.1808–1810)

White thighs, lily-white bellies and red buttocks were all to become central themes for aficionados of the birch, along with bizarre leitmotifs of flagellation such as purple gloves and monstrous nosegays. Interest in flagellation was so keen in the eighteenth century that it was evident in every type of printed matter from broadsheets, plays and poems to the gilt-edged calf-backed memoirs of the female flagellant. Whipping was a common sight in everyday eighteenth-century life. Servants were flogged in the household; criminals were publicly whipped through the streets. It was considered an acceptable punishment for a number of misdemeanours, from upsetting one's master to prostitution, as well as a cure for impotence. Flogging was practised by working-class whores in the brothels of Soho and Covent Garden and it was used as both a punishment and a sexual activity between couples in their homes.[1]

Keeping It in the Family

A woman, a dog and a walnut tree
The more you beat them, the better they be.[2]

In 1749, Sir Francis Blake-Delaval of Seaton Delaval in Northumberland, on being told that his mistress was in bed with an Italian eunuch, seized a horsewhip and dashed off with one of his chair-men in order to surprise them. On his arrival, he instructed the chair-man to hold down his mistress while he flogged her, and then to hold down the eunuch while he sodomized him.[3] Such incidents of correction of adulterous wives, along with sordid revelations of bloodied flogging of servants and children, had became common currency.

Flogging one's wife was perfectly acceptable to the run-of-the-mill family man. He considered himself master of his household and entitled to correct his family and servants as he saw fit. Indeed, the law supported this idea, giving a man property rights over his wife's body. In 1728, Daniel Defoe was to complain,

> There ought to be a shorter way, and when a man had beaten his wife (which by the bye is a most unmanly action, and great sign of cowardice), it behoves every neighbour who has the least humanity or compassion, to complain to the next Justices of the Peace, who should be impowered [*sic*] to set him in the stocks for the first offence; to have him well scourged at the whipping-post for the second; and if he persisted in his barbarous abuse of the holy marriage state, to send him to the house of correction till he should learn to use more mercy to his yoke-fellow.[4]

Women, however, had very few legal rights. One woman complained in 1735, 'Our law gives the husband the entire disposal of his wife's person, but she does not seem to retain any property in his.'[5] The truth of her claim can be seen in the apparent reluctance of the law to prosecute men who abused their wives. A thirty-eight-year-old Scot, William Thompson, was brought to Newgate on 28 January 1792 for beating his wife but he was discharged only two days later.[6]

Men of the law, far from hesitating to interfere in cases of wife-beating,[7] were only too willing to advise husbands on how flogging should be undertaken. In 1782, one Judge Buller went so far as to specify the appropriate size of the stick to be used, declaring that a man could legally beat his wife with it as long as it was no thicker than the width of his thumb.[8] Gentlemen's magazines seized on this ruling to exemplify the further benefits of a good birching. One piece in the *Rambler's Magazine* for the year 1783 entitled 'The Laws of Flagellation' highlighted the issue: 'The master, says lord Coke, is allowed by law to chastise his *Wife*, or *any other Servant* with moderation.' The *Rambler's* author ruminated, 'It is hoped that our modern lawyers have more politeness than to follow Lord Coke's example, by classifying a man's wife with his servants.' He continued:

> The ladies ought, however, to be very happy in this consideration, that though they are legally obliged to suffer the discipline of the *Thumb-Flick*, they are totally excused and exculpated from circumstances of a much more disagreeable nature. A married woman, for example, cannot be arrested for any debt contracted whether before or after her marriage; but in either of these cases, the husband is liable to be arrested, dragged to a spunging-house, and perhaps, from thence to a prison. A very dear purchase indeed for the satisfaction of exercising the Thumb-stick![9]

The idea of wife-beating and the furore caused by the case of Lord Coke, who had mistreated his wife, even inspired a popular song about the episode:

> *Since Judges, high grac'd, with learning and taste,*
> *Examples and precepts bring home,*
> *Says Hodge,* on my life, I will chastise my wife,*
> *With a weapon as thick as my thumb.*
> *Toll de roll, &c.*
>
> *'As Thick as My Thumb Song'*[10]

In 1767, a serious incident of servant-flogging came to light which was highly suggestive of being sexually motivated.[11] Mrs Brownrigg, a parish nurse who attended women in childbirth during the early part of the reign of George III, made a great point of appearing a sober and religious woman. She had employed three parish girls as apprentices – Mary Mitchell, Mary

---

* Hodge = A typical English agricultural labourer, *OED*; an abbreviation of Roger: a general name for a country booby, *The 1811 Dictionary of Vulgar Tongue*.

Jones and Mary Clifford in her house at Flower-de-Luce Court on the east-side of Fetter Lane. Her method of training was to whip them as hard as she could, assisted on occasion by her elder son. Mary Jones was often made to lie across two kitchen chairs and whipped mercilessly. She managed to escape but Mary Clifford continued to be constantly stripped and beaten with a cane, a hearth broom and a horsewhip. The girls were kept in the coal-hole, sleeping on straw and living on bread and water. When their clothes were torn, they were tied up and kept naked for several days. After Clifford had been stripped and tied up five times and beaten with the butt-end of a whip while Mitchell was made to look on, neighbours eventually raised the alarm and she was taken to hospital where she died a few days later. On 14 September 1767, Mrs Brownrigg was hanged at Tyburn for the murder of her female apprentice. Her husband and son were given only six months' imprisonment for their involvement.

In the latter half of the eighteenth century, Lady Anne Lindsay writing of her childhood recalled the whipping she and her sisters experienced at the hands of her governess. Her mother had also inflicted chastizement upon them: 'had she [her mother] only endeavoured to prevent our errors instead of correcting them, by the judicious advice which the early knowledge of our various dispositions might have suggested, how much better would it not have been.'[12]

School Discipline

In January 1735, the *Gentleman's Magazine* published a satirical piece entitled 'A Dissertation upon Flogging' which considered the precise way a good beating should be inflicted: 'Flogging is an art which teaches us to draw blood from a person's posteriors in such a manner as may twinge him most severely without danger of mortification.'[13] For the best administration, the author advised, the birch should be held at an angle of 45 degrees as a perpendicular movement was too violent. Sexual stimulation from flagellation was seen as the result of blood rushing to the brain: 'a proper application made to the posteriors draws the stupefying humours from the *cranium*, thoroughly purges the brain, and quickens the fancy wonderfully.' The author alleged that flagellation was practised frequently, 'now as much as ever', and the people to whom he referred were male flagellants at colleges and schools. He testified, 'I have seen a professor foam with ecstasy at the sight of a jolly pair of buttocks.'[14]

Birching for the purpose of discipline was common practice in public schools. Sometimes the boys would take the rod into their own hands. Edmund Curll, publisher of erotica, received a birching from the boys of Westminster School after printing a copy of the oration given at the funeral service of Robert South the prebendary of the school, without the author's consent. During the 1790s, Francis Fortescue Turville, a member of an aristocratic Catholic family, sent his two sons to boarding school. The master complained that Turville's son, Charles, had 'practised indecencies in word and deed, which he admitted were common in his former school', presumably masturbation, and as a method of correction he whipped the boy until he bled.[15] In 1815, Lt-Gen. Sir Eyre Coote (1762–1823) was charged with indecent conduct after having been caught in a boys' school with his breeches down, asking the boys to birch him.[16] Anecdotes of punishments meted out at public schools included notorious whippings by Dr Busby of Westminster (**FIG. 40**); in 1813, Dr Wool of Rugby allegedly flogged thirty-eight boys in a quarter of an hour; and Dr Keate of Eton, who reigned from 1809 to 1834, undertook the flogging of eighty boys in one go for collective absence at roll-call.[17] By all accounts, girls were whipped with the same frequency as boys. During the 1770s, allegedly at a charity school in East Barkham run by one Lady Marjory,* the girls were whipped soundly for any misdemeanour. In one alleged incident involving the whipping of a schoolgirl, Betty Brown, the girl was made to kiss the rod before its application, 'one of the new notions she [the governess] had brought from France'.[18]

Meanwhile, serious discussions on the necessity for discipline in schools were taking place, as seen in a 31-page sixpenny pamphlet, *The Benefit of School Discipline* (1741),[19] a response to an earlier pamphlet *The Shameful Discipline of the Schools Exposed*. The author confessed to being 'a Lover of Decency and Order in Youth' and provided a reasoned argument for the

* The author uses pseudonyms supposedly to hide the true identities of the people and places involved.

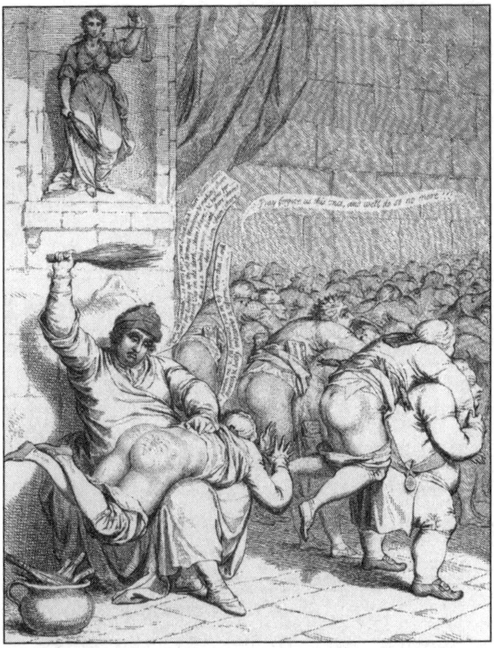

FIG. 40 James Gillray, *Westminster School, Or Dr Busby Settling Accounts with Master Billy and his Playmates*, 1785

punishment of schoolchildren. Books on the subject were advertised in *The Times* on 1 January 1785, such as *The Governess; or the Boarding-School Dissected*, which exposed 'the Errors in the present Mode of Female Education, and a Method of correcting them . . .'[20] The debate continued in an exchange of letters in *The Times* in July 1788 on the virtues and vices of public schools.[21] The lack of discipline in female boarding schools was even blamed for nurturing fledgeling prostitutes, as seen in a letter in *The Times* on 18 September 1788 from 'A Good Father':

> It is not only at Greenwich that seminaries, under the denomination of boarding-school, are opened for the reception of handsome children from indigent parents by fashionable bawds – they are to be found in almost every quarter around this extensive metropolis. They increase daily to the disgrace of our Government and the ruin both in soul and body, of many an unfortunate female.[22]

Boarding schools were seen to sow the seeds of debauchery, encouraging girls to shirk their domestic duties in the pursuit of an extravagant lifestyle. (**FIG. 41**). As a result, these girls would ultimately find themselves turning to prostitution.

> Miss now, as soon as she is proper to leave home, is sent to a boarding-school and taught French, before she understands English. Her mind is turned from domestic matters to a routine of high life – when she has finished her stitches, she returns to her father's poor cot, where the picture of industry and labour not suiting those notions she had at school, she throws herself into the arms of the first fellow she meets, and commencing prostitution, figures a way for a few butterfly months, just tasting the sweets of her summer, and then thrown upon the town, perishes in a garret, or dies on a dunghill.[23]

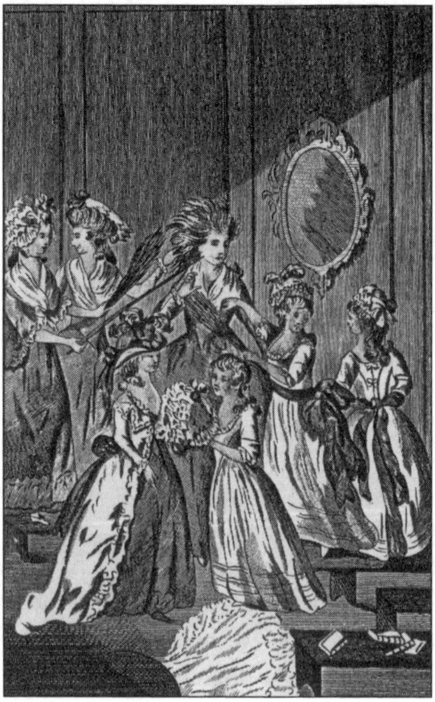

FIG. 41 *The Boarding School*, *Rambler's Magazine*, vol. I, 1783

Even the theatre picked up on school discipline as a sexually titillating topic in *The Boarding-School; or the Sham Captain*, an opera performed at the Theatre Royal in Drury Lane around 1732:

> *While she is stripping to get a good whipping.*
> *I'll away, dance and play,*
> *Yes, I will, that I will;*
> *While she is stripping to get a good whipping,*
> *I'll go and romp with the Girls and the Boys, &c.*[24]

Flogging Female Felons

Flogging had been advocated in the Bible as a punishment for women guilty of sexual demeanours: 'And whosoever lieth carnally with a woman, that is a bondmaid, betrothed to an husband, and not at all redeemed, nor freedom given her; she shall be scourged' (Leviticus 19: 20). The penalty was most frequently employed for petty larceny and vagrancy but also on unmarried mothers and transgressors of sexual morality, usually with a cat-o'-nine-tails and often with the added stipulation that blood should be drawn. The sentence was generally carried out in public, with the offender tied either to a whipping-post or the end of a cart, or whipped through the streets. In 1680, at Durham, Eleanor Wilson 'was publicly whipped in the market-place, between the hours of eleven and twelve o'clock' for being drunk on a Sunday. The town council of Great Staughton in Cambridgeshire paid 8s 6d for the whipping of a female lunatic. The infamous Judge Jeffreys called upon the executioner, about to flog one female criminal, 'Hangman, I charge you to pay particular attention to this lady. Scourge her soundly, man: scourge her til her blood drips down! It is Christmas, a cold time for madam to strip. See that you warm her shoulders thoroughly.'[25] British travellers were accustomed to similar spectacles in Europe. Thomas Coryate saw 'a fellow whipped openly in the streets of Lyons'. Lauder mentions that robbers and thieves were whipped through the town with a fleur de lis burned into their cheek with a branding iron.[26] Pierre de Brantôme's *Memoirs* relate the tale of the whipping of Mademoiselle de Limeuil, a

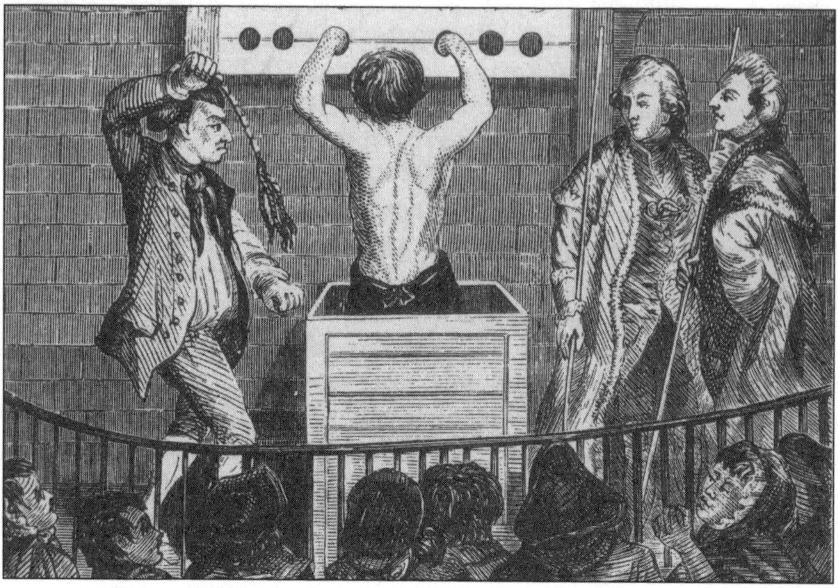

FIG. 42 *Whipping in the London Sessions House Yard*, 1745

member of the French court and maid of honour to the Queen, for writing satirical verse.

In England, Bridewell was intended as a House of Correction 'for the strumpet and idle person, for the rioter that consumeth all, and for the vagabond that will abide in no place'. In *Mr William Fuller's Trip to Bridewell* (1703), the author's account of what happened to him while serving his sentence exposed the common usage of the whip (**FIG. 42**). Not only were prostitutes flogged, but the men caught in the act with them were similarly corrected in Bridewell: 'one poor old Man I heard was there for being found in Bed with 2 young Whores, two too many for the Temper I myself was in at the time.'[27] For this crime he had to endure sixty lashes and was ordered to do hard labour.

The public flagellation of prostitutes through the streets of London was a common sight throughout the eighteenth century. The journalist Ned Ward, in his *London Spy*, related how parties of young men made excursions to witness the public flogging of whores.[28] Action against prostitutes taken by the Society for the Reformation of Manners resulted in eleven of them being publicly whipped in 1762 after being arrested for street-walking.[29] In his account of cross-dressing in *The Female Husband* (1746), Henry Fielding regaled the reader with images of the bleeding Mary Hamilton after having received punishment by flogging, reporting 'so lovely a skin sacrificed with rods, in such a manner that her back was almost flaed'.[30]

By the end of the century, female offenders were flogged in private; at Launceston in 1792, a female thief was ordered 'to be stripped to the bare back, and privately whip'd until she be bloody'; at the same time a man was given a similar sentence but to take place 'in the public street'.[31] There was no government regulation regarding this punishment and it was left to the discretion of the local authorities. The abolition of public flogging took place only in 1862, although this had been preceded by the Whipping of Female Offenders Abolition Act which had prohibited the flogging of women prisoners either in public or in private.[32] This use of flogging as a punishment for crimes would be adapted in erotica to form a sexualized discipline, introducing a structured kind of carnal sado-masochism.

Sex with 'Birchen Twigs'

In *The London Spy*, Ned Ward related a visit to a flagellation brothel in 1709. He had overheard a bawd, Mother Beelzebub, asking whether there were any rods in the house, to which a wench answered, 'Yes, yes. You know you fetched sixpennyworth but yesterday.' He asked a friend what this meant and he replied, 'That sober-seeming saint . . . is one of that class in the black school of sodomy, who are called by learned students in the science of debauchery, flogging-cullies. This unnatural beast gives money to those strumpets which you saw, and they down with his breeches and scourge his privities till they have laid his lechery. He, all the time, begs their mercy, like an offender at a whipping-post, and beseeches their forbearance. But the more importunate he seems for their favourable usage the severer vapulation they are to exercise upon him, till they find by his beastly ecstasy when to withhold their weapons.'[33]

Flagellatory practices with a sexual context were highlighted in pictures: Hogarth's harlot in *A Harlot's Progress, Plate III* (**FIG. 43**) is depicted with

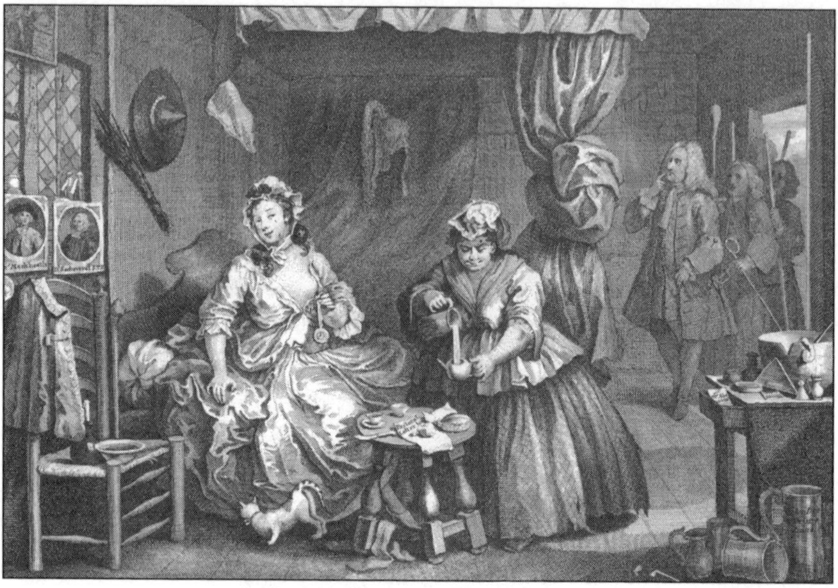

A Harlot's Progress, Plate III, 1732

a birch hanging above her bed, indicating that she would indulge in flagellation with her customers. Factual reports came through contemporary magazines and trials. The *London Journal* for 14 May 1726 referred to whores who provided a flagellation service.[34] In April 1718, Amy Warrington of St Giles-in-the-Fields was tried for having broken a broom over the back of Bernard Kemble during a session involving two other prostitutes, for which he paid ten shillings. The trial of Mary Wood in September 1719 involved John Tenants who had supplied his own rods when he paid her to whip him in front and behind.[35] Likewise, Susan Brockway related how John Richmond offered her ten shillings if she would get a pennyworth of rods to whip him 'and make him a good boy'.[36]

Sexual flagellation was thought to have been a vice which originated in France. Jean-Jacques Rousseau, although known mainly as a French philosopher who influenced virtually every major political development of the time, gave a vivid account of his life and sexual preferences in his *Confessions*. His autobiography revealed the pleasure he gained at an early age through the tender beatings of his governess:

> As Mademoiselle Lambercier had the affection of a mother for us, she also exercised the authority of one, and sometimes carried it so far as to inflict upon us the punishment of children when we had deserved it. For some time she was content with threats, and this threat of a punishment that was quite new to me appeared very terrible; but, after it had been carried out, I found the reality less terrible than the expectation; and, what was still more strange, this chastisement made me still more devoted to her who had inflicted it. It needed all the strength of this devotion and all my natural docility to keep myself from doing something which would have deservedly brought me a repetition of it; and I found in the pain, even in the disgrace, a mixture of sensuality which had left me less afraid than desirous of experiencing it again from the same hand.[37]

Rousseau confessed that these nursery punishments led to a sexual predilection which he found difficult to satiate. The long-lasting consequences of such flogging were all too evident: 'Who would believe that this childish punishment, inflicted upon me when only eight years old by a woman of thirty, disposed of my tastes, my desires, my passions, and my own self for the remainder of my life, and that in a manner exactly contrary to that which should have been the natural result? When my feelings were once inflamed, my desires went so astray that, limited to what they had already felt, they did not trouble themselves to look for anything else.'[38]

Much of the early French pornography was to influence eighteenth-century English erotica, its flagellation scenarios derived from the practices of Catholic penitents. Books such as *Venus dans la Cloître*, *Thérèse Philosophe* and *Histoire de Dom B* would set their scenes within nunneries or monasteries to enable the arena of religious flagellation to develop into a sexual one. British flagellation material developed its own ruses, one of which was to introduce the sado-masochistic British reader to the pains and pleasures of the birch through the memoirs of the prostitute female flagellant.

Memoirs of a Female Flagellant

> At last, he twigg'd me so smartly as to fetch blood in more than one lash: at sight of which he flung down the rod, flew to me, kissed away the starting drops, and, sucking the wounds, eased away a good deal of pain.
>
> John Cleland, *Memoirs of a Woman of Pleasure*[39]

In *Memoirs of a Woman of Pleasure* (1749),[40] the fictitious whore Fanny Hill experimented with flagellation within the course of her sexual career. Prior to this book, there had been little fictional exploration of flogging for sexual pleasure in British erotic writing.[41] Yet from the 1770s onwards, a new line in English pornography developed which included *Venus School-Mistress* (*c*.1808–1810), a whore's memoirs completely devoted to flagellation. According to Henry Spencer Ashbee, the expert Victorian bibliographer of erotica, this book was written by Theresa Berkeley who was herself a notorious flagellant.

The preface to the 1830 reprint of the book described the brothels of the Regency period, an addition probably made by its publisher, George Canon. The book itself acted as an advertisement for these sumptuously furnished sex establishments, including addresses where flagellation practices took place: Mrs Emma Lee could be found at No. 50 Margaret Place, Regent Street; Mrs Phillips at No. 11 Upper Belgrave Place, Pimlico; Mrs. Shepherd at No. 25 Gilbert Street; and Mrs Sarah Potter, alias Stewart, at various addresses.

Theresa Berkeley ran her whipping parlour from No. 28 Charlotte Street, and stood out as the exemplar of her trade. Theresa's clientele came from all walks of life. Some were worn-out old men in need of invigoration:

> It is true that there are innumerable generals, admirals, colonels, and captains, as well as bishops, judges, barristers, m'lords, commoners, and physicians, who periodically go to be whipped, merely because it warms the blood, and keeps up a little agreeable excitement in their systems long after the power of enjoying the opposite sex has failed them.[42]

According to the preface to her memoirs, her personal papers included a letter written from Dublin in January 1834 by 'a very good-humoured and tolerant Catholic'. He described to her at length the severity and professional manner of each of the female flagellants whom he had visited: Mrs Brown had been recommended to him and he found her to have 'a pretty strong arm'; Mrs Wilson of Marylebone 'was no chicken at all' and Mrs Chalmers was 'a very experienced hand'. But even Mrs Noyeau with 'her tall and robust figure could not make a sufficient impression on my backside'. Unfortunately, Mrs Jones of London Street and all her assistants 'were too drunk to break a rod on me'; Betsy Burgess had left the 'Diable au Corps' [i.e. quit flogging]; and to his distress, Mrs Gordon, to whom he had been sent by Lord A——y had 'lost Mrs Potter's address and was out of rods'.[43] Luckily, he managed to find relief at the hands of Mrs Collet and Mrs Beverly, 'as knowing dames as any in London'. However, as a customer, he was a hard man to satisfy as 'even their united energies have left me unconquered'.

Theresa Berkeley aroused her clients not just through whipping them with birches and the cat-o'-nine-tails but by means of various contraptions designed specifically for this purpose. One was 'a hook and pulley attached to the ceiling by which she could draw a man up by the hands'. Another was called the Berkeley horse (**FIG. 44**):[44]

> A machine was invented for Mrs Berkeley to flog gentlemen upon, in the Spring of 1828. It is capable of being opened to a considerable extent (so as to bring the body to any angle which might be desirable). In the original memoirs, there was apparently a print representing a naked man upon the machine being worked upon by a woman sitting in a chair exactly under it, with her bosom, belly, and bush exposed whilst Mrs Berkeley birched his posteriors.[45]

When the new flogging machine was invented, its designer told Theresa Berkeley that it would bring her fame. Indeed, it brought her a great deal of business until her death in September 1836, when the horse was presented to the Society of Arts at the Adelphi.[46] Another flagellation machine, designed by Chase Price, could take care of no less than forty

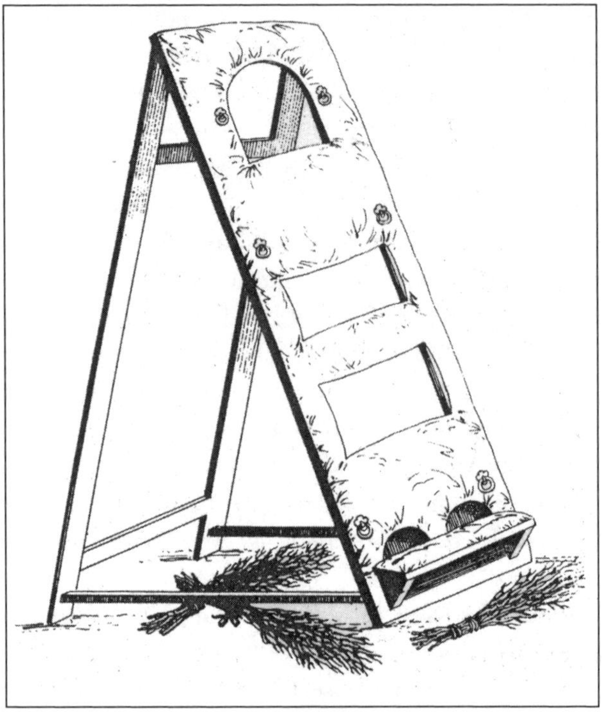

FIG. 44 Theresa Berkeley's Flogging Machine

victims at once. The famous actor Samuel Foote had a long debate with the inventor of this contraption in the brothel of Charlotte Hayes, a machine Price wanted to patent.[47]

The Birchen Bouquet

From the 1770s, new images appeared in fictional pornography, most notably that of the female dominatrix. This figure was not a leather-clad woman wielding a whip over a subservient male but a refined, upper-middle-class woman who enjoyed whipping. Although such women here not entirely averse to beating pubescent males, the focus – initially, at least – was on young women. Early books, such as *Exhibition of Female Flagellants* (1777), feature scene upon scene of women whipping young girls over sofas, chairs or laps. By the time *Exhibition of Female Flagellants*

Part II (1785) was published, men were making the occasional appearance to oversee the action. Grown men were only gradually introduced to erotic flagellation scenes. In later books, flagellation would be followed by scenarios of sexual intercourse, with whipping being part of the build-up to the whole experience. Within this pornography, the dominatrix's dress is described in great detail: her hair was coiffed in a stylish understated way, her shoes had shiny buckles and her dresses were tightly laced. One of the most significant characteristics of the heroines in these porngraphic novellas is that they all wore huge nosegays – enormous clutches of heavily scented flowers – on their lapels.

One such pornographic novella, *The Birchen Bouquet*, which was previously thought to be from the Victorian era, actually dates back to 1770 or 1790.[48] Part of the appeal in this erotica was the detailed images of young governesses. The book describes one young woman accompanying a pupil to school: 'her skin was as fair as alabaster, her hair of a fine auburn flowing in natural ringlets over her shoulders, rather full-chested for her age, which was turned fifteen; delicately shaped, and very slender in the waist, with firm round hips, rising elegantly, and terminating in a pouting bum, that provoked a desire to see it uncovered.'[49] The fashionable refined young woman, Charlotte, was the central character and the book affirms the flagellant's delight in flogging young people,

> . . . that a number of ladies take a secret pleasure in whipping children with a birch rod, particularly grown-up boys and girls, is too well credited to need comment, nor are the ladies singularly culpable of this propensity. Several gentlemen experience a similar satisfaction in seeing correction administered by a fair hand on the posteriors of a bold boy or impertinent miss.

One of the main governess characters in *The Birchen Bouquet,* Mrs Vaux, runs a fashionable school for young ladies at Greenwich. The themes follow the pattern of other flagellation material of the last decades of the eighteenth century, concentrating on the colour and texture of the female posterior ('dazzling white buttocks', 'rising plumpness and beautiful roundness'); on the types of whips ('almost green, and made out of two swinging rods'); and on details of underwear ('taking up at the same time her frock and petticoats in the most deliberate manner, and at length her shift, which she pinned to her shoulders'). Contraptions similar to Theresa Berkeley's horse were used to tie the girls up. The descriptions also contain details about bodily fluids such as blood and 'emissions'. Mrs Vaux, after beating Harriet, was surprised to find 'Her thighs and part of the bed, were covered with that precious liquid which is never spent'.

Nosegays in pornography were part of the dress code of a female flagellant. A nosegay worn on the lapel was a blatant indication of the wearer's predilection for flagellation. Charlotte, in *The Birchen Bouquet*, brings up the subject of flowers while whipping her male guardian: 'Now I think of it, did you order the bouquet of artificial flowers you are to present me on my birthday, did you, did you, did you? Now mind that the flowers will be scented, and the nosegay as big as a broom, just like this I have got in my bosom, otherwise you may depend upon another good whipping'; and again, after the flogging as he is about to take her, her breasts jutting out of her loose chemise, 'on the left side of which she wore a large nosegay, whose luscious fragrance excited the most voluptuous sensations'. Later, he made the most of the scent, 'kissing her bosom and smelling the bouquet alternately'.[50] Flowers induce a state of euphoria and ecstasy: 'But to see Charlotte in the act of coition, her pretty face half buried in her nosegay, her eyes twinkling, her mouth a little open, as in the paroxysm of fainting . . . one arm and its fair hand thrown round the back of the partner of her joys, the other still grasping the birching sceptre.'[51]

Nosegays added an air of elegance to a woman, and made her more desirable: 'When a lady is tolerable [*sic*] handsome, with a good bosom, such a nosegay completes her dress, and gives her that bewitching, nay, lascivious look, which should be the study of a knowing women always to have.'[52] Having witnessed Charlotte and her lover together, Harriet decided to entice the music master, with the nosegay as the main lure. 'She had purposely that day in her bosom an elegant nosegay, uncommonly large, she asked him if he was fond of the sweet scent of flowers, he replied in the affirmative, and soliciting her permission to smell them, she complied and showed him the finest breast in the universe.'[53] Harriet's lover becomes fired up with passion at the fragrance of her nosegay, which suggests that flowers were worn for their aphrodisiacal effects as well as being part of the flagellant's dress code: 'The ladies on the Continent generally wear those large nosegays at their weddings, at their balls, public places, &c, and many when they perform the rites of Venus, having found not only that they excite libidinous desires, but also aggravate very much venereal enjoyment.'

Unusually for this type of erotica, there is a case of incestual buggery in *The Birchen Bouquet* which was probably an addition by its nineteenth-century publisher. However, it continues with the themes of nosegays: Harriet, peering through the keyhole, saw a beautiful young girl, 'her sweet face buried in a nosegay, her legs extended, her clothes turned up behind, and Maria's brother with his little pintle in his hand, trying to enter by the back avenue.'[54]

The Bagnio Miscellany, although imprinted with the date '1792', was in fact published by George Canon in 1830, along with lascivious engravings by Siddon who had engraved *The Accomplished Whore* (1827). This book also engages with the nosegay motif, the male protagonist declaring to the female flagellant, 'And sweet Lizzy, what a lovely nosegay! Allow me to smell it.'[55] The names of the characters had become decidedly less twee and more obscene: Miss Sophy Frigger, Lucy Rose-cunt, Amelia Shoveitin, Betsy Suckprick and Emily Longslit. Scenes now involve pupils from the nearby boys' school and the male characters have become more domineering, setting the trend for later material in this genre: 'He then stript her of the blue silk, unlaced her stays, and in a few minutes not one of her ravishing charms were hid.' Many of the light analogies and niceties of *The Birchen Bouquet* had given way to more brutal talk. Whereas, the flagellation pornography of the 1770s had featured many scenes between women, as in *Exhibition of Female Flagellants* (1777), male ravishers were now increasingly being introduced. Thus the beginning of the nineteenth century witnessed the beginning of a more aggressive form of pornography.

*

Specific areas of the lascivious body had become important for those with an interest in sexual flagellation: thighs, upper arms, breasts and, most of all, buttocks. The flagellant's dress code, with its huge nosegay, had become a known indicator for those with similar tastes.

Whipping was a common spectacle in the eighteenth century, as seen in household punishments dispensed to wives and servants. The enforcement of school discipline and public punishments meted out by the courts were topics continually discussed in magazines and newspapers. Specialized brothels as well as middle-class homes were becoming sites for more private flagellation. Towards the end of the century, punishments were also increasingly being made private and flagellation itself became infused with an erotic value. In fact, carnal flagellation in British pornography from the 1770s onwards was merely the sexualization of an existing practice. With the explosion of print culture, writers of erotica were playing with objects and scenarios that were already sexually wrought, and stretching the imagination to experiment with flagellation in fantasies.

British flagellation scenes were initially set in nurseries, parlours boarding schools, the stronghold of the middle class which perpetuated the domestic sexual strait-jacket. Catholic pornographers had chosen their own areas of taboo for their flagellation scenarios – that of the nunneries and monasteries. In their attack on the morally pious, the writers were venturing into prohibited areas in a bid to make the material sexually exciting. These early stories would pave the way for greater exploration of sexual diversions by the master of sadism, Marquis de Sade, and later experimenters in pain and sexual pleasure.

CHAPTER TWELVE

Unnatural Lewdness

'[Potter] lived in most infandous Buggeries for no less than fifty years together, and now at the gallows there were killed before his eyes a cow, two heifers, three sheep and two sows, with all of which he had committed his brutalities. His wife had seen him confounding himself with a bitch ten years before; and he then excused himself as well as he could, but conjured her to keep it a secret.'

Cotton Mather, *Magnalia Christi Americana*[1] (1702)

Bestiality was seen as a sodomitical act, a felony which incurred the death penalty on conviction in the eighteenth century[2] and was comparable in its wickedness to sodomitical acts between men. Most of the cases of bestiality are known because the trial reports were printed for an inquisitive reading public. In the trials, the activities always involved men, women were never involved. Yet in erotic fiction, this trend was reversed; women were described as becoming highly aroused by watching animals mating and having sex with them; men's bestial activity was never mentioned. The type of animal involved varied depending on whether the bestiality occurred in fact or fiction. In reality, men might bugger cows and mares, as well as dogs, but in erotic fiction, women rarely took on anything bigger than cats and dogs – although in the following century, one female character was depicted as having sex with a baboon.[3]

Bestiality was just one of the many 'unnatural lusts' of the long eighteenth century. Other curious inclinations were remarked upon in *The Wandering Whore* (1660), particularly those involving men who 'will not be contented with doing the business', or having straight sex, but apparently were in need of other stimulation. One man wanted to be under a table snarling like a dog as if he would bite the 'whibb-bobs' off the girls around him; another 'will needs shite in one of our wenches mouth's'; the third 'will needs be whipt to raise lechery and cause a standing prick'.[4] Some sixty-odd years later, Daniel Defoe described London's debaucheries in much the same vein, relating how 'many old lechers (beasts as they are) steal from their families, and seek these harlots' lurking holes, to practice their unaccountable schemes of new invented lewdness: Some half hang themselves, others are whipt, some lie under a table and gnaw bones that are thrown 'em, while others stand slaving among a parcel of drabs at a washing-tub.'[5] Strange activities were taking place among the more adventurous members of the public, despite conventional moralists stressing that sex was to be practised between a man and a woman within marriage, and then only in order to conceive children. These types of sexual behaviour were viewed as 'abnormal' in the eighteenth century, with some rated as worse offences than others.

From the 1770s onwards, experiments with electricity in the scientific world inspired the erotic industry to try out novel remedies for a flaccid penis using shock therapies. Impotent men might, with the assistance of London whores, also try hanging themselves to encourage ejaculation, sometimes to the fatal end of the practitioner. The fascination with attempting to obtain an erect penis meant that the castrati, and their genitals, became the subject of much curiosity and speculation. An interest in female underwear and small feet were considered acceptable, if not condoned. Bestiality, incest, masturbation, group sex, oral and anal sex, however, were regarded as repugnant. All of these practices would be discussed, experimented with and pornographically described, showing just how diverse the sexual activities of the eighteenth century really were.

'The Sin of Uncleanliness with a Cow and Other Creatures'

Bestiality was considered a particularly horrendous crime, the Bible specifying the punishment for its practice: 'And if a man lie with a beast, he shall surely be put to death: and ye shall slay the beast' (Leviticus 20:15). However, there was a change in early attitudes towards bestiality: the seventeenth-century accounts of it were closely associated with witchcraft[6] and political subversion. By the eighteenth century, it was more likely to be viewed purely as an abominable crime committed by people with unnatural lusts.

An earlier case involving bestiality and religion was that of a preacher who was executed for 'an attempt which he made on the Sacred Person of the Archbishop of St Andrews'. This was related in a 'small and curious volume', *Ravillac Redivivus, Being the Narrative of the late Tryal of Mr James Mitchell* (1678),[7] to which was attached an account of the trial of Major Thomas Weir, executed for adultery, incest and bestiality. Both these accounts were connected to controversies looming in the Scottish Church.

With his 'unnatural Lusts', Weir was compared to Tiberius and was seventy years old when he came to trial on 9 April 1670. He was accused on four counts: firstly, of incest with his German sister, Jane Weir (when she was ten, again at sixteen, and then at forty years old, at which time he lived with her); secondly, of incest with his daughter; thirdly, of a series of adulterous acts with married and unmarried women, particularly with his servant, Bessy Weems; and finally 'to his Fornications, Adulteries, and Incests, he proceeded to add the unnatural Sin of Bestiality in lying with Mares and Cows, particularly polluting himself with a Mare, upon which he rode into the West Country near *New Mills*.'

Various witnesses gave evidence at Weir's trial, including his wife, Margaret, who had caught him lying with his sister in the barn near her house at Wickenshaw, stating 'that they were both naked in the bed together, and that she was above him, and that the Bed did shake, and that she heard some scandalous Language between them, in particular that his sister said, she was confident she should prove with Child.'[8] Most damning of all was Weir's admission to copulating with a mare. One John Alexander recounted how Weir had been questioned about his act of bestiality and had responded, 'That a Gentleman having given him the Mare, he rode upon her into the *West* Country to see some Friends, and dealt with her near *New Mills*, and that a Woman saw him in the act, and complained to Mr John Nave the Minister of *New Mills*.'

These accusations of bestial activities were a subversive attack on dissenters rather than merely sexual revelations, the most pertinent aspects being the political and religious issues. Weir belonged to a Scottish religious sect and seems to have upset his political colleagues. The accusations of magic and consorting with the Devil appear to have been a method by which his political adversaries could rid themselves of a troublesome man. Initially, Weir's actions were not considered credible, being too gross and indecent for contemplation. Eventually, it was alleged, his guilty conscience led him to admit to the crimes: 'the terrour of God which were upon his Soul, urg'd him to confess, and accuse himself'. He was convicted and sentenced to be strangled and his body to be burned at the stake; his sister was sentenced to hang, having admitted complicity, telling of their 'Compact with the Devil' and the use of his 'Magical Staff' which 'he received it of the Devil' and with which he could do 'wondrous things'. Bestiality was still associated with sorcery and pacts with the Devil, a 'transgressional' act. This was commonly suggested in cases of heresy or treason[9] but, in the case of Weir, accusation of bestiality also served religious and political ends.

By the early eighteenth century, titillating accounts of cases of bestiality and sodomy were being appropriated purely to provide sexual entertainment. In 1710, Edmund Curll printed *The Case of John Atherton, Bishop of Waterford in Ireland, who was Convicted of the Sin of Uncleanliness with a Cow and other Creatures, for which he was Hang'd at Dublin*. The preface to the pamphlet stated the motive for publication of such trial reports:

> The publisher had better have told us that the profit of the edition was the true reason for the publication. And that the readers may infer so much from the bottom of the title paper, where he tells us the price is one shilling, which is very high for a pamphlet of about four sheets. The novelty of so rare a subject and scandalous story (he thought) would not fail of alluring buyers at any rate . . .[10]

Thus Curll was well aware that reports of bestiality would fetch a high price, such was the curiosity of the public. Bishop Atherton had been hanged for buggery on 5 December 1640. The chief witness against the bishop had been a robber, 'a most profligate and wicked fellow' who, at his own execution, admitted the bishop's innocence. The High Sheriff of the County, though, was already prejudiced against the bishop and had great influence with the jury. Both Atherton's case and another seventeenth-century trial, that of Lord Audley who had been hanged for sodomy, were rehashed by Curll under the title of *The Cases of Unnatural Lewdness*, selling for three shillings.[11]

Bestiality appears to have become a lesser crime towards the end of the century, as sentencing became less harsh. In 1791, a red-haired twenty-three-year-old tailor, of sallow complexion, Matthew Mubrie, succumbed to the attractions of a cow at Tothilfields where he committed the crime of bestiality for which he was imprisoned at Newgate for two years.[12] Previously, bestiality had been seen as such a horrific sin that the animal had been burned alive in front of the sinner before he was hanged.

Bestiality was taken as seriously abroad as it was in England. One perpetrator came to the notice of the public in New Haven, Connecticut, in 1662. A member of the Church, the sixty-year-old Potter was executed for 'damnable Bestialities'. He had apparently been practising these abominations since he was ten years old. Another well-practised sodomite 'who had been wont to defile himself with greyhounds, cows, swine, sheep and all manner of beasts' was brought to trial at Wünschelburg in Silesia. He and his horse were found guilty and both were punished by being burned alive, although some animals might on occasion be executed (**FIG.** 45).[13] Similar cases were reported in France. In 1721, a young Catholic, François, was caught 'behind a mare with his apron raised, extremely aroused'. The witness waited a few moments, wondering what he should do, and then seeing 'the said [François] standing on his tiptoes and making all the movements proper to the consummation of his pernicious act, he made some noise'.[14] François was sensible enough to make good his escape when the witness went off to fetch the master, and the case never came to trial. In Vanves in 1750, Jacques Ferron was sentenced to death for having intercourse with a she-ass. Because it was deemed that the ass did not co-operate, having no free will in the activities, she was acquitted. The inhabitants of the area, along with the priest of the parish, signed a statement verifying that they had known the ass for many years and they could vouch for her virtue and previous good behaviour, she being 'a most honest creature'.[15]

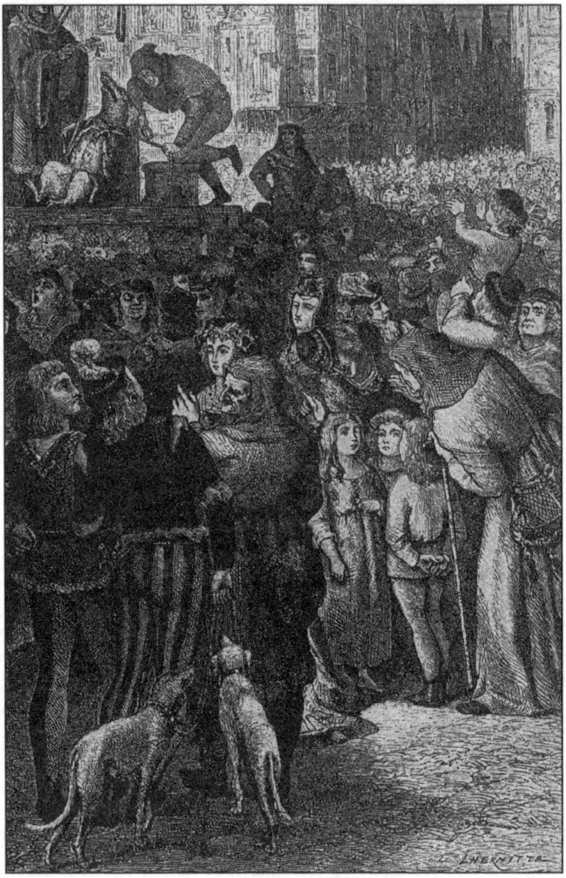

FIG. 45 Execution of a Sow

At the same time as these activities were taking place, publishers of erotica were making further inroads into bestiality as a sensuous pleasure. French erotica had already tested the potential of animal involvement in *Les Egaremens de Julie*, where the heroine spies on an older girl masturbating. She, in turn, tries the experiment for herself with her cat.[16] The protagonist in *Le Diable au corps* similarly experiments with her dog (**FIG. 46**). British erotica would not be slow to catch on to the appeal of animal sexuality. Bestiality had been touched on in *A New Atlantis for the Year 1758*, introducing a dog which 'sipped up many a lady's privacy'. The dog was prone to licking itself, 'his long red indelicacy used to spontaneously unsheath [*sic*] itself'; Tonzenie, the heroine, delighted in this and 'impelled by instinct, and to ease the itching of her fingers, immediately fell a tickling it: pug grinned'. She also swooned at the sight of bulls and horses copulating.[17] Similarly, in *New Atlantis for the Year 1762*, the tale of Henry and Emma reiterated the educative value of watching animals;

> Well, all this while nature does not fail to act her part, to raise in her little fluttering heart such commotions as excite her curiosity to know how she came into the world. She sees the lambs, the birds, nay every animal creature, speak a sensible passion. She watches them, observes a converse between them, pleasing, though unintelligible to her: – She sees the bulls and the heifers wanton with their mates in a more striking manner.[18]

Accounts of bestial voyeurism had already appeared in John Aubrey's *Brief*

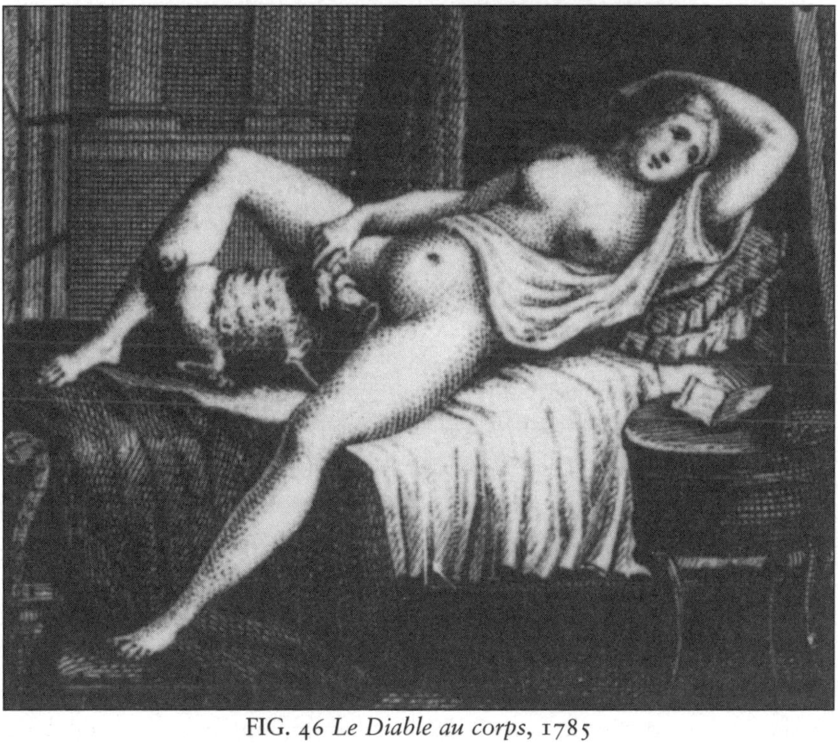

FIG. 46 *Le Diable au corps*, 1785

Lives of Contemporaries between 1669 and 1696. Popular throughout the eighteenth century, it related the story of Lady Mary Herbert, sister of the poet Philip Sidney, becoming sexually excited while watching horses:

> She was very salacious, and she had a contrivance that in the spring of the year, when the stallions were to leap the mares, they were to be brought before such a part of the house, where she had a *vidette* [a hole to peep out at] to looke on them and please herself with their sport; and then she would act the like sport herselfe with *her* stallions.[19]

Bestial voyeurism was thought to contain an instructive quality, at the same time as encouraging natural female sexual feelings to spring forth. Watching animals copulate initiated a woman into the world of sex; the reading of romantic novels finished the job, as seen in the case of Lady Mary: 'The seeds of corruption having been thus sown, they are brought to maturity by novels and romances, which soon excite her.'[20]

Eunuchism Display'd

The fact that Italian opera singers had their testicles cut off when young to ensure the continuation of a falsetto voice post puberty was anathema to the English. Because of this, there was a decided curiosity about eunuchs and their genitalia (or lack of them). Moreover, stories of Turkish harems overseen by eunuchs in erotic stories such as *Arabian Nights Entertainments* (1713) were extremely popular, and were reprinted steadily throughout the eighteenth century. One such pamphlet, thought to be lost, was being sought through a series of advertisements carried in *The Country Journal: Or, The Craftsman* from August through to December 1735. This missing pamphlet, *Curious Letters*, carried a 'most curious Account of the *Turkish* Women in General. Of their Wives and Concubines, Of the Grand Signior's *Seraglio*, and his Ladies in it. Of the Two Sorts of Eunuchs who have but half Cut off, and Those who have all Clean Cut off. How and why they are made so.'[21]

These stories connected eunuchs to lascivious women and all things exotic. Edmund Curll, never one to miss an opportunity, stimulated interest in the topic of eunuchs with his publication of Charles Ancillon's *Traité des Eunuques*, translated as *Eunuchism Display'd* (1718). In it, he described

> all the different Sorts of Eunuchs; The Esteem they have met with in the World, and how they came to be made so. Wherein principally is examin'd, whether they are capable of Marriage, and if they ought to be suffer'd to enter into that State . . . Also a Comparison between Signor *Nicolini, Pasqualini, Pauluccio* and *Jeronimo* or *Morro*: With several Observations on Modern Eunuchs. Occasion'd by a young Lady's falling in Love with *Nicoloni*, who sung in the Opera at the *Haymarket*, and to whom she had like to have been Married.[22]

Eunuchs were described as having soft squeaky voices, a female complexion, soft down for a beard and lacking in courage or bravery, their ways and manners considered entirely effeminate. Yet Italian opera singers had become popular entertainment. The famous castrati, Valentino Urbani, performed at Drury Lane Theatre in 1707; a year later, the admired bass-baritone Nicolino sang at the Queen's Theatre; Handel employed Senesino to perform his operas, staying in London for eleven years such was his reputation; and Farinelli, his rival, took his own troupe to the King's Theatre in Lincoln's Inn Fields. Curll was obviously keen to cash in on the contemporary public interest in operatic castrati as well as continuing with his usual business of promoting sex.

Avid female fans of the Italian opera singers gave rise to male jealousies. Warnings were given about how easily women fell in love with these 'creatures'. Eunuchs were seen as particularly dangerous as they could satisfy a woman's lust without the fear of pregnancy, thus women could have sex with them with impunity. In his *Traité des Eunuques*, Ancillon declared, 'It is certain, however, that a eunuch can only satisfy the desires of the flesh, sensuality, passion, debauchery, impurity, voluptuousness and lechery. Since they are not capable of engendering children they are more sought after by debauched women, because they provide them with the pleasures of marriage unaccompanied by any of its risks.'[23] Usually they only had their testicles removed but could still obtain an erection and ejaculate. Castrati were known to have affairs with women and even marry. In 1766, the great sopranist, Tenducci, fell in love with an Irish girl and married her in the face of great hostility and opposition from her family. When she amazed everyone by falling pregnant Tenducci rejected her, believing she had been unfaithful. In his memoirs, Casanova speculated that Tenducci had, in fact, been born with three testicles and therefore, if only two had been removed, he would have still been capable of paternity.[24]

So strong was the sexual power of castrati that falling in love with them could have horrendous and even fatal side effects. So said the satirical *An Epistle to the most learned doctor W—d—d from a Prude that was unfortunate Metamorphos'd on Saturday December 29 1722*. It related an incident in which, during a visit to the opera, one women who was deeply attracted to the opera singer, became so overcome that she experienced an attack of the vapours and had to leave for home. Such were the consequences of her lust for the castrato that a penis fell from inside her body and she turned into a hermaphrodite. Indirectly, these joking anecdotes expressed underlying anxieties about fears of male incapacity and female lasciviousness. Although this fictitious rendition was relatively harmless, the dangers of falling for a castrato could be much more lethal. In a later story by Balzac, a French sculptor, Sarrasine, fell in love with what he thought was a young girl. 'She' turned out to be the male love object of Cardinal Cicognara, who promptly had the sculptor murdered.

In a display of antagonism towards Roman Catholics, castration was advocated for its priests. British Protestants believed Catholics to be sexually lascivious hypocrites and their priests to be evil corruptors of their womenfolk. The threat of these perceived sexual aggressors ran so deep in British culture that an array of anti-Catholic literature was published, calling for the castration of priests and the Pope. Under such titles as *Reasons Humbly Offer'd for a Law to enact the Castration of Popish Ecclesiastics* (1700) and *The Priest Gelded: Or, Popery At The Last Gasp Shewing* (1747), Italy was blamed for initiating the practice of castration. The operation involved the removal of the male genitals in order to create better voices for opera singers; it was believed to be common practice in

Italy and other Popish countries 'to *Geld* their own Sons to make the better Market of them for Singing-Boys, and Musicians, or to be Calamities to Cardinals, and other Dignitaries of the Romish Church.'[25]

Electricity and Impotence

As a result of a burst of scientific interest in electrical experiments in the 1770s, electricity quickly came to have relevance in sexual matters. Notorious quack Dr James Graham devised an electric bed which allegedly had rejuvenating qualities. 'The Celestial Bed' had an electrical mattress which he purported increased the potential fertility of barren couples; it was supposed to add vigour to sexual activities and to assist in conception. Hired out to couples at fifty pounds a night, it sent out electrical vibrations which allegedly aided procreation. One wit remarked, 'That *extraordinary Physician* and *natural Philosopher*, Dr Graham in his sublime theories of generation, was perhaps the first who informed mankind that *certain aids* were necessary, even in the most athletic and vigorous constitutions, to enlarge and enrapture the practice.'[26] His Temple of Health opened at the popular Adelphi in the Strand, full of electrical conductors, Leyden jars and attention-grabbing apparatus. From here, he gave lectures and promoted his new electrical therapies. Graham was known to have had a violent disagreement with Dr Gustavus Katterfelto, a fellow scientist, because of his assertions about the properties of electricity. In a hoax, a poem was created based on Katterfelto disingenuously effusing about the greatness of Graham's bliss-inducing love machine:

> *Long had Pandora's ills, &c. &c. —*
> *When thou eccentric! thou celestial ray!*
> *Whose dictums, sense and nature obey:*
> *Appolo sent, to succour* feeble *man,*
> *His joys to heighten, and* extend *his* span.

The poem extolled Dr Graham for creating systems to improve the species. The antagonism between the pair was satirized in a cartoon depicting each of them astride phallic-looking electrical conductors (**FIG. 47**), a symbol of their egotistical boastings about increasing men's virility.

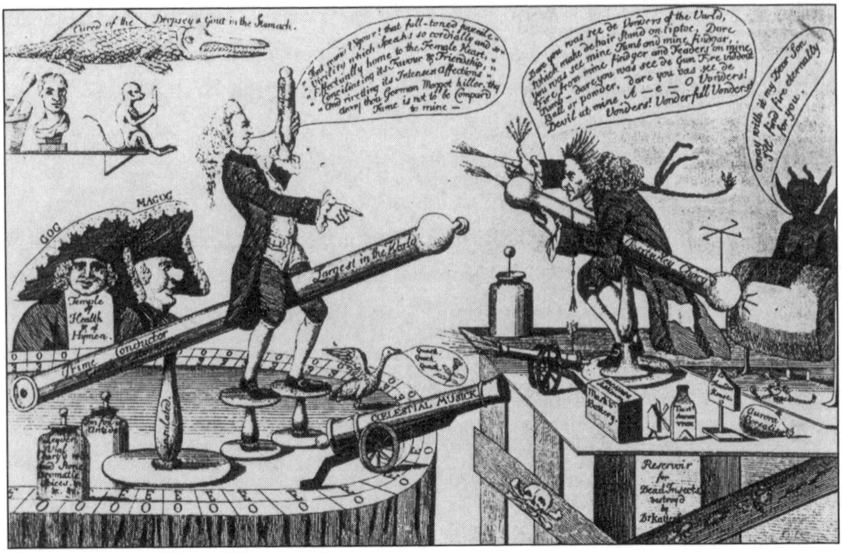
Cured of the Dropsey & Gout in the Stomach.
Virility which speaks so cordially and Effectually home to the Female Heart, Conciliating its Favour & Friendship, And rivetting its Intensest affections damn thou German Maggot killer, thy Fame is not to be Compar'd to mine —
Dare you was see de Vonders of the Vorld, which make de hair stand on tiptoe, Dare you was see mine Tumb and mine finger, Fire from mine finger and Feaders on mine Tumb — dare you was see de Gun Fire vidout Ball or powder, Dare you vas see de Devil at mine, A — e — O Vonders! Vonders! Vonderfull Vonders!
my Dear Son find fire eternally for you.
GOG
MAGOG
Temple of Health & of Hymen.
Largest in the World
Prime Conductor
CELESTIAL MUSICK
Reservoir for Dead Insects destroyed by Dr Katterfelto

FIG. 47 James Graham and Gustavus Katterfelto, *The Quack's*, 1783

Tales proliferated expounding the problems of impotence and its remedies, most notably jocular warnings about sexual excess in old men. One ancient general with a young wife was unable to gain an erection. Try as he might, he could by no means 'render him agreeable to the rights of Hymen'. He finally managed to penetrate his young bride 'by a wonderful metamorphosis' brought about by the imbibing of a quack medicine. Unfortunately, the astonishing feats he then performed subsequently killed him off. Similarly, a General S., also lacking 'any power over a certain corporeal debility', was attracted by the possibility of his impotence being rectified with the help of London whores and so made his way to a well-known brothel in Lisle Street, Soho. On entering the bagnio, he took a love potion but, due to the ecstatic effects of the drug, he became 'overcharged' and 'burst in the explosion' and died.[27]

The Amorous Art of Strangling

Auto-asphyxiation, or self-strangulation, was another sexual divergence that proved a popular topic of discussion and experimentation for the inquisitive during the 1790s. One particular case came to the attention of the public at the Old Bailey on Friday, 16 September 1791, when a prostitute, Susannah Hill, was charged with the hanging of Franz Kotzwara, a popular composer. He had visited Hill's lodgings in Vine Street two weeks earlier and hired her services to fulfil his strange request; he asked her to put a rope round his neck to effect an erection. They had gone into the back room which Hill rented, where several acts of gross indecency had taken place:

> in particular he pressed her to cut off the means of generation, and expressly wished to have it cut in two. But this she refused. He then said he should like to be *Hanged* for *five* minutes; and while he gave her the money to buy the cord, observed, that *hanging* would *raise* his passions – that it would produce all he wanted.[28]

It seemed that Kotzwara had heard about the practice of asphyxiation and had gone to London particularly for the purpose of trying it out. He had previously visited a brothel in Charlotte Street, telling the whore about his infirmity and the method he had resolved upon to remedy the evil – all this, in order 'to possess her lovely person with all the fullness of enjoyment'.[29]

Counsel for the prosecution, Mr Garrow, lamented the fact that certain men were prepared to go to such extreme lengths to satisfy their lust. He noted that the case had started a dangerous curiosity 'which by no means tended to advance the morals of the welfare of society'. The way to check such immoralities, he declared, was to punish the women who prostituted themselves in this way. 'The prisoner could not be a stranger to the probable consequence that might ensue from such a mode of suspension', the barrister argued, and therefore could not be seen as wholly innocent. Hill had run from the house, exclaiming to the neighbours that she had hanged a man, 'but feared she had hung him too long!' Elizabeth Dalton, a sworn witness at the trial, attested to her respectability, affirming that she was neatly dressed in common apparel, and that there was nothing in her countenance that seemed to indicate 'a rooted depravity'.[30]

Prostitutes were being blamed for the spread of vice at this time rather than the men who sought out their services. The prosecution intended to make an example of Hill in order that 'it might deter the depraved part of mankind from seeking indecent stimulatives', and that 'it might also deter the abandoned part of the female sex from lending themselves for hire, to purposes so vile'.[31] Hill was eventually dismissed but the incident attracted much satirical comment in Grub Street.[32]

Incidents of strangulation had provoked so much curiosity that they were still being discussed in the November 1793 issue of *Bon Ton*. One anecdote referred to in an anonymous essay, *Modern Propensities*, was recounted virtually verbatim in an article entitled 'The Origin of Amorous Strangulation'. In *Bon Ton* in March 1793 a Doctor 'Manacle' had discovered the effects of auto-asphyxiation: 'Though the Reverend Parson Manacle might not have been the first discoverer of the wonderful effects of strangulation, he certainly was the first who ever put it into practice.'[33] So interesting was the story that it ran into further editions; by April, it was reported that a Mrs Birdlime* was sentenced to hang after being caught stealing when 'a pair of rich point ruffles happened unfortunately to stick to her hands in a shop in Tavistock-street'. Parson Manacle, determined to show her how painless hanging could be, persuaded her to indulge him in his fantasy. To this end, the good doctor fixed the noose around his neck, and fastened the other end to his penis. His intention, readers were led to believe, was to allay her fears at her impending death sentence.

> . . . the Doctor Manacle raised his feet from the floor, and to the incredible astonishment of his fair assistant, actually hung for one or two minutes with infinite composure. At length, observing his breast begin to heave, and that he still made no effort to relieve himself, she readily performed the remainder of the agreement, and cut the instrument which might otherwise have proved fatal.[34]

So delighted was he by the desired effect that he clasped Mrs Birdlime in his arms 'in a transport of ecstasy' and finished off what the strangulation had started.[35] Parson Manacle became extremely fond of the practice but on one occasion enjoyed himself a little too long and inadvertently expired.

* Birdlime was slang for 'thief'.

The unfortunate Mrs Birdlime was taken off to be hanged at Tyburn the following day.

Warnings were given against practising strangulation too frequently for fear of the potentially fatal effects. Gentlemen were cautioned that, if they were determined to use this method to acquire the powers of erection, they should devise some means of checking its progress. To this end, it was suggested that a machine should be invented:

> There is no medical or surgical artist better calculated than the celebrated Patent Inventor of Spring Bands in Mount-street, who, from his wonderful improvements in surgery and mechanics, could very probably invent not only a safe but an agreeable and graceful mode of suspension, in which the gentle undulations of the body vibrating with reciprocal motion to the action and re-actions of elastic powers, might communicate a softer degree of pressure to the jugular muscles.[36]

Until this apparatus was invented, however, the safest bet was to stick to medicinal remedies for impotence, such as Dr Vanbutchell's 'great, wonderful, and astonishing Nostrum' allegedly approved of by the surgeon John Hunter. According to an advertisement in *Bon Ton* magazine, the tincture was said to preserve wives from corruption and produce children with true athletic stamina.

Love of the Dead

Dead bodies were often on open view in eighteenth-century England. Watching the execution of criminals was a popular pastime, with hundreds of people turning up to witness the proceedings at the public gallows at Tyburn, commonly known as 'the Hanging Tree'. The public dissection of criminals had been allowed since 1564 and, by the eighteenth century, the anatomy theatre acted as a display case for splayed bodies. As executions were gradually withdrawn from public view, images of them in print were more widely dispersed than ever.[37] In some cases, this morbid obsession with dead bodies had a sexual basis, as in the case of thirty-five-year-old John Curtis from Wiltshire. Although the courts were aware of necrophilia, it was not in fact a crime in itself. Instead Curtis was delivered to the New Compter, being accused of rape on the body of one Sarah Tippel. However, the crime was not verified and he was found not guilty at his trial on 23 February 1793.[38]

George Selwyn, a friend and member of the social circle of Caroline and Henry Fox, developed various sexual oddities, one being a morbid obsession with corpses and executions. Rumoured to enjoy dressing up as a woman, he was equally interested in young men, two of whom were the Earls of March and Carlisle. One account related how Lord Holland, on his death-bed, when asked by the servant whether he should show Selwyn up to the bedroom, answered, 'If I am alive I will be delighted to see him; and if I am dead, he would like to see me.'[39] Selwyn's fascination for watching executions was a standing joke with his friends, as was his aversion to women and his passionate fondness for other people's children. His necrophilia was denied by a Dr Warner in a letter to the *Gentleman's Magazine* shortly after Selwyn's death – but it was Warner who had so eagerly called at the Shakespear Tavern to catch a glimpse of the body of Miss Martha Reay, murdered by her lover Hackman, in order to report details back to Selwyn. Selwyn was away in France at the time of her death and had ordered at least three friends to send him information after sighting the corpse. Indeed, Lord Carlisle asserted that he had also attended Hackman's execution, not to fulfil his own curiosity but in order to forward the account to Selwyn. After a murder at nearby Castle Howard, Lord Carlisle had taken the trouble to write to Selwyn to affirm that he would find him the best viewing position for the execution. In 1746, when rebel lords were to be executed on Tower Hill, Selwyn not only obtained a ticket but made attempts to secure the head of one of the corpses. 'I can with great pleasure inform you, my dear Selwyn,' wrote his friend Phillips, 'that the head is ordered to be delivered on the first application made on your part. The expense is little more than a guinea. The person who calls for it should pay it.'[40]

A Revd T. Heppel, who travelled and preached during 1793–4 in the northern counties of England under the name Miss Jane Davison, was accused of seducing and robbing several girls, and eventually transported to Australia for stealing dead bodies at York.[41] *The Crimes of the Clergy*

(1823) related the story of the unusual transgressions he had committed but we are not told whether he had stolen the corpses with the intention of using them for necrophilia or of selling them for dissection. Unfortunately, there has been little research into the practice of necrophilia and its full extent in the eighteenth century is simply not known.

Lovely Legs and Pretty Toes

Admiration of ladies' feet was commonplace in eighteenth-century England. The sight of a well-turned foot was recognized as an object of desire and something in which men might take a keen interest. Sally Salisbury's legs and feet drew many admirers, it being said that 'her Leg and foot having Powers to excite, like the Face and Voice of others'.[42]

After the marriage in 1791 of Frederick Augustus, Duke of York and Albany (1763–1827), to Frederica Charlotte Ulrica Catherine, newspaper reports were eager to respond to public excitement about the wedding. Since the duchess was rather plain, they expounded on the attractiveness of her feet rather than her face, complimenting her gracefulness, the smallness of her foot and the elegance of her diamond-encrusted shoes. The *Morning Post* of 7 January 1792 commented, 'A foreigner would suppose that several of our flimsy prints were conducted by shoe-makers . . . so much have they said about the Duchess of York's slippers.' The affair was captured in a print by James Gillray, *Fashionable Contrasts; or, The Duchess's Little Shoe yielding to the Magnitude of the Duke's Foot* (**FIG. 48**), his foot a jocular metaphor for his penis.

Courtesan Harriette Wilson's small feet were esteemed by her paramours. Julia, her rival, admitted, 'the pretty little feet of Harriette Wilson, which Dukes were so proud to admire were often tripping down the merry dance, to the tune of a Jew's harp . . .'[43] Harriette herself admired a handsome foot in others. Commenting on the feet of her lover's wife, Lady Jersey, she remarked, 'She possesses all the beauty of all the Jerseys . . . and what a pretty little foot! This I had observed as she got out of her carriage in Curzon Street.' Of her lover, she noted, 'His Lordship really loved me, and, above all, he loved my foot. I was never, in his opinion, *assez bien chasseurs* [well-shod], therefore, he used to go about town with

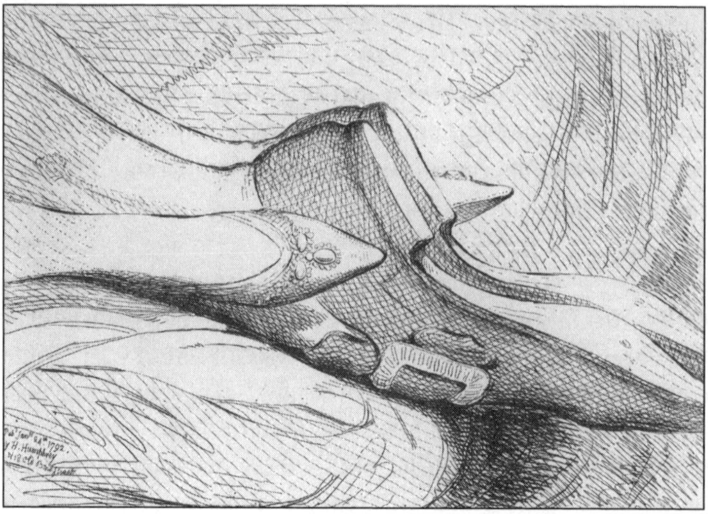

FIG. 48 James Gillray, *Fashionable Contrasts; or The Duchess's Little Shoe Yielding to the Magnitude of the Duke's Foot*, 1792

one of my shoes in his pockets, as a pattern to guide him in his constant search after pretty shoes for me.'[44]

Obsessions with a lady's feet also appeared in the memoirs of the notorious Irish courtesan Mrs Leeson, a.k.a peg Plunkett. One of Leeson's friends was conducting an intrigue with a marquis, who was interested only in her feet. Surprisingly, 'she had in all that time no sort of connection with him'; in other words, they did not have sexual intercourse. When asked by her astonished friend as to why he kept her, she replied archly, 'of picking, washing and cleaning my pretty little toes, which he took great delight in, and in which pleasurable, innocent, and inoffensive pastime he has often spent hours; 'twas the greatest gratification to him on earth, nor did he (said she) indulge in any other in all the time we spent together, he never was even rude enough to give me a kiss'.[45] The marquis was obviously smitten by his lover's feet as the affair continued for many years.

The interest in feet was pandered to in the directory of whores, *Harris's List Of Covent Garden Ladies* (1788), which recommended one prostitute as 'Her leg and foot is particularly graceful, always ornamented with a white silk stocking, and a neat shoe'. Indeed, the thought of white stockings on beautiful legs could well give a man near-apoplexy. White stockings had a perilous effect, as the *Universal Spectator* in 1737 admitted, 'A lady's leg is a dangerous sight in whatever colour it appears, but when it is enclosed in white, it makes an irresistible attack upon us.'[46] Even the sober Dr Samuel Johnson was to declare to David Garrick after a visit to the theatre, 'I'll come no more behind your scenes, David; for the silk stockings and white bosoms of your actresses excite my amorous propensities.'[47]

The Earl of Kildare, husband of Emily Lennox, was immensely fond of purchasing stockings for his wife's lovely legs. She particularly liked ones which had been 'clocked' or embroidered with silk. After over-spending on stockings for her, he wrote excitedly, 'I bespoke two pairs with bright blue, two pairs with green and two pairs with pink clocks . . . I am sure when you have them on, your dear legs will set them off. I will bespoke you six more pairs with white clocks; you mean to have them embroidered I suppose, therefore [I] shall make you a present of the dozen. The writing about your stockings and dear, pretty legs makes me feel what is not to be expressed.'[48]

Different sexual inclinations and 'fetishes' only began to be categorized by the sexologists at the end of the nineteenth century. It was suggested that the emotional key to such attractions can be traced to the deprivations or traumas in childhood. 'Conversely, some have claimed that, after a favourable childhood experience, a fixation takes place and associations are maintained into adulthood. However, fixations with underwear and feet occurred well before they were labelled as fetishisms. Possibly, since bosoms and arms were on display but legs were not, feet peeping out invitingly from beneath long dresses appeared tantalizingly seductive. Being well-shod was part of a woman's deshabillé; buckled and highly ornamented shoes gave a decided air of *je ne sais quoi*, so much talked about in gentlemen's magazines and among the *bon ton*.

The More the Merrier

The notion of group sex was not uncommon; various British and French pornographic books of the 1700s were full of pictures of men and women in communal sex activities (**FIG. 49**). People wanting to engage in group

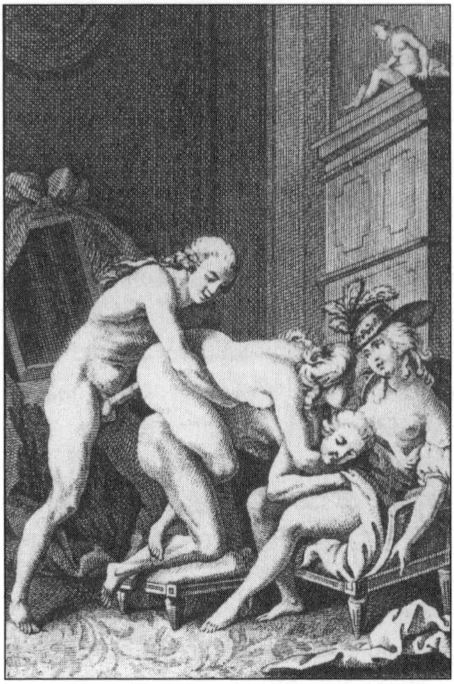

FIG. 49 Group Sex in *Memoirs of a Woman of Pleasure*, 1776

sex might go to a brothel to hire out a couple of prostitutes, or attend an orgy. Alternatively, men and women might gather at home. The fictitious Fanny Hill describes taking part in an orgy in a room full of gallants enjoying themselves with the women from the brothel: '. . . the table was remov'd from the middle, and became a side-board; a couch was brought into its place, of which when I whisperingly inquired the reason of my particular [her regular customer], he told me that as it was chiefly on my account that this convention was met, the parties intended at once to humour their taste of variety in pleasures, and by an open public enjoyment, to see me broke of any taint of reserve or modesty . . .'[50]

In 1706, a group of experimenters among the middling sort in Norwich are known to have engaged in various sexual activities which included flagellation and the cutting of pubic hair.[51] Boswell had sex with more than one woman at a time, as did Casanova, who also attended occasional full-blown orgies. Multiple sex encounters were often stimulated by drinking. In 1751, the novelist Henry Fielding blamed the gin-shops for most of society's ills: 'Gin-shops', he proclaimed, 'are undoubtedly the Nurseries of all manner of Vice and Wickedness.' Indeed, in June 1743, the gin was blamed after Daniel Flannigal bought twopence halfpenny worth for two women, intending to spend the night with them. When they demanded a higher payment, he obliged with another halfpenny worth of gin, but one of the women insisted on 'a Present of something else' – intent on procuring his shoe buckles. In another incident, after enjoying a pint or two of wine with Elizabeth Jerron, on being joined by another woman, it all became too much for Robert Stafford who 'let down his Breeches, pull'd up his Shirt, and bid them see what he had got'.[52] Thus, although there is still not a great deal of evidence for group sex in the eighteenth century, there is reason to believe that it was indeed taking place.

Taking It in Hand

Masturbation was often condemned as sinful with references made to the biblical story of Onan who 'spilled his seed on the ground' (Genesis 38: verse 8–10).[53] The act was condemned by the Church as it wasted sperm intended for procreation. Yet, prior to the eighteenth-century, masturbation had not been identified as a problem to one's health. Indeed, some medics positively advocated it as a cure for certain ailments.

Galen, the second-century Greek physician, advised women that gentle rubbing on the clitoris would relieve tension. His knowledge was strongly influenced by Hippocrates, whose ideas dominated medical theories for the next 1,700 years. Thus, right up until the 1700s, female masturbation was seen as having beneficial effects. Women were thought to suffer from depression if they did not have sexual intercourse frequently enough. In response, Robert Burton in his *Anatomy of Melancholy* (1621) advocated masturbation for the ease of female melancholy brought on by lack of sex.[54] Physicians and midwives might even stimulate their female patients to release any 'blockages' which might be the cause of illness. Meanwhile, medical writings advocated masturbation for men to alleviate a build-up of 'seed' or semen.[55]

From the beginning of the new century, anti-masturbation literature exploded on the scene with *Onania, Or the Heinous Sin of Self Pollution, and all its Frightful Consequences in both Sexes Considered* (*c*.1712), a work which shattered all preconceptions about masturbation and laid the foundations for a new-found fear of its adverse effects on health. Masturbation, it was now claimed, could cause epilepsy, spinal tuberculosis, wasting and madness. Fear-mongering around masturbation was continued in Samuel Tissot's *Onanism: or, a Treatise upon the Disorders Produced by Masturbation* (1760) and, J. T. de Bienville's *Nymphomanie, ou Traité de la Fureur Utérine* (1771). Both provided lurid details of the afflictions which would beset the male and female body if subjected to prolonged masturbation.[56] Jean-Jacques Rousseau shared Tissot's view that onania was a threat to health, vigour and life, and saw masturbation as a self-polluting 'solitary vice'. Dr James Graham joined the tirade against masturbation. He warned that masturbation would lead to 'debility of body and mind – infecundity – epilepsy – loss of memory – sight, and hearing-distortion of the eyes, mouth and face – feeble harsh and squeaking voice, pale sallow and blemished complexion'.

Confusion was also arising as to the moral implications of masturbation. In a letter published in Daniel Defoe's journal, *The Review*, in 1704, one gentleman enquired as to whether self-pollution was a mortal sin or not, to which Defoe answered in the affirmative. The French philosopher Diderot described one of the three definitions of 'pollution' in his *Encylopédie* (1745–72) as the effusion of seed, outside of marriage. He indicated that the defilement was in the waste of semen rather than the act of masturbation itself – in other words, it was not being used for the purpose of procreation.

This change in attitude towards masturbation – that it was no longer acceptable – can been in seen in the differing reactions of seventeenth-century Samuel Pepys and John Cannon and the eighteenth-century James Boswell. Pepys masturbated anywhere and everywhere, even in church, without much evidence of guilt. Although he burned the book *L'Escole des Filles* immediately after reading it, this was out of fear of being caught in possession of pornography rather than of being found masturbating. John Cannon recalled a childhood incident in his diary: how a boy at a party 'took his privy member in his hand rubbing it up and down till it was erected and in short measure followed Emission'. The other boys were told that this was a good way to deal with 'lustful venereal thoughts'. For James Boswell though, masturbation continued to be something he felt he should not be doing. Feeling guilty about it, he promised to stop masturbating and 'never pleasure but with a woman's aid'.[57]

Reading erotica was also seen as harmful, particularly for women. Rousseau famously commented: 'I was thirty years old before I set eyes on any of those dangerous books which a fine lady finds inconvenient because they can only be read with one hand',[58] indicating that women would read pornography while masturbating. The dangers of the imagination were exemplified in his novel *Emile*: 'As I have said a thousand times, it is by the imagination alone that the senses are awakened.'[59] Philosophers and physicians alike were concerned about the effects of reading on the imagination and contradictory arguments emerged.[60] Etienne Bonnot de Condillac wrote of the advantages of the imagination in *Essays on the Origin of Human Understanding* (1746), but by the second half of the eighteenth century, physicians were representing the imagination as a dangerous site where unnatural associations took hold.[61] The imagination was particularly susceptible to erotica, enticing people to lascivious thoughts and encouraging masturbation. Thus readers were made aware that reading was potentially bad for their health, pornography being the worst culprit.

Wicked Nasty Books

Pornographic images and texts involving masturbation were commonplace. Self-abusers were portrayed using all sorts of devices: genteel young ladies with fake penises in *Le Portier de Chartreux* (**FIG. 50**); nuns with candles in *Venus in the Cloister*; and scullery-maids with carrots in *Voyage to Lethe* (1741). Even mainstream novels such as *Tristram Shandy* carried depictions of women having injections thrust into them (**FIG. 51**). Oral sex was presented in Cleland's *Memoirs of a Woman of Pleasure*, when Polly, a young prostitute, performs fellatio on her young foreign client in order to 'keep it [his penis] in good humour, stroking it, with her head down, and

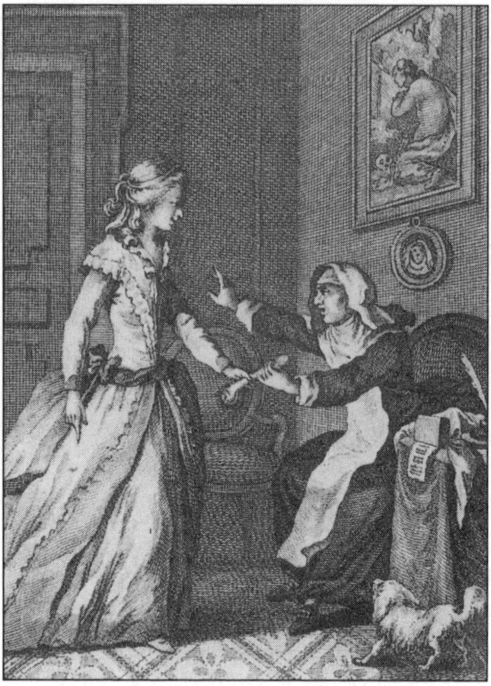

FIG. 50 *Le Portier des Chartreux*, 1787

received even its velvet tip between the lips of not its proper mouth' to provide lubrication and effect an easier entrance.[62]

Because of the threat to the innocence of young boys and girls, there was an attempt to ban certain lewd books while others, curiously, escaped the censor's notice. Pornography which described unusual sexual practices was regarded with particular suspicion and considered even more likely to corrupt the mind. In 1788, John Morgan of Hanover Square was taken to court for 'most lawfully wickedly and impiously devising contriving and intending to vitiate and corrupt the morals of all the subjects'. His crime was the publication of 'a certain wicked nasty filthy Bawdy and obscene Libel' entitled *The Battle of Venus* which described a sex act that was considered a novelty, even in pornography, and therefore deemed worthy of detailed discussion:

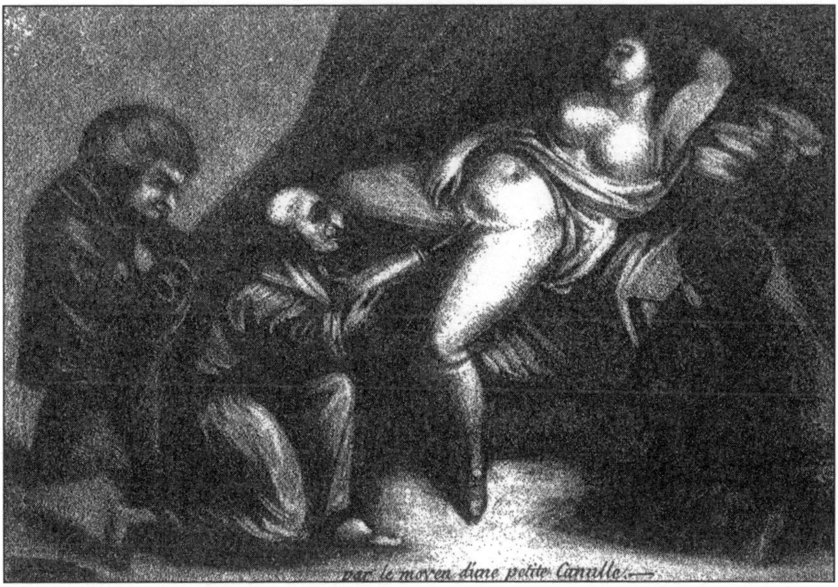

FIG. 51 Scene from *Tristram Shandy*

> The woman in front must lie straight on either side and the Man who attacks her in front must after entering her lift her uppermost leg on his Buttock. The antagonist in the rear must accommodate himself to her Posture, and glide in likewise. The Men may knock her as hard as they will; so long as the Woman is careful to keep herself exactly straight and not to withdraw from one or the other their violent shocks will only serve to make her more fixed and steady. But in this Contrivance the chief pleasure is undoubtedly the novelty and the idea and sensation of two Persons besides oneself uniting in the Act of Coition.[63]

The act of anal and vaginal sex occurring at the same time, between a woman and two men (known as 'sandwiching' in more recent terms) – one in the front and one in the rear – obviously upset the censors.[64]

Another court case some years later related to the publication of material which contained both sodomy and bestiality. On 2 July 1809, Edward Rich the younger, a Soho publisher, was accused of being '. . . most wicked lewd lascivious depraved and abandoned . . .' The charges again related to the corruption of the morals of 'our subjects', attempting to incite and encourage them to indecent practices, and to engage in 'crimes against nature'. The book *A Feast for all. Choice Spirits who love uncommon Frolicks in the Comical Way* contained prints of naked men and women in 'indecent filthy unnatural and bestial situations attitudes and practices'.[65] Rich was sentenced to the pillory at Charing Cross, imprisonment in the House of Correction at Clerkenwell and two years' hard labour. Some books were considered so obscene that they corrupted the minds of their readers while others, just as explicit, escaped prosecution altogether. To this extent, the regulation of pornography in the hands of the censors was an arbitrary process.

*

The association of men and women in relation to sex with animals tended to be gendered. The act of bestiality, from the evidence in trial reports, was always committed by men. In erotic tales, women were more often portrayed as taking pleasure in watching animals copulate. These female voyeurs of animals were perceived as lascivious yet shown to have normal, healthy sexual urges, unlike men who, in the trial reports, were seen as filthy as the beasts they played with.

Of the various sexual practices that were regarded as unusual, some were viewed with distaste, others as most heinous crimes. Sodomy and bestiality were considered most 'unnatural' and therefore condemned as 'vile abominations'. Masturbation was an activity previously thought to be beneficial to the physical health of both women and men but, by the eighteenth century, had come to be seen as harmful. Yet some sex-related practices which might be regarded as abnormal were *de rigueur* during this period: the admiration of a pretty foot was commonplace. Other interests, such as strangling, were more likely to be mocked than taken seriously, judging from the reports in pamphlets and magazines. And despite opposition from the sexually conservative to such novel practices as a threesome involving 'sandwiching', it is clear that, regardless of the censors, the more adventurous experimenters would continue to try any sex act or explore any fetish which captured their imagination.

Conclusion

Eighteenth-century London was a rumbustious town which acted as a magnet for those seeking opportunity. Some, like Wilkes and Boswell, enjoyed London for its sheer exuberance. Backed by their fathers' money, they could indulge in all the diversions the city had to offer. Those unable to make a living in rural England went to the metropolis to forge their careers. Those less fortunate, both male and female, fell into prostitution to earn their keep. Prettier or more intelligent women would aim, where possible, to become courtesans, gratifying the whims of the rich and powerful. The more wily among them might juggle a number of patrons in an attempt to avoid the insecurity of relying on just one man. Young mollies might earn a little money from prostitution but were less likely to find a rich long-tern protector. However, it was easier for men than women to make their way in life, with greater employment opportunities available to them and higher wages paid for their jobs. Few people, if sexually active, would have escaped without becoming afflicted with one venereal disease or another. Some men and women were lucky enough to avoid the moral reformers responsible for securing prison sentences for homosexual men and forcing poor female prostitutes into Magdalen institutions.

A person's sexual inclination depended as much on individual choice as on opportunity; in turn, opportunity depended on how much money a person had, where they lived, whether they were male or female and whether they were heterosexual or homosexual. Within this world, sex was a commodity to be bought and sold, as well as an expression of love, whether inside or outside marriage. People experimented with different forms of sexual pleasure: heterosexual men visited prostitutes to try out flagellation practices; they formed groups involving sexual activities in order to promote business deals; and homosexual men established clubs for enacting rituals which reinforced and celebrated their sexual difference. Meanwhile, female prostitutes were selling sex to the highest bidder, or seeking out other women for sexual pleasure through their female networks.

Despite proscriptive advice in the literature of the day, and warnings in letters to sons and daughters, lewd behaviour continued to flourish. The married elite were busy carrying on their affairs; the middling sort were engaging in love matches, and the labouring poor were undertaking marriages through promise. No doubt many were carrying on mundane sex lives, but the Christian notion of the ideal sexually restrained man and woman was only one of the images circulated in the eighteenth century, and was often a far cry from some of the others that were being promoted. An ideal sexual relationship for the male reader of erotica, for example, might have been a lusty whore hell-bent on whipping the daylights out of a subservient man.

Women were to be seen in businesses, running coffee-houses or brothels, or working in a variety of retail jobs that often involved them in sexual matters. They frequented the same places as men – the streets, the theatres, the parks and pleasure gardens, playing an active part in the social whirl where sex was on offer. Libertine men were writing about their conquests in diaries and memoirs – expounding the virtues of the whores in London. In reality, courtesans were enjoying sex a lot less than men (unless they were in love), and were sometimes resentful of the lives they were forced to lead. These women sought financial independence but were frequently let down by the men they had serviced. They were, however, both ruthless and resourceful enough to fight back.

Clubs and coffee-houses thrived all over London, not just for the heterosexual middle-class libertine but for aristocrats such as Sir Francis, Dashwood. Whereas men tended to congregate in clubs and secret societies based around sexual enjoyment, but which also provided a political and financial network for their members, female friendships operated on a less formal basis. With some notable exceptions such as the female flagellants' club in Jermyn Street, women were less inclined than men to form secret societies to share an interest in sex. When they wanted to exchange experiences, it was in the form of gossip in the intimate company of their female friends, as seen in the case of Harriette Wilson and her circle, and they would often bail out a courtesan or fellow prostitute in time of trouble.

Mollies tended to pick up men in the street or in known private rooms or molly-houses. Women with Sapphic tendencies tended to form relationships within their established female network. Women who had sex with other women were seen to be more threatening to the status quo than those who merely professed love for each other – after all, love between women was understood to be a typically feminine characteristic, in keeping with the role which society had created for them. The greatest threat was perceived to be from those women who dressed as men and took on a man's role, and even married another woman, thus aping their 'superiors' and challenging the true hierarchical order. None the less, lesbians in Britain enjoyed greater freedom than their sisters on the Continent and did not suffer the severity of punishment exacted in Germany and Holland. Nor did they endure the relentless persecution of the male sodomites who suffered more than any other transgressive group in the eighteenth century.

Sapphist subcultures did exist – Anne Lister was never short of a place to find women, mainly introduced through her female friends. Lesbian relationships have a history of long-term commitment, as in the case of the Ladies of Llangollen, but this was not always so. Lister spoke of her own flightiness, even though she had some lasting relationships. She was a great flirt and recklessly lusted after other women. From her diaries, it is clear that she saw herself as part of such a subgroup: both she and her friends knew themselves to be 'too fond of women', yet did not identify themselves with men.

Although the racy tales of female cross dressers were meant to provide entertainment, they also carried warnings against ungovernable women. Autonomous women were seen to be impossible to control, and as such, a danger to society, not least because other women might follow their example, causing disruption to the whole hierarchy of male authority. However, in cases where it was recognised that women might have to dress as men to find work, in the army or at sea, they were frequently – if grudgingly – shown respect. Meanwhile, rich men who dressed in women's clothes, such as D'Eon and De Choisy, met with more acceptance and less antagonism than the English mollies, which suggested that tolerance of sexual deviation to a large extent depended on wealth and class. Just as male sodomy was regarded as more of a threat than tribadism, so cross-dressing for men posed a greater threat than female cross-dressing. Society might understand a woman disguising herself to seek employment in a man's world; but there was no excuse for a man to ape his 'inferiors'. Although female husbands were seen as a problem, part of society still revelled in watching women dressing in breeches in the theatre. Those who came off worst were the plebeian male cross-dressing mollies who would be persecuted remorselessly.

During the course of the long eighteenth century, a re-categorization of sex was taking place. New fears and anxieties developed, particularly concerning masturbation and homosexuality, while other forms of sexual activity, such as group sex and flagellation, were more acceptable because they led to 'normal' heterosexual intercourse. Indeed, flagellation had been deemed a cure for impotence and was therefore a boon, since it led indirectly to procreation, which was not the case with masturbation and sodomy. Mutual masturbation would continue to feature in pornographic books, but this would generally involve two women rather than a woman and a man, and was more in the way of an introduction to sex, a warm-up for the 'proper' heterosexual intercourse to be experienced later.

Even bestiality became less of a threat to the nation during the eighteenth century, with fewer burnings or hangings for such offences. Whereas previously it had been connected to devil worship and was therefore perceived to threaten religion, with the declining importance of magic and the Church this practice slipped down the list of demonized vices. As suggested, medical science now began to have more influence over which forms of sex were good and which were bad. A prime example of this can be seen in the attacks on masturbation by Tissot and Bienville. What was once condemned by the clergy was now also being condemned by the medics, science serving as a new reinforcer of sexual morality.

New ways, and reasons, were being devised to re-categorize sexual activities in relation to rational ideas, with sexual boundaries becoming more fluid and changes in perception dictating what was acceptable or unacceptable. Yet the sheer diversity of sexual activity was astonishing. People were trying out all kinds of libidinous experiments and, despite attempts to contain them, eighteenth-century lascivious bodies would continue to indulge in new forms of sexual experiences and enjoyments.

APPENDIX

The Gender-Sex Debate: A Historiography

Debates surrounding the study of the history of sexuality have spawned enough books to furnish a library, with scholars making and destroying new theories with apparent abandon. I offer only a simplified outline of some of the complex arguments, with a guide to further material for the interested reader on pages 320–37.

The history of sexuality emerged in the late 1970s and early 1980s with the work of a group of historians in various monographs and a handful of editions of collected essays and it is still expanding.[1] Around the same time, women's history was similarly emerging, and by the late 1980s and into the 1990s, historians were asserting a multiplicity of frameworks, from 'separate spheres' to 'golden ages', with arguments about the disparity of the sexes stretching from total dominance of men over women as a result of patriarchy, at one extreme, to the belief in a 'rough-and-ready equality' between men and women at the other.[2] Meanwhile, discussions were raging as to whether there was a traceable continuity through history, or detectable change.[3] After much construction, deconstruction and reconstruction of various models, women's history mutated into gender history in the final decade of the twentieth century.[4] This allowed frameworks already in use to include the study of men, using interdisciplinary methods to uncover a multiplicity of male roles – fops, dandies, macaronis, libertines, beaux – as well as the emergence of the 'manly' man.[5]

From the study of masculinity, it was argued that prior to the eighteenth century, or thereabouts, effeminate men had been seen to enjoy women as well as boys, but effeminacy increasingly came to be associated with the adult male sodomite. Although effeminate dressing had been thought to undermine manly qualities, reinforcing an allegedly female penchant for gossip and self-indulgence in fashion, it had not previously been regarded as a sexual threat. A proper man was seen to be a heterosexual (preferably married) 'manly' man, one who should do his duty by ruling with an iron rod over his wife, his children and his servants; an effeminate man was considered unable to fulfil this role.

Having 'rediscovered' homosexuals in history, a highly charged debate began, involving both historians and sociologists, as to how best to 'see' or understand them. Although this is a radical oversimplification, studies on male homosexuality initially fell into two positions: one group called 'contructionalists' (or those who see homosexuality as being 'made up', or constructed, by society), and the opposing team called determinists or 'essentialists' (those who see homosexuality as an intrinsic part of a person's character or biology).

A long tussle between historians took place, as well as a fierce political debate, regarding the categorization of people according to their sexual inclinations (homosexual, lesbian, heterosexual, bisexual, etc). This set off a long chain of discussions about anachronism and problems with applied terminology. Much energy was exerted against the use of the terms 'homosexuality', 'lesbianism', 'transvestism' and 'bisexual', all of which have meanings and connotations that were not present in the eighteenth century. Contructionalists themselves even quibbled about when the homosexual was actually constructed.[6] For some historians, the essentiality of self-identity and consciousness of an individual was necessary for a man to be considered a homosexual. Others still have examined subcultures and friendships between men.[7] Meanwhile, lesbian history began to create its own furore based on much the same arguments regarding terminology and categorization, and whether lesbianism can be said to have actually existed at an earlier period in history.[8] Yet others have found ample evidence of both lesbian identities and lesbians' self-identity (as indeed we can see with Anne Lister and her group) throughout the eighteenth century.[9] The final entrants into the fray are the queer theorists who have added psychoanalysis to the exploration in an attempt to obtain an individualistic approach.

Quite correctly, some of these historians (myself included) are asking why we should be taking heterosexuality as normative in history. Indeed, the whole area of reading sexuality into a historical text is, in itself, problematic. In a sense, history constructs its own archive from the reading material; the historian is merely a decoder and an interpreter of the written word. He or she interprets the material selectively, and thus the archive varies according to the reader. Despite the attempts by historians to be unbiased, this is impossible because each person has their own leaning and experiences, or 'tools' with which to interpret the material. Also, historians are naturally inclined to retain the parts which reinforce the point they are trying to make, leaving us with the fact that a complex process of formulating meaning exists in which the concepts are unstable. An example of this can be seen in the historical examination of heterosexual men, women and their relationships. While it has been 'assumed' that married people are heterosexual, unless proof of their non-heterosexual behaviour is uncovered or becomes evident, this assumption does not work in reverse. But the proof of sexual behaviour is only ever deemed to be necessary in sexual relationships that were previously perceived as 'abnormal'. Historians do not ask themselves if a married couple were in fact having sex in order to 'prove' their heterosexuality, yet, in historical examinations of male and female homosexuals, sexual activity appears to be essential in so defining them. The 'standard of proof' is not equally applied[10] but there should be a standard way of understanding sexuality across the whole of the spectrum.

The notion of social construction of categories of sexuality (heterosexuality, homosexuality, hermaphrodism, lesbianism) sees sexuality as constructed at the level of culture and history through complex machinations. But the fact remains that, even if specific sexualities had different ways of showing itself at different times in history, feelings no doubt existed between people and these sexual feelings were also subjective and cannot be relegated to the realms of mere social conditioning. History as seen through the eyes of the social contructionalists merely becomes a history of labelling which, on its own, is not enough to provide insights into what people thought about their own sexual predilections. Such deviations were often labelled as 'perversions', according to what was deemed unnatural by society at any given time, but it is important to see how the individual or group saw themselves.

There is no one homogeneous group called 'homosexuals' or 'lesbians' any more than there is a homogeneous group of 'heterosexuals'. It is more or less accepted now that neither the purely socially constructed theory nor the deterministic or essentialist theory is enough on its own to offer a full explanation of any sort of sexuality in history. We need to assume a more fluid sexual framework in order to understand diversification and multiplicities within history. If we accept this then maybe the way forward is to look at sexuality *en masse*, rather than in four or five labelled boxes (lesbian, homosexual, heterosexual, etc), and attempt to pick out each strand of differing sexualities in order to build up a sexual map (rather like DNA strands in the genetic code, only on a social, cultural and individualistic level). This would incorporate the huge variations in the ways in which men and women saw themselves, and how others perceived them in different periods in history. It would also show how these perceptions can change over time, both internally, through any one individual's feelings and urges; and through the external restrictions or freedoms existing in any particular society.

Notes

List of Abbreviations

Ashbee, Vol. I	Fraxi, Pisanus [Henry Spencer Ashbee], *Index Librorum Prohibitorum*
Ashbee, Vol. II	Fraxi, Pisanus [Henry Spencer Ashbee], *Centuria Librorum Absconditorum*
Ashbee, Vol. III	Fraxi, Pisanus [Henry Spencer Ashbee], *Catena Librorum Tacendorum* (London, privately printed, 1877)

All reprinted as *Bibliography of Forbidden Books* (New York, Jack Brussel, 1962).

BL	British Library
DNB	Dictionary of National Biography
KB	King's Bench Records
MSS	Manuscripts
PRO	Public Records Office

One: The Streets of London

1. Peter Wagner, 'The Discourse on Sex – or Sex as Discourse: Eighteenth-Century Medical Paramedical Erotica', in G. S. Rousseau and Roy Porter (eds.), *Sexual Underworlds of the Enlightenment* (Manchester, Manchester University Press, 1987), pp. 46–68; see pp. 52–3.

2. Tony Henderson, *Disorderly Women in Eighteenth-Century London. Prostitution and Control in the Metropolis, 1730–1830* (London, Longman, 1999), p. 45.

3. Roy Porter, *A Social History* (London, Penguin, 1996), p. 152; M. Dorothy George, *London Life in the Eighteenth Century* (1925; repr., London Penguin, 1992).

4. Porter, *Social History*, p. 153.

5. Mary King was one of nine people named among the organizations for vitualling licences in the London borough of Westminster in 1728. See Helen Berry, 'Rethinking Politeness in Eighteenth-Century England: Moll King's Coffee House and the Significance of Flash Talk', in *Royal Historical Society Transactions*, 2001, pp. 65–81.

6. Roy Porter, *English Society in the Eighteenth Century* (London, Penguin, 1990), p. 31.

7. Lisa Picard, *Dr Johnson's London: Life in London, 1740–1770* (London, Weidenfeld & Nicolson, 2000), p. 200. See also Marie-Mulvey Roberts, 'Pleasures Engendered by Gender: Homosociality and the Club', in Roy Porter and Marie-Mulvey Roberts, *Pleasure in the Eighteenth Century* (Basingstoke, Macmillan, 1996), pp. 48–76.

8. Porter, *Social History*, p. 170.

9. Anon, *The Case Between the Proprietors of Newspapers, and the Coffee-Men of London & Westminster* (London, R. Walker, n.d., *c.*1750), p. 13. Price 6d.

10. Julie Johnstone, *Confessions of Julia Johnstone . . . in contradiction of the fables of Harriette Wilson* (London, Benbow, 1825).

11. *British Magazine*, vol. 3, September 1748, pp. 391–2.

12. *Historical Collections Relating to Ranelagh* in collection of pamphlets in BL, MSS CUP 401 k 8, pp. 179–91.

13. Collection of Tracts in BL (1690 816 m 19 (44)).

14. Grace E. Thompson, *The Cyprian. The Life of a Covent Garden Lady* (London, Hutchinson, 1932), p. 122.

15. See newspaper clipping inserted into *The Midnight Ramble, Or, The Adventures of Two Noble Females; Being A true and impartial Account of their late excursion through the Streets of London and Westminster* (London, B. Dickson, 1754).

16. W. Speck, 'The Harlot's Progress in Eighteenth-Century England', *British Eighteenth-Century Studies*, vol. 3 (1980), pp. 127–39.

17. Saunders Welch, *A Proposal To Render Effectual A Plan To Remove The Nuisance Of Common Prostitutes From The Street Of This Metropolis* (London, 1758). The real extent of prostitution was difficult to assess because much of it was seasonal employment affected by the agricultural cycle.

18. Henderson, op. cit., pp. 55, 345.

19. P. J. Grosley, *A Tour to London* (London, 1772).

20. Boswell's *London Journal, 1762–1763* ed. Frederick A. Pottle (repr., Harmondsworth, Penguin, 1966), pp. 264, 278–9.

21. Ibid., 14 December 1762.

22. M. D.'Archenholz, *A Picture of England; Containing a Description of the Laws, Customs and Manners of England* (Dublin, P. Byre, 1790), p. 189.

23. 'A Monk of the Order of Saint Francis', *Nocturnal Revels, Or the History of the King's Palace and other Modern Nunneries* (London, M. Goadby, 1779).

24. Grosley, op. cit.

25. Ibid.

26. Anon, *Harris's List Of Covent Garden Ladies, Or Man Of Pleasure's Kalander For The Year 1788* (London, H. Ranger, 1788), pp. 18–35.

27. Ibid., pp. 19–20.

28. Lawrence Stone, *The Family, Sex and Marriage in England 1500–1800* (London, Weidenfeld & Nicolson, 1977), p. 305.

29. Anon, *Prostitutes of Quality; or Adultery à-la-mode. Being Authentic Memoirs of several person of the Highest Quality* (J. Cook & J. Coote, London, 1757).

30. Joanna Innes, 'Politics and Morals: the Reformation of Manners Movement in Later Eighteenth-Century England', in Eckhart Hellmuth (ed.), *The Transformation of Political Culture: England and Germany in the Late Eighteenth Century* (1990); M. J. D. Roberts, 'The Society for the Suppression of Vice and its Early Critics, 1802–1812', *Historical Journal*, vol. 26, pp. 159–76.

31. Speck, op cit.

32. Quoted in ibid.

33. V. Bullough, 'Prostitution and Reform in Eighteenth-Century England', in R. P. Maccubbin (ed.), *'Tis Nature's Fault. Unauthorized Sexuality During the Enlightenment* (Cambridge, Cambridge University Press, 1987); Special Issue of *Eighteenth Century Life*, vol. 9, no. 3 (1989), p. 71; S. Nash, 'Prostitution and Charity: the Magdalene Hospital, a case study', *Journal of Social* History, 17 (1984), p. 624.

34. Although some time later William Ewart Gladstone, the Victorian prime minister, is a fine example of apparent mixed motives. He chose to seek out prostitutes whilst wearing a hair shirt to allay any sexual thoughts, rather than undertake any other charitable work; his almost complete lack of success in their salvation did not deter him. He was also known to scourge himself for reading pornography. See chapter on 'Ladies of the Night' in Roy Jenkins, *Gladstone* (London, Macmillan, 1995), pp. 100–15.

35. Victorian female sex reformers caught on later, e.g. Josephine Butler, Annie Besant, Marie Stopes et al.

36. 'M. Ludovicus', *A Particular but Melancholy Account of the Great Hardships, Difficulties and Miseries, That Those Unhappy and Much-To-Be Pitied Creatures, The Common Women of the Town, Are Plung'd into at this Juncture* (London, 1752).

Initially babies had to be under two months old and pass a health inspection but by 1756, government subsidies were raised on the basis that the services were open to the public. On 2 June 1756, the first day of this new arrangement, 117 babies were deposited on the doorstep of the hospital. *Britain in the Hanoverian Age, 1714–1837*, p. 264.

37. Stanley D. Nash on Prostitution in *Britain in the Hanoverian Age, 1714–1837. An Encyclopaedia* (NY and London, Garland Publishing, 1997), pp. 570–2.

38. Anon, *Memoirs of the Celebrated Miss Fanny Murray* (London, J. Scott, 1759), p. 113.

39. Defoe, *Augusta Triumphans*, p. 409.

40. Stone, *Family*, p. 378.

41. Ned Ward, *The History of the London Clubs* (London, n.p., 1709).

42. John Marten, *A Treatise of all the Degrees and Symptoms of the Venereal Disease* (London, 1704), p. 68.

43. Alexander Pope, *The Second Satire of Dr John Donne, Versifyed* (1733).

44. Numerous clippings have been inserted into the book, Anon, *The Romance of a Night. Or A Covent-Garden Adventure, The Reverie: Or, A Flight to the Paradise of Fools, Nocturnal Revels; or, A Universal Dream-Book* (1744) in the BL.

45. Roy Porter and Dorothy Porter, *In Sickness and in Health: The British Experience, 1650–1850* (London, Fourth Estate, 1988), p. 106.

46. Linda E. Merians (ed.), *The Secret Malady: Venereal Disease in Eighteenth Century Britain and France* (Lexington, University Press of Kentucky, 1996), particularly ch. 9, Betty Rizzo, 'Decorums', pp. 149–67.

47. See the second case in *Trials for Adultery, or the History of Divorces . . . From 1760, to the Present Time* (London, S. Bladon, 1779–80).

48. Stone, *Family*, pp. 379–80.

49. Merians (ed.), op. cit.

50. Angus McLaren, *Reproductive Rituals. The Perception of Fertility in England from the Sixteenth to the Nineteenth Century* (London, Methuen, 1984), p. 85; Stone, *Family*, p. 334.

Two: Love, Honour and Betrayal

1. James Boswell, *The Life of Samuel Johnson* (Calcutta, British India Publishing Company, n.d.), vol. IV, p. 219.

2. Lord Halifax, *The Lady's New Year Gift: or advice to a Daughter 1688* (London, 1688).

3. Lord Chesterfield, *Letters to His Sons and Others* (1774, repr., London, Everyman, 1984), p. 106.

4. *The Works of Hannah More* (London, 1801), pp. 221–2.

5. *Eclectic Review*, October 1806, II, pt 2, pp. 813–14, quoted in Eric Trudgill, *Madonnas and Magdalens: the Origins and Development of Victorian Sexual Attitudes* (London, Heinemann, 1976).

6. KB 28/347/4 Michaelmas Term 1788.

7. Alice Browne, *The Eighteenth Century Feminist Mind* (Brighton, Harvester Press, 1987), p. 47.

8. *The Society for the Suppression of Vice Report*, 1825, pp. 29–31, 39.

9. Keith Thomas, 'The Double Standard', *Journal of the History of Ideas*, 20 (1959), pp. 195–216; Laura Gowing, 'Gender and the Language of Insult in Early Modern London', *History Workshop Journal*, 35 (1993); Gowing 'Language,

Power and the Law: Women's Slander Litigation in Early Modern London', in J. Kermode and G. Walker (eds.), *Women, Crime and the Courts in Early Modern England* (London, UCL Press, 1994).

10. David Turner, '"Nothing is so secret but shall be revealed": the Scandalous Life of Robert Foulkes', in Tim Hitchcock and Michèle Cohen (eds.), *English Masculinities, 1660–1800* (London, Longman, 1999), pp. 169–92. For the connection between honour and sex, see Elizabeth A. Foyster, *Manhood in Early Modern England. Honour, Sex and Marriage* (London, Longman, 1999).

11. Sir William Blackstone. *Commentaries on the Laws of England*, 12th edn., 4 vols. (London, 1793–5), vol. I, p. 445; and Anna Clark's *Women's Silence, Men's Violence. Sexual Assault in England 1770–1845* (Pandora Press, 1987).

12. Anthony E. Simpson, 'Vulnerability and the Age of Female Consent: Legal Innovation and its Effect on Prosecution for Rape in Eighteenth-Century London', in Rousseau and Porter (eds.), op. cit., pp. 181–205.

13. Harriette Wilson, *The Interesting Memoirs and Amorous Adventures of Harriette Wilson* (1825), p. 161.

14. Chesterfield, op. cit., p. 158.

15. Boswell quoted in Stone, *Family*, pp. 352–3.

16. For a summary of women's place in the eighteenth century, see Katherine M. Rogers, *Feminism in the Eighteenth Century* (Brighton, Harvester Press, 1982); Browne, op. cit.; an anthology by Vivien Jones (ed.), *Women in the Eighteenth Century* (London, Routledge, 1990).

17. E. A. Wrigley and R. S. Schofield, *The Population History of England, 1541–1871* (London, Edward Arnold, 1981).

18. Lawrence Stone, *Road to Divorce, England 1530–1987* (Oxford, Clarendon Press, 1990), p. 61.

19. Stella Tillyard, *Aristocrats* (London, Vintage, 1995), p. 58.

20. To Wortley (5 May 1710), Robert Halsband (ed.), *The Complete Letters of Lady Wortley Montagu* (Oxford, Clarendon Press, 1965), vol. I, p. 35.

21. Isabel Grundy, *Lady Mary Wortley Montagu. Comet of the Enlightenment* (Oxford, OUP, 1999), pp. 61, 360–1.

22. Stone, *Family*, pp. 217–18.

23. Rogers, *Feminism*, p. 2.

24. Anon, *The Case Between the Proprietors of Newspapers, and the Coffee-men of London and Westminster*, pp. 2–4.

25. Anon, *Proposal For The Erecting A Protestant Nunnery In The City Of Dublin Utterly* rejecting and renouncing *The New Game of Quadrille*, 'By the Ladies' (Dublin, E. Waters, 1726).

26. Anon, *Kick Him Jenny* (London, W. France, 1737), pp. 10–19. It sold for 6d.

27. Anon, *The Court Jester, or Lady's and Gentleman's Treasure of Wit, Humour, and Amusement* (London, Britannia Printing Office, J. Roach, n.d., 12314 c 35 (2)). Price 6d.

28. Anon, *A New Atlantis for the Year One Thousand Seven Hundred and Fifty-Eight* (2nd edn., London, 1758), pp. 40, 46–7, 92.

29. Ibid., p. 113.

30. Foyster, op. cit., p. 70.

31. E. P. Thompson, *Customs in Common* (London, Penguin, 1993), pp. 467–538.

32. Although single women and widows could own property, make wills and conduct business, for a married woman the system was more complex. Under common law, all her property, including her earnings, belonged to her husband. See Lee Holcombe, *Wives and Property: Reform of the Married Woman's Property Law in Nineteenth-Century England* (Oxford, Martin Robertson, 1983).

33. Evidence of these agreements can be found in toll-books such as that at the Bell Inn, Edgbaston Street, Birmingham; E.P. Thompson, *Customs*, pp. 404–66.

Three: Men of Pleasure

1. Porter, *English Society*, p. 258.

2. Roy Porter and Lesley Hall, *Facts of Life: The Creation of Sexual Knowledge in Britain, 1650–1950* (New Haven, Yale University Press, 1995), p. 116.

3. Roy Porter, 'Mixed Feelings: The Enlightenment and Sexuality' in Paul-Gabriel Boucé (ed.), *Sexuality in Eighteenth-Century Britain* (Manchester, Manchester University Press, 1982), pp. 1–27.

4. James G. Turner, 'The Properties of Libertinism', *Eighteenth-Century Life*, vol. IX (1989), pp. 75–87.

5. See Michel Fener's 'Libertinisms', introduction to *The Libertine Reader. Eroticism and Enlightenment in Eighteenth-Century France* (New York, Zone Books, 1997), pp. 10–47.

6. Ibid.

7. Peter Quennell (ed.), *Memoirs of William Hickey* (London, Routledge & Kegan Paul, 1975), p. 8.

8. Ibid., pp. 19, 21, 23–4.

9. George, op. cit., p. 95.

10. Ibid., p. 23.

11. See Angus McLaren, *Reproductive Rituals: The Perception of Fertility in England from the Sixteenth to the Nineteenth Century* (London, Methuen, 1984), pp. 57–87.

12. Quennell (ed.), *Hickey*, p. 31.

13. Ibid., pp. 64–5.

14. Ibid., pp. 48, 50.

15. Ibid., p. 58.

16. Ibid., p. 160.

17. Ibid., p. 437.

18. Peter Quennell, *The Profane Virtues. Four Studies of the Eighteenth Century* (1905; repr., CT, Greenwood Press, 1945), pp. 1–63.

19. Adam Sissman, *Boswell's Presumptuous Task. Writing the Life of Mr Johnson* (London, Penguin, 2000), p. 11.

20. The Scottish Beggar's Benison and Wig Club for 1783 list an Earl of Eglinton as a member. St Andrews University Muniments, MS 38351.

21. Peter Martin, *A Life of James Boswell* (London, Weidenfeld & Nicolson, 1999), p. 75.

22. Ibid., p. 94.

23. Ibid., pp. 59, 94, 97.

24. Boswell, *London Journal*, 21 November 1762.

25. Ibid., 25 November 1762.

26. Ibid., 2 December 1762.

27. Ibid., 11 December 1762.

28. Diary entries for 14, 16, 17, 18, 19, 20, 22, 24, 30, 31 December 1762.

29. Diary entries for 1, 2, 3, 4, 5, 7, 11, 12, 15,16, 18 January 1763.

30. Martin, op. cit., p. 212.

31. Boswell, *Journal*, 10–11 January 1765.

32. Ibid., 1 September 1764.

33. J. Rives Childs, *Casanova, A New Perspective* (London Constable, 1989), p. 37; John Masters, *Casanova* (London, Michael Joseph, 1969), pp. 48, 154, 224–5.

34. Childs, op. cit., p. 13.

35. Martin Green (ed.), *The Further Memoirs of Casanova. Casanova in London* (London, Mayflower, 1969), p. 129.

36. Ibid., p. 116.

37. Casanova here means legitimate children; he did have two children by Thérèse.

Four: Memoirs of a Courtesan

1. I have used Mary Lyon's edition of *The Memoirs of Mrs Leeson, Madam, 1727–1797* (Dublin, Lilliput Press, 1995) and have examined first editions of Harriette Wilson and Julia Johnstone's memoirs, both held in the British Library;

Harriette Wilson, *The Interesting Memoirs and Amorous Adventures of Harriette Wilson* (London, W. Chubb, T. Blacketer, and T. Reed, 1825); Julia Johnstone, *Confessions of Julia Johnstone, Written by Herself* (London, Benbow, 1825). Harriette Wilson's memoirs have been reprinted in Lesley Blanch (ed.), *The Game of Hearts. Harriette Wilson and Her Memoirs* (London, Gryphon Books, 1957).

2. Joanna Richardson provides a description of the French courtesan of nineteenth-century France which fits well with the eighteenth-century English courtesan in *The Courtesans: The Demi-Monde in Nineteenth-Century France* (London, Weidenfeld & Nicolson, 1967).

3. M. D.'Archenholz, *A Picture of England; Containing a Description of the Laws, Customs and Manners of England* (Dublin, P. Byre, 1790), p. 189.

4. Lyons (ed.), op. cit., p. 204.

5. Ibid., pp. 3–4.

6. Ibid., pp. 6, 10, 13, 15.

7. Ibid., p. 13.

8. Ibid., p. 19.

9. Ibid., p. 5.

10. Boris Ford (ed.), *Cambridge Cultural History of Britain: Eighteenth Century* (Cambridge, Cambridge University Press, 1992), p. 32.

11. Lyons (ed.), op. cit., p. 40.

12. Ibid., p. 49, 53.

13. Ibid., p. 72.

14. Ibid., p. 73.

15. Ibid., pp. 88–90.

16. Ibid., pp. 80, 86, 92, 143.

17. Ibid., p. 146.

18. Johnstone, *Confessions*, pp. 45–6.

19. Ibid., p. 74.

20. Walter Scott, *Journal*, 9 December 1825.

21. Ibid., p. 115.

22. Blanch (ed.), op. cit., pp. 73–4. This contains a reprint of Harriette Wilson, *The Interesting Memoirs and Amorous Adventures of Harriette Wilson* (London, William Stockdale, 1925).

23. Wilson, *Memoirs*, p. 5. For recent biographies, see Valerie Grosvenor Myer, *Harriette Wilson, Lady of Pleasure* (Ely, Fern House, 1999); Katie Hickman, *Courtesans* (London, HarperCollins, 2003); Frances Wilson, *The Courtesan's Revenge* (London, Faber, 2003).

24. Johnstone, *Confessions*, pp. 45–6.

25. Blanch (ed.), op. cit., p. 177.

26. Johnstone, *Confessions*, p. 173.

27. Ibid., p. 47.

28. Ibid., p. 106.

29. Blanch (ed.), op. cit., p. 97.

30. Johnstone, *Confessions*, pp. 301–2.

31. Blanch (ed.), pp. 103–5.

32. Ibid., pp. 129–31.

33. 'By a student of the inner temple', *A Commentary in the Licentious Liberty of the Press In which the recent publication, entitled 'Memoirs of Harriette Wilson' is severely censured* (London, 1825), pp. 10, 21.

34. *Stockdale's Budget*, no. III, Wednesday 27 December 1826.

35. Johnstone, *Confessions*, p. 3.

36. Ibid., p. 5.

37. Ibid., p. 8.

38. Ibid., pp. 9–12.

39. Ibid., pp. 12–13, 50.

40. Ibid., p. 50.

41. Blanch (ed.), pp. 87, 117.

42. Ibid., p. 52.

43. Blanch (ed.), p. 133.

44. Johnstone, *Confessions*, pp. 41–2.

45. Ibid., p. 57.

46. Ibid., p. 90.

47. Ibid., p. 207.

48. Ibid., pp. 94–5.

Five: The Monks of Medmenham

1. Quoted in Geoffrey Ash, *The Hell-Fire Club. A History of Anti-Morality* (1974; repr., Stroud, Alan Sutton, 2000), p. 129.

2. Sir Francis Dashwood, *The Dashwoods of West Wycombe* (London, Aurum Press, 1987), p. 18. For other main bibliographies of Sir Francis Dashwood, see Ronald Fuller, *Hell-Fire Francis* (London, Chatto & Windus, 1939); Donald McCormack, *The Hellfire Club* (Jarrolds, 1958), Daniel P. Mannix, *The Hell-Fire Club* (London, New English Library, 1964); Betty Kemp, *Sir Francis Dashwood: an eighteenth-century independent* (London, Macmillan, 1967); Eric Towers,

Dashwood. The Man and the Myth (Wellingborough, Crucible, 1986); Gerald Suster, *The Hell-fire Friars. Sex, Politics and Religion* (London, Robson, 2000). These biographies are of varying quality, some based on fact, some apparently complete fabrication. Ash states that 'The Order has no documented history', p. 119. However, written documents about the meetings, including letters, cellar books and inventories, do exist in the private papers of the twentieth-century Sir Francis Dashwood who was kind enough to let me research them. I use both Dashwood's original Private Papers and the more spurious contemporary revelations to provide an overview of both the factual events and the gossip surrounding the Medmenham set.

3. An earlier version of the society had been established in 1707 but floundered; a form of the society still exists today.

4. Walpole, *Memoirs of King George III* (London, Colburn 1847, 4 vols.), vol. I, p. 309.

5. These pictures still hang in the Dashwood Estate, West Wycombe.

6. Dashwood, Private Papers.

7. Philip Henry Stanhope, *History of England* (London, 1836–54, 7 vols.).

8. Dashwood, Private Papers.

9. Towers, op. cit., pp. 17–18. Charles Johnstone (1719–1800?) was a lawyer of Scottish descent, born in Ireland and educated in Dublin. Deafness made it impossible for him to practise so he turned to writing. Johnstone was never invited to Medmenham, a snub which might have had something to do with his defamation of Dashwood and his friends.

10. Charles Johnstone, *Chrysal; or the Adventures of a Guinea* (London, 1760), pp. 186, 192. The author remarked upon Dashwood's mocking of religion from an early age, relating a tale in which his tutor took Dashwood to witness a miracle at the shrine of a saint; 'The absurdity was too striking to escape his observation. He turned it into the most poignant ridicule, in spite of all his tutor's pains to defend it', p. 195.

11. Anon, *The Fruitshop* (London, C. Moran, 1765), p. 99.

12. Ibid., p. 22.

13. 'By A Monk Of The Order Of St Frances', *Nocturnal Revels, Or, The History Of King's-Palace and Other Modern Nunneries* Containing Their Mysteries, Devotions And Sacrifices. Comprising Also, The Ancient And Present State Of Promiscuous Gallantry: With The Portraits Of The Most Celebrated Demireps And Courtezans Of This Period: As Well As Sketches Of Their Professional And Occasional Admirers. In Two Volumes (London, M. Goadby, 1779). The book was published under the name of Goadby and describes the West End brothel, Mrs Goadby's, in Berwick Street, Soho. It was translated into French as *Les Sérails de Londres* (1801). pp. A2, A5.

14. Ibid., p. A5–6.

15. Ibid., p. A7.

16. James Boswell, *London Journal*, 27 November 1762.

17. Benjamin Franklin, *Old Mistresses Apologue, or Advice to a Young Man on the Choice of a Mistress* (sometimes referred to as *A Letter on Marriage*).

18. McCormack, op. cit., p. 32.

19. *DNB*. Also see his *Genuine Memoirs* (London, 1765). Charles Churchill (1731–64) was disqualified from Oxford, probably due to a Fleet marriage at the age of seventeen years with a Westminster girl called Scot. He took up his father's curacy at Rainham, and composed *Rosciad* (1761), a satire on Pope's *Dunciad* and Byron's *English Bards*. Churchill seduced the daughter of a tradesman but kept her until his death.

20. Dashwood, Private Papers.

21. Ibid.

22. Ibid.

23. John Hall-Stevenson, *Confessions of Sir Francis and Lady Mary his wife in Crazy Tales* (1762), BL: 1081.h.6-8.

24. Thomas Yoseloff, *Laurence Sterne, A Fellow of Infinite Jest* (London, Francis Aldor, 1948), p. 55.

25. See 'Anthony's Tale; or the Boarding-school Tale' in *Crazy Tales*; quoting from *Works of John Hall Stevenson*, in 3 vols., 1795, vol. 3, p. 20.

26. In his *New Crazy Tales*, Hall Stevenson described *The Wonderful Grot*:

> Beneath a chalky cliff is found,
> Nor in the air, nor in the ground
> A Grot! There Cupid keeps his court.
> There Venus and her nymphs resort.
> Close shaded, it on pillar stands;
> Pillars ne'er raised by mortal hands.
>
> John Hall Stevenson, *New Crazy Tales, Or Ludicrous Strokes* (Mulberry Hill, Printed at Crazy Castle, 1783).

27. Frank Brady and Frederick A. Pottle (eds.), *Boswell on the Grand Tour* (London, Heinemann, 1955), p. 58.

28. Add MSS 30872, fo. 92–3.

29. Dashwood, Private Papers, p. 37.

30. H. Bleackley, *Life of John Wilkes* (London, John Lane, 1917), p. 69.

31. Ibid., pp. 178–9.

32. BL Add. Mss 30867, fo. 65, quoted in Peter D. G. Thomas, *John Wilkes. A Friend to Liberty* (Oxford, Clarendon Press, 1996), p. 4.

33. Ibid., p. 18.

34. Adrian Hamilton, *The Infamous Essay on Woman, or, John Wilkes seated between Vice and Virtue* (André Deutsch, 1972), p, 54.

35. Raymond Postgate, *That Devil Wilkes* (1930; repr., London, Dobson, 1956), p. 95. See Wilkes's autobiography, Add MSS. 300865.

36. Quennell, *Profane Virtues*, p. 205.

37. The political arguments are argued in depth elsewhere; Hamilton, op. cit.

38. Some historians have been misled into thinking the poem was not the sole or main author; see Thomas, *John Wilkes*, p. 230.

39. Ashbee, vol. I, p. 207.

40. *Gentleman's Magazine* (1763), vol. 33, p. 526.

41. Ibid., vol. 34, p. 580.

42. There were two Mrs Phillips and a Mary Perkins who were vendors of condoms in the eighteenth century; McLaren, op. cit.; Peter Fryer, *The Birth Controllers* (London, Secker & Warburg, 1965) – both cite F. Gross, *Guide to Health and Beauty*, 1783.

43. For a fuller account of her life, see Janet Camden Lucey, *Lovely Peggy. The Life and Times of Margaret Woffington* (London, Hurst & Blackett, 1952); Hamilton, op. cit., p. 221.

44. John Wilkes, *An Essay on Woman* (Aberdeen, James Hay, 1788), p. 21. Ashbee believes this is *not* the original version since it has too many mistakes on the title page; it concludes with 'The end of Mr Wilkes's Book', it had no design on the title page and it is not printed in red. It does, however, appear to have been printed at the same time, from the original edition, but no authentic copy is believed to exist. See Ashbee, vol. I, p. 201.

45. Hamilton, op. cit., p. 230.

46. *The North Briton*, no. 1, Saturday 5 June, 1762.

47. Anon, *The Life, Adventures, Intrigues, and Amours of the Celebrated Jemmy Twitcher* (London, Jonathan Brough, 1770).

48. C. B. Lucas (ed.), *Letters of Horace Walpole* (London, George Newnes, 1904), p. 35.

49. Grundy, op. cit.

50. Ibid., p. 35.

51. E. J. Burford, *Wits, Wenches and Wantons. London's Low Life: Covent Garden in the Eighteenth Century* (London, Robert Hale, 1986), pp. 118, 120, 121.

52. Anon, *Memoirs of the Celebrated Miss Fanny Murray*, op. cit.

53. Ibid., p. 13.

54. *Nocturnal Revels*, op. cit., pp. 141–2.

55. Ibid., p. 162.

56. Anon, *Kitty's Atlantis for the Year 1766*, (London, J. Harrison, 1766), pp. 4–29.

57. N. A. M. Rogers, *The Insatiable Earl. A Life of John Montagu, 4th Earl of Sandwich* (London, W. W. Norton, 1994), pp. 122–3.

58. Anon, *The Case and Memoirs of the late Rev. Mr James Hackman* (London, G. Kearsly, 1779).

Six: Scottish Secret Sex Societies

1. *Notes on 'The Records of the Beggar's Benison Society and Merryland of Anstruther, Fife, 1739–1836'* (Anstruther, Printed for Private Circulation, 1892), St Andrews University Muniments, MSS 38351. This is said to be a typewritten copy of a short history of a late nineteenth-century revived version of the order as written by a member, but looks like proofs, with additions, to Smithers's edition of the book.

2. David Stevenson, *The Beggar's Benison. Sex Clubs of Enlightenment. Scotland and their Rituals* (East Linton, Tuckwell Press, 2001), p. 8.

3. Tobias Smollett, *The Expedition of Humphry Clinker* (repr. London, Everyman, 1966), pp. 215–17.

4. Lyons (ed.), op. cit., p. xvi.

5. Ibid., p. 169.

6. Stevenson, op. cit., p. 125.

7. Alan, Bold (ed.) *Records of the Most Ancient and Puissant Order of the Beggars Benison and Merryland, Anstruther* (London, Paul Harris, 1982), p. 7.

8. This was rediscovered in a pawn shop in 1823 in Edinburgh.

9. Stevenson believes Robert Cleland, listed as a member of Beggar's Benison records, is no relation to John Cleland. Stevenson, op. cit., p. 42.

10. Alongside is an emblem of a ship surrounded by the words 'Success to The United States of America'. Also (scratched rather than engraved, which indicates a later graffiti) are the words in capital letters: 'MANY A SIX INCH LONG PRICK, IN FULL BLOOM AND STATURE OF FIERY BEGOT IN SUITABLE CUNT DRIPPING WITH JUICE HAS BEEN BRANDERED HEREUPON' – this also believed to be a later addition.

11. According to *Notes on 'The Records of the Beggar's Benison Society and Merryland of Anstruther, Fife, 1739–1836'*, op. cit., also extant is a copy of the diploma of Thomas, Earl of Kellie, carrying the distinctive insignia of anchor and castle. St Andrews University Muniments 38351, p. 4.

12. H. A. Cockburn, 'An Account of the Friday Club' in *Book of the Old Edinburgh Club* (1910).

13. *Minutes of the Wig Club 1775*.

14. The word 'caddie' was formerly in common use in Scotland for errand-boy's

odd-job men, chair-men, etc. Brewer's *Dictionary of Phrase and Fable* (London, Cassell, 1957).

15. *Minutes of the Wig Club for 5 February 1776.*

16. *Minutes of the Wig Club for 27 November 1777.*

17. A list of all the members appear at the back of the minute book.

18. This source is early twentieth century, written by Robert Maxwell Canach Kanavegh, MSS 38351. Yet Stevenson found proof of only one member connected to both clubs, Stevenson, op. cit., p. 201; see also MSS notes of R.M.C. Kavaugh's *Army Book 135 – The United Service Club, Edinburgh*, providing a list of members of both clubs.

19. *Minutes of the Wig Club, 1775*, p. 3.

20. *Minutes of the Wig Club for 5 February 1776.*

21. C. Willett Cunnington and Phillis Cunnington, *Handbook of English Costume in the Eighteenth Century* (London, Faber & Faber, 1957), pp. 241–58.

22. *Minutes of the Wig Club for 5 February 1776.*

23. *Minutes of the Wig Club, 1775.*

24. *Minutes of the Wig Club for 29 February 1776.*

25. Brewer's *Dictionary of Phrase and Fable*, p. 447.

26. *Minutes of the Wig Club*, 11 January 1792.

27. St. Andrews University Muniments MSS 38351, *no. 2 minutes of the Wig Club for 13 April 1801.*

28. St. Andrews University Muniments MSS 38351, *nos. 3 and 4 minutes of the Wig Club for 18 July 1801, 9 January 1802.*

29. MSS 38351.

30. MSS. 38351, *no. 7 Minutes of the Wig Club for 8 April 1805* (with seal MS 38351). The minutes of this meeting still contain the stamp from a seal, one which is no longer extant in the artefacts collection. The seal is of a bird-like penis inserted into a bird-like vagina (this seal is not in the collection).

31. MSS 38351.

32. Anon, *Records Of The Most Ancient And Puissant Order Of The Beggar's Benison And Merryland, Anstruther and Supplement To The Historical Portion Of The 'Records Of The Most Ancient And Puissant Order Of The Beggar's Benison And Merryland, Anstruther', Being An Account Of The Proceedings At The Meeting Of The Society, Together With Excerpts, Stories, Bon-Mots, Speeches, And Songs Delivered Thereat* (Anstruther, Printed for Private Distribution, 1892).

33. Peter Wagner and David Stevenson are also tentative about the veracity of the minutes.

34. MSS 38351.

Seven: Sodomy: 'A Monstrous Sin Against Nature'

1. Alan Bray, *Homosexuality in Renaissance England* (New York, Columbia University Press, 1982), p. 14.

2. Robert Latham and William Matthews (ed.), *The Diary of Samuel Pepys* (London, George Bell, 1971), vol. 4, pp. 209–10.

3. Randolph Trumbach (ed.), Anon, *the Wandering Whore* (London 1660–3), 6 pts, pt 3, p. 9; (repr., New York, Garland, 1986).

4. Quoted by Jeremy Black, *The British Abroad: Grand Tour in the Eighteenth Century* (Stroud, Alan Sutton, 1992), p. 201.

5. Anon, *A Flaming Whip for Lechery: or the Whoremaster's Speculum* (London, Elizabeth Harris, 1700), p. 15.

6. Anon, *The Priest Gelded: Or, Popery At The Last Gasp Shewing* (London, 1747), p. 13.

7. *London Journal*, 7 May 1726, quoted in Rictor Norton, *Mother Clap's Molly House: The Gay Subculture 1700–1830* (London, GMP, 1992), p. 67.

8. Anon, *Plain Reasons for the Growth of Sodomy* (London, A. Dodd and E. Nutt, 1728), pp. 7–11.

9. Ibid., p. 11.

10. A. D. Harvey, Prosecutions for Sodomy in England at the Beginning of the Nineteenth Century', *Historical Journal*, 21 (1978), pp. 939–48; Netta Murray Goldsmith, *The Worst of Crimes: Homosexuality and the Law in Eighteenth-Century London* (Aldershot, Ashgate, 1998).

11. *Gentleman's Magazine*, 1762, p. 549.

12. Stone, *Road to Divorce*, p. 193.

13. Edmund Curll, *Curlicism Display'd: or, an Appeal to the Church. Being just observations upon the books publish'd by Mr. Curll* (London, Curll, 1718).

14. *Select Trials for Murders, Robberies, Rapes, Sodomy, Coining, Frauds and Other Offences at the Sessions-House in the Old Bailey from 1724–1732* (London, J. Wilford, 1735), vol. II.

15. *The New Newgate Calendar* (London, 1818), vol. II, p. 49. For further information on some of the sodomites mentioned here, see Rictor Norton's detailed and lively accounts in *Mother Clap's Molly House*.

16. A. R. Henderson, *Female Prostitution, 1730–1830*, RHBNC, PhD thesis, 1982. Taken from CLRO 204B GJRM/9 sitting 25–26 July 1780.

17. PRO, Register of all the Prisoners of the Gaol of Newgate from 28 September 1793, HO26/3.

18. See Colin Spencer, *Homosexuality, A History* (London, Fourth Estate, 1995), pp. 186–8.

19. See collection of Tracts in BL (816m19).

20. Stanley D. M. Carpenter, 'The Army', in *Britain in the Hanoverian Age, 1714–1837*, ed. Gerald Newman (London, Garland, 1997), pp. 27–9.

21. Ned Ward, *The London Spy*, ed. Paul Hyland (repr. from 4th edn. of 1709, East Lansing, Colleagues Press, 1993), p. 281.

22. For cases of buggery in the navy, see A. N. Gilbert, 'Buggery and the British Navy, 1700–1861', *Journal of Social History*, vol. X, no. 1 (1978), pp. 71–98; and his 'Conceptions of Homosexuality and Sodomy in Western History', *Journals of Homosexuality*, vol. VI (1980/81), pp. 57–68.

23. *The Proceedings on the King's Commissions of the Peace, Oyer and Terminer, and Gaol Delivery for the City of London; And also the Gaol Delivery for the County of Middlesex, held at Justice-Hall in the Old-Bailey, on Wednesday the 10th, and Thursday the 11th of July [1745]* (London: Printed, and sold by M. Cooper, at the Globe in Paternoster Row, 1745), pp. 186–7. For this and many other interesting cases, see Rictor Norton's website, www.infopt.demon.co.uk.

24. The clipping is glued into p. 8 of *The Midnight Ramble, Or, The Adventures of Two Noble Females, Being a true and impartial account of their late excursion through the streets of London and Westminster* (London, B. Dickson, 1754).

25. Goldsmith, op. cit., p. 34.

26. Gilbert, 'Buggery and the British Navy', op. cit., pp. 71–98.

27. *London Chronicle*, 7–9 June, 1764.

28. Gilbert, 'Buggery and the British Navy', and 'Conceptions of Homosexuality', pp. 57–68.

29. Ashbee, vol. II, p. xxxviii, quoting *Monasticon Anglicanum* (London, William Dugdale, '1718'), p. 181: 1718 is likely to be the original date; the reprint made by Dugdale was at the beginning of the nineteenth century.

30. Vivian Green, *The Madness of Kings. Personal Trauma and the Fate of Nations* (Stroud, Alan Sutton, 1993), p. 246. Harvey, op. cit., also mentions the case.

31. Picard, op. cit., pp. 67, 178.

32. *Select Trials for Murders, Robberies, Rapes, Sodomy, Coining, Frauds . . .* vol II.

33. The poem is taken from *College Sharpen'd: Or, the Head of a House with, A Sting in the Tail* (London, 1739).

34. 'A Faithful Narrative Of The Proceedings In a late Affair between The Rev. Mr John Swinton, and Mr George Baker, Both of *Wadham* College, *OXFORD* wherein the Reasons, that induced Mr Baker to accuse Mr Swinton of sodomitical Practices, and the Terms, upon which he signed the recantation . . . To which is prefix'd a Particular Account of the Proceedings against Robert Thistlethwayte, Late Doctor of Divinity, and Warden of Wadham College, For a Sodomitical Attempt upon Mr W. French, Commoner of the same College' (London, n.p., 1739), p. 4.

35. Ibid., pp. 16–18.

36. *The Trial of Richard Branson for An Attempt to Commit Sodomy on the Body of James Fassett* (London, H. Serjeant and T. Drake, 1760).

37. Ned Ward, *History of the London Clubs*, p. 284.

38. Ibid., p. 288.

39. *A Genuine Narrative of All the Street Robberies Committed since October last, by James Dalton and his Accomplices* (London, 1728). Also on this case, see Norton, *Mother Clap's Molly House.*

40. *Select Trials for Murders . . . Old Bailey from 1724–1732.*

41. Ibid.

42. My thanks to Rictor Norton for this information.

43. Proceedings from the Old Bailey, 11 July 1726.

44. Anon, *The Phoenix of Sodom, or the Vere Street Coterie. Being an Exhibition of the Gambols Practised by ancient Lechers of Sodom and Gomorrah embellished and improved with the Modern Refinements in Sodomitical Practices, by the members of the Vere Street Coterie, of detestable memory* (London, Holloway Printers, 1813), p. 23.

45. Ibid.; KB/28/445/10, 1813.

46. Rochester kidnapped Elizabeth Malet, a wealthy heiress, whom he married in 1667 and proved to be an attentive husband. He subsequently had an affair with the celebrated actress Elizabeth Barry. His works include, *Senior Dildo*, *A Ramble in St James Park* and *The Maimed Debauchee*, and he was to influence Pope. *Poems on Several Occasions*, previously ascribed to Rochester, has, however, been found to include works by Aphra Behn, among other poets. See Ian Ousby, *The Cambridge Guide to English Literature* (Cambridge, Cambridge University Press, 1998).

47. *New Atlantis for The Year 1758*, pp. ii, 44. Not to be confused with Delariviere Manley's *The New Atlantis* (London, 1709).

48. David Foxon, *Libertine Literature in England 1660–1745* (New York, University Books, 1965).

49. Henry Merritt, 'A Biographical Note on John Cleland', *Notes and Queries*, no. 226 (1981), pp. 305–6, quoted in Trumbach, 'Sex, Gender and Sexual Identity in Modern Culture', *Journal of the History of Sexuality*, vol. 2 (1991), no. 2.

50. 'Bumper Allright, Esq.', *The Honest Fellow, Or Reveller's Memorandum-Book* (London, 1790), selling at an expensive 4s 4d.

51. Anon, *A Spy On Mother Midnight, Or The Templar Metamorphos'd, Being A Lying-In Conversation with a Curious Adventure* (London, E. Penn, 1748). Sold for 9d.

52. H. G. Cocks, *Nameless Offences. Homosexual Desire in the Nineteenth Century* (London, I. B. Tauris, 2003), p. 7.

Eight: Tribadism: 'A New Sort of Sin'

1. S. Bladdon, *The Adulteress* (London, 1773), pp. 25–6.

2. G. P. S. Bianchi, *An Historical and Physical Dissertation on the Case of Catherine Vizzani, containing the adventures of a young woman who for eight years poised in the habit of a man . . . with some curious and anatomical remarks on the nature and existence of the hymen . . . On which are added certain needful remarks by the English editor* (London, 1751); *The True History and Adventures of Catherine Vizzani* (London, W. Reeve and C. Sympson, 1755). Price 1s 0d.

3. Alice Domurat Dreger, *Hermaphrodites and the Medical Invention of Sex* (Cambridge, MA, Harvard University Press, 1998).

4. Anon, *Rare Verities. The Cabinet of Venus Unlocked and Her Secrets laid open* (London, P. Brigg, 1657), pp. 12–13.

5. Jeremy Black, *Illustrated History of Britain, 1688–1793* (Manchester, Manchester University Press, 1996), p. 64.

6. James Parsons, *A Mechanical and Critical Enquiry into the Nature of Hermaphrodites* (London, J. Walthoe, 1741).

7. Emma Donoghue, *Passions Between Women: British Lesbian Culture, 1668–1801* (London, Scarlet Press, 1993), p. 6.

8. Anon, *Plain Reasons for the Growth of Sodomy*, p. 11.

9. Katharine C. Balderston (ed.), *Thraliana. The Diary of Mrs Hester Lynch Thrale, 1776–1809* (Oxford, Clarendon Press, 1951), pp. 740, 770, 949.

10. Vern and Bonnie Bullough, *Sin, Sickness and Sanity* (New York, New American Library, 1977).

11. Judith Brown 'Lesbian Sexuality in Renaissance Italy: The Case of Sister Benedetta Carlini, *Signs*, Summer 1984, pp. 751–8.

12. Brigette Eriksson, 'A Lesbian Execution in Germany, 1721. The Trial Records', *Journal of Homosexuality*, vol. 6, no. 1–2 (1980/81), pp. 27–40.

13. Frank McLynn, *Crime and Punishment in the Eighteenth Century* (Oxford, OUP, 1991), p. 130.

14. Bonnie Blackwell has pointed to the significance of the names of both 'Miss Ivythorn' and 'Mrs. Baytree' mentioned in Fielding's *The Female Husband*, connecting them to herbs given as asexual cures for green sickness. This was a malady which afflicted pubescent girls and was seen to be related to sexual abstinence, leaving them pallid and weak. In fact, it was probably an iron deficiency. Bonnie Blackwell, '"An Infallible Nostrum": Female Husbands and Greensick Girls in Eighteenth-Century England' in *Literature and Medicine*, vol. 21, no. 1 (Spring 2002), pp. 56–77.

15. Henry Fielding, *The Female Husband: or the Surprising History of Mrs Mary, alias George Hamilton* (London, M. Cooper, 1746), p. 1.

16. Lillian Faderman, *Surpassing the Love of Men. Romantic Friendship and Love*

Between Women from the Renaissance to the Present (London, Junction Books, 1981).

17. 'Extraordinary Female Affection', *General Evening Post*, 24 July 1790.

18. Journals and letters of Eleanor Butler and Sarah Ponsonby quoted in Elizabeth Mavor, *The Ladies of Llangollen* (Harmondsworth, Penguin, 1973), pp. 28, 36, 74, 95, 98.

19. Anne Lister's diary entry for 29 January 1821. See Helena Whitbread (ed.), '"*I Know My Own Heart*"': *The Diaries of Anne Lister 1791–1840* (New York, New York University Press, 1992).

20. Ibid., Tuesday 5 December 1820.

21. Ibid., Monday 30 June 1817. Anne was eventually to visit Llangollen and meet with Sarah Ponsonby – Eleanor was ill at the time.

22. Ibid., Saturday 13 September 1817.

23. Ibid., 18 November 1819.

24. Ibid., Wednesday 29 April, Sunday 28 June, 18 August, 23 August, 26 August 1818.

25. Ibid., 4, 10, 11 August 1820.

26. The last two reports are cited in Donoghue, op. cit., p. 69.

27. Theo van der Meer, 'Tribades on Trial: Female Same-Sex Offenders in Late Eighteenth-Century Amsterdam', in *Forbidden History*, ed. John C. Fout (Chicago, Chicago University Press, 1992), pp. 189–210.

28. For a fuller investigation, see Julie Peakman, *Mighty Lewd Books: The Development of Pornography in Eighteenth-Century England* (London, Palgrave, 2003). For tribadism in mainstream literature, see Lisa A. Moore, *Dangerous Intimacies. Towards a Sapphic History of the British Novel* (London, Duke University Press, 1997).

29. John Cleland, *Memoirs of a Woman of Pleasure* (London, G. Fenton, 1749), p. 20.

30. *New Atlantis for the Year 1758*, pp. 52–3.

31. Martha Vicinus, '"They Wonder to Which Sex I Belong": The Historical Roots of the Modern Lesbian Identity', in Dennis Altman et al., *Which Homosexuality?* (London, GMP, 1989), pp. 171–98.

Nine: 'Strength to Wear a Dress'

1. Chevalier quoted his mother in his memoirs; see Gary Kates, *Monsieur D'Eon Is a Woman. A Tale of Political Intrigue and Sexual Masquerade* (HarperCollins, 1995), p. 15.

2. The quotes are taken from R. H. F. Scott (ed.), *The Transvestite Memoirs of the*

Abbé De Choisy (London, Peter Owen, 1973). The memoirs were expropriated from De Choisy's executor who had loaned them to a female family member, and then to Abbé Olivet; also on De Choisy, see Vern L Bullough & Bonnie Bullough, *Sin, Sickness and Sanity*, p. 70.

3. Bullough & Bullough, *Sin, Sickness, and Sanity*, pp. 76–83. See Marjorie B. Garber, *Vested Interests. Cross-dressing and Cultural Anxiety* (London, Routledge, 1992).

4. John Dollimore, *Sexual Dissidence. Augustine to Wilde, Freud to Foucault* (Oxford, Clarendon Press, 1991), p. 291; see chapter 'Early Modern: Cross-Dressing in Early Modern England', pp. 284–306.

5. Randolph Trumbach, 'Sodomy Transformed: Aristocratic Libertinage, Public Reputation and the Gender Revolution of the Eighteenth Century, *Journal of Homosexuality*, vol. 19, no. 3 (1990), pp. 105–24.

6. Norton, op. cit., pp. 96–7.

7. De Choisy, *Memoirs*, p. 27.

8. Ibid., p. 80.

9. Ibid., p. 99.

10. Ibid., p. 28.

11. Ibid., p. 29.

12. Ibid., p. 32.

13. Ibid., p. 33.

14. Ibid., p. 36.

15. Ibid., pp. 41–2.

16. Ibid., p. 49.

17. Ibid., p. 50.

18. Dr Robert Baldrick (ed.), Fredéric Gaillardet, *Memoirs of the Chevalier D'Eon* (London, Anthony Blond, 1970), pp. xv–xvi. This book is useful for its introduction by the editor but for little else. They are not, in fact, D'Eon's memoirs and Gaillardet, the author, admitted that a large proportion of the biography was fiction.

19. Kates, op. cit., pp. 37, 183.

20. Gaillardet, *D'Eon Memoirs*, quoted by Kates, op. cit., p. 13.

21. Ibid., p. 18.

22. Ibid., p. 27.

23. For example, Kates believes that D'Eon fabricated the tale but Edna Nixon believed it; *Royal Spy* (London, Heinemann, 1966).

24. Gaillardet, *D'Con Memoirs*, p. 312.

25. Martin Green (ed.), *Further Memoirs of Casanova*, pp. 115–16.

Ten: Women in Breeches

1. George Colman quoted in Kristina Straub, 'The Guilty Pleasures of Female Theatrical Cross-Dressing and the Autobiography of Charlotte Charke', in Julia Epstein and Kristine Straub, *Body Guards: The Politics of Gender Ambiguity* (London, Routledge, 1991), p. 153.

2. John Aston, *Chapbooks of the Eighteenth Century* (1882; repr., London, Skoob Books, n.d.), p. 334.

3. Roger Thomson, *Samuel Pepys' Penny Merriments* (London, Constable, 1976), pp. 50–3.

4. Anon, *The Lives and Adventures of a German Princess, Mary Read, Anne Bonny, Joan Philips* . . . etc. (London, M. Cooper, W. Reeve and C. Sympson, 1755). Price 1s 0d.

5. Nadezhda Durova, *The Cavalry Maiden. Journals of a Female Russian Officer in the Napoleonic Wars* (London, Angel Books, 1988); Julie Wheelwright, *Amazons and Military Maids* (London, Pandora Press, 1989); Suzanne J. Stark, *Female Tars. Women Aboard Ship in the Age of Sail* (London, Constable, 1996), pp. 102–7.

6. Pat Rogers, 'The Breeches Part' in Boucé, op. cit., pp. 244–58.; Lucey, op. cit.

7. Fidelis Morgan, *The Well-Known Trouble-maker: A Life of Charlotte Charke* (London, Faber & Faber, 1988). This is a reprint of Charke's autobiography, *A Narrative of the Life of Charlotte Charke.*

8. Anon, *The Nun in the Cloister or, the Amours, Intrigues and Adventures of the Marchioness of Beauville* (London, W. Dugdale, 1828), p. 56.

9. Rudolph M. Dekker and Lotte C. van de Pol in *The Tradition of Female Transvestism in Early Modern Europe* (Basingstoke, Macmillan, 1989) have argued that most people were ignorant of tribadism, or lesbianism; and that no networks or subculture existed and so women would therefore identify themselves as men when cross-dressing, following the reasoning, 'If I covet a woman, I must be a man'. But these assumptions can be rejected as there are ample examples of the lesbian affairs of cross-dressers rendered public through songs, court cases, pornographic pictures, medical books and endless gossip-relating anecdotes. Apart from those already mentioned in the chapter on tribades, also see Vern L. Bullough, *Cross Dressing, Sex and Gender* (Philadelphia, University of Pennsylvania Press, 1993).

10. Faderman, op. cit.

11. Anon, *Hic Mulier, The Man–Woman Being a Medicine to cure the Coltish Disease of the Staggers in the Masculine-Feminines of our Times* (London, 1620?).

12. *Female Tatler*, no. 37, 28–30 September 1709.

13. *Gentleman's Magazine*, July 1732.

14. Marcus Rediker, 'Liberty Beneath the Jolly Roger. The Lives of Anne Bonny

and Mary Read, Pirates' and Dianne Dugdaw 'Female Sailors Bold' in Margaret S. Creighton and Lisa Norling, *Iron Men, Wooden Women. Gender and Seafaring in the Atlantic World, 1700–1920* (Baltimore, John Hopkins Press, 1996), p. 5.

15. John Gillis, *For Better For Worse: British Marriages, 1600 to the Present* (New York, OUP, 1985), pp. 13–18, 84–99.

16. For the original accounts, see Anon, *A General History of the Pyrates* (London, 1724), Anon, *Lives and Adventures of a German Princess* . . . and Anon, *A History of Lives of the following Notorious Pirates* (London, T. Hughes, 1806). Price 6d. There are some variations in accounts; in one version, Mary's mother had gone with her son to live with her mother-in-law after the death of her husband. When she fell pregnant again, she hurried back to England to hide her state, but the boy died whilst there and Mary's mother was obliged to disguise Mary as the deceased son. The ruse was uncovered when the mother-in-law heard about the intended switch from gossip from a returning ship and she refused to send any more money.

17. Jock Haswell, *The British Army. A Concise History* (London, Thames & Hudson, 1975), pp. 28–9.

18. *Annual Register*, 19 June 1773, p. 111; 5 July 1777, pp. 191–2; 1 September 1815, p. 64; see also Stark, op. cit., pp. 83–4.

19. As with many of these tales, this account was prone to exaggeration; Anon, *The Life and Adventures of Hannah Snell* (London, R. Walker, 1755).

20. Menie Muriel Dowie (ed.), *Women Adventurers* (London, 1893), pp. 97–8.

21. Stark, op. cit., pp. 102–7.

22. Anon, *The Life and Extraordinary Adventures of Susanna Cope. The Female British Soldier* (Banbury, 1810).

Eleven: Pains and Pleasures of the Birch

1. Lawrence Stone, 'Libertine Sexuality in Post-Restoration England: Group Sex and Flagellation among the Middling Sort in Norwich in 1706–7', *Journal of the History of Sexuality*, vol. 2, no. 4 (1992), pp. 511–25.

2. *Brewer's Dictionary of Phrase and Fable.*

3. Stone, *Road to Divorce*, pp. 240–1.

4. Defoe, *Augusta Triumphans*.

5. Ibid., p. 242.

6. Old Bailey February Session, 1792.

7. Anna Clark, 'Humanity or Justice? Wife-beating and the Law in the Eighteenth and Nineteenth Centuries; in Carol Smart (ed.), *Regulating Womanhood. Historical Essays on Marriage, Motherhood and Sexuality* (London, Routledge, 1992), pp. 187–206.

8. Simpson states that this was not a legal precedent but a phrase that merely

reflected the judge's general attitude. A. Simpson, *Biographical Dictionary of Common Law* (London, Butterworth, 1984), p. 88.

9. *Rambler's Magazine*, January 1783, vol. 1. pp. 10–11.

10. *Rambler's Magazine*, January 1783, vol. 1, p. 35.

11. The incident, with its sadistic erotic undertones, scored in the public imagination. Pandering to the broad morbid interest, numerous accounts were published selling for between 6d. and 1s. 6d. See Anon, *An Appeal to Humanity in an Account of the Life and Cruel Actions of Elizabeth Brownrigg* (London, Harrison & Ward, 1767); Anon, *The Whole Proceeding on the King's Commission of the Peace, Oyer and Terminer, and Gaol Delivery for the City of London; Old Bailey* no. VII, pt I (London, J. Wilkins, 1767), pp. 258–76. Elizabeth Brownrigg, *Genuine and Authentic Account of the Life, Trial and Execution of Elizabeth Brownrigg who was executed for the Barbarous Murder of Mary Clifford. Together with the Sufferings of Mary Mitchell and Mary Jones* (London, R. Richards, 1767). There are many more pamphlets on the case in the British Library.

12. Lord Lindsay, *Lives of the Lindsays: or a Memoir of the Houses of Crawford and Blacarres* (London, John Murray, 1849), vol. II, p. 304.

13. 'A Dissertation upon Flogging', *Gentleman's Magazine*, January 1735, vol. I, pp. 17–18.

14. Ibid.

15. Mark Bence-Jones, *The Catholic Families* (London, Constable, 1992), p. 84.

16. Maj.-Gen. Frank M. Richardson, *Mars Without Venus: a Study of Some Homosexual Generals* (London, Blackwood, 1981).

17. Rev. William M. Cooper, *Flagellation and the Flagellants. A History of the Rod* (London, William Reeves, 1870), pp. 430–5.

18. Ibid., p. 419. This nineteenth-century recollection of incidents is frequently fanciful, and not all incidents appear to be from trustworthy sources.

19. Anon, *The Benefit of School Discipline* (London, R. Minors, 1741).

20. *The Times*, 1 January 1785.

21. *The Times*, 2, 3, 4 July 1788.

22. *The Times*, 18 September 1788.

23. Ibid.

24. Charles Coffey, *The Boarding-School; or the Sham Captain. An Opera. As it is Perform'd at the Theatre-Royal in Drury-Lane By His Majesty's Servant* (London, J. Watts, 1732). Coffey (d. 1745) was an Irish dramatist who also wrote the better-known *Devil upon Two Sticks*. He had his plays performed in London theatres but without much success.

25. George Ryley Scott, *The History of Corporal Punishment* (London, Tallis, 1968), pp. 41–2.

26. John Lough, *French Travellers in the Seventeenth Century by British Travellers* (London, Oriel Press, 1985), p. 109.

27. William Fuller, *Mr William Fuller's Trip to Bridewell* (London, n.p., 1703), p. 1. Price 6d.

28. Ward, *London Spy*, p. 110.

29. Trumbach, *Sex and the Gender Revolution. Heterosexuality and the Third Gender in Enlightenment London* (Chicago and London, Chicago University Press, 1998), pp. 192–4.

30. Fielding, op. cit.

31. The Whipping of Female Offenders Abolition Act 1820 prohibited the flogging of female offenders both publicly and privately; Riley Scott, op. cit., p. 45.

32. Ibid., p. 54; J. A. Sharpe, *Judicial Punishment in England* (London, Faber & Faber, 1990), pp. 23–4. See also McLynn, op. cit.

33. Ward, *London Spy*.

34. *London Journal*, 14 May 1726.

35. Henderson, *Female Prostitution*, p. 72.

36. Trumbach, *Sex and the Gender Revolution*, p. 158.

37. Jean-Jacques Rousseau, *Confessions* (repr., London, Everyman, 1931), pp. 10–11.

38. Ibid., p. 11.

39. Cleland, *Woman of Pleasure*, vol. II, pp. 155–6.

40. Julie Peakman, 'Initiation, Defloration and Flagellation: Sexual Propensities in *Memoirs of a Woman of Pleasure*', in Patsy Fowler and Alan Jackson (eds.), *This Launch into the Wide World: Essays on Fanny Hill* (New York, AMS Press, 2003).

41. For an in-depth exploration of the development of eighteenth-century pornography, see Peakman, *Mighty Lewd Books* (London, Palgrave, 2004).

42. 'Theresa Berkeley', *Venus School-Mistress, Or Birchen Sports* ('Reprinted from the edition of 1788, with a Preface by Mary Wilson'; London, *c.*1808–10 repr. *c.*1917). p. x. The date of 1788 is false.

43. Ibid., pp. XIV–XV.

44. A picture of the machine is printed in Ashbee, vol. I (1877).

45. Berkeley, *Venus School-Mistress*, pp. IX–XIII.

46. Ibid., p. XIV. For more on the Society of Arts, see John Brewer, *The Pleasures of the Imagination. English Culture in the Eighteenth Century* (London, HarperCollins, 1997), pp. 229, 232, 274, 290, 296, 514, 596.

47. Iwan Bloch, *Sexual Life in England* (Royston, Oracle, 1996), pp. 207–8.

48. *The Birchen Bouquet* was republished by George Canon in 1826, 1860 and 1881; Ashbee, vol. III, pp. 242–3.

49. Ibid., pp. 1–9.

50. Ibid., pp. 18–19.

51. Ibid., p. 20.

52. Ibid.

53. Ibid., p. 22.

54. Ibid., p. 27.

55. Anon, *The Bagnio Miscellany* (London, 'Printed by John Jones, in the Whitefriars, 1792'; Canon, 1830).

Twelve: 'Unnatural Lewdness'

1. Quoted in E. P. Evans, *The Criminal Prosecution and Capital Punishment of Animals. The Lost History of Europe's Animal Trials* (1906, repr., London, Faber & Faber, 1987), pp. 147–53.

2. Patricia Crawford, 'Sexual Knowledge in England, 1500–1750', in Roy Porter and Mikulás Teich, *Sexual Knowledge and Sexual Science. The History of Attitudes to Sexuality* (Cambridge, Cambridge University Press, 1994), p. 90.

3. See Anon, *Nunnery Tales* (London, *c.*1888).

4. Trumbach (ed.), *Wandering Whore*, pt III, p. 9.

5. Defoe, *Augusta Triumphans*.

6. Liliequist has already made comparisons between trials for bestiality in Sweden and later witch trials; Jonas Liliequist, 'Peasants against Nature: Crossing the Boundaries between Man and Animal in Seventeenth- and Eighteenth-Century Sweden', in John C. Fout (ed.), *Forbidden History. The State, Society and the Regulation of Sexuality in Modern Europe* (Chicago, Chicago University Press, 1990), pp. 57–87.

7. G. Hickes, *Rabillac Redivivus* (London, Henry Hills, 1678). Also see Ashbee, vol. II, pp. 51–61.

8. One inadvertent revelation here is evidence that some sexually active women went 'on top', not always adhering to the standard 'missionary' position.

9. For examples, see H. A. Kelly, 'English Kings and the Fear of Sorcery', in *Mediaeval Studies*, vol. 39, 1977, pp. 206–38; Paul Strohm, *Hochon's Arrow. The Social Imagination of Fourteenth-Century Texts* (Princeton, NJ., Princeton University Press, 1992), particularly ch. 6, 'Treason in the Household', pp. 121–44.

10. Anon, *The Case of John Atherton, Bishop of Waterford in Ireland* (London, Curll, 1710), preface.

11. Straus, Ralph, *The Unspeakable Curll* (London, Chapman & Hall, 1927), p. 211.

12. *Criminal Register for Middlesex*, 1791, HO 26/2.

13. Evans, op. cit., pp. 148–9.

14. William Naphy, *Sex Crimes. From Renaissance to Enlightenment* (Stroud, Tempus, 2002), p. 163.

15. Ibid.

16. Dorelies Kraakman, 'A Critical History of Sexual Knowledge for Girls in French Erotic Fiction, 1750–1840', *Journal of the History of Sexuality*, vol. 4, no. 4 (1994), pp. 517–48.

17. Anon, *New Atlantis for the Year 1758*, pp. 48–50.

18. Quoted from Ashbee, vol. 3, pp. 268–79.

19. John Aubrey, *Brief Lives* (repr., Bury St Edmunds, Boydell Press, 1998), pp. 138–9.

20. Ibid., p. 272.

21. Francis Doherty, *A Study in Eighteenth-Century Advertising Methods: the Anodyne Necklace* (New York, Edwin Mellen Press, 1992), p. 396.

22. Anon [Charles Ancillon], *Eunuchism Display'd* (London, Curll, 1718).

23. Ibid.

24. Patrick Barbier, *The World of the Castrati. The History of an Extraordinary Operatic Phenomenon* (London, Souvenir Press, 1996), pp. 12–13, 142–3, 152.

25. Anon, *Priest Gelded*, p. 18.

26. Anon, *Modern Propensities; Or An Essay On The Art Of Strangling, &C. Illustrated With Several Anecdotes. With Memoirs Of Susannah Hill* (London, J. Dawson, 1791), pp. 8–11.

27. Ibid.

28. Ibid., p. 44.

29. *Bon Ton*, November 1793, p. 242.

30. Anon, *Modern Propensities*, pp. 41–5.

31. Ibid.

32. For other comments on the case, see Peter Wagner, 'The Discourse on Sex – or Sex as Discourse. Eighteenth Century and Paramedical Erotica', in Rousseau and Porter (eds.), op. cit., p. 52; Peter Wagner, 'The Hang-up of Franz Kotzwara and its Relationship to Sexual Quackery in Late Eighteenth Century London', in H. T. Mason (ed.), *Sex and Eighteenth-Century English Culture, Studies on Voltaire and the Eighteenth Century*, vol. CCXXVIII (1984), pp. 47–67; William B. Ober, *Bottoms Up! A Pathologist's Essays on Medicine and Humanities* (London, Alison & Busby, 1987).

33. *Bon Ton*, March 1793, p. 27.

34. *Bon Ton*, April, 1793, p. 27

35. Ibid., pp. 24–5

36. Ibid., p. 50.

37. Roy Porter, *Bodies Politic. Disease, Death and Doctors in Britain, 1650–1900* (London, Reaktion, 2001), p. 48.

38. Middlesex Sessions, February 1792.

39. Tillyard, op. cit., p. 306.

40. John Fyvie, *Wits, Beaux and Beauties of the Georgian Era* (London, John Lane, 1909), pp. 162–4.

41. Ashbee, vol. II, p. 48.

42. Anon, *The Genuine History of Mrs. Sarah Prydden*, pp. 11–15.

43. Johnstone, *Confessions*, p. 87.

44. Blanch (ed.), op. cit., pp. 135, 158.

45. Lyon (ed.), op. cit., pp., 176–7.

46. C. Willet Cunnington and Phillis Cunnington, *Handbook of English Costume in the Eighteenth Century* (London, Faber & Faber, 1957), p. 174.

47. Boswell, *Life of Johnson*, p. 82.

48. Tillyard, op. cit., p. 66.

49. Louise Kaplan, *Female Perversions: The Temptations of Madame Bovary* (London, Penguin, 1991), p. 138.

50. Cleland, *Woman of Pleasure*, p. 138.

51. Lawrence Stone, 'Libertine Sexuality', pp. 551–525.

52. Jessica Warner, *Craze. Gin and Debauchery in an Age of Reason* (New York, Four Walls, Eight Windows, 2002), pp. 56–8, 63.

53. Yet this reference does not in fact refer to masturbation but to *coitus interruptus*; even then, the act itself was not the sin but the fact than Onan was refusing to carryout his duty to his brother's wife in making her pregnant.

54. Roy Porter (ed.), *Cambridge Illustrated History of Medicine* (Cambridge, Cambridge University Press, 1996), p. 62. Thomas W. Laqueur, *Solitary Sex. A Cultural History of Masturbation* (New York, Zone Books, 2003), pp. 95, 168.

55. Patricia Crawford, 'Sexual Knowledge', pp. 82–106.

56. Laqueur, *Solitary Sex*.

57. Quoted in ibid., pp. 182, 255.

58. Rousseau, *Confessions*, pp. 34, 126.

59. Rousseau, *Emile* (1762), p. 106.

60. Vernow A. Rosario, *The Erotic Imagination. French Histories of Perversity* (Oxford, OUP, 1997), p. 185. See ch. 1, 'Onanists: The Public Threat of Phantastical Pollutions', pp. 13–43.

61. Ibid., p. 28.

62. *Memoirs of a Woman of Pleasure*, p. 45.

63. KB 28/347/4 MICHAELMAS Term 1788.

64. Although this came to trial in 1788, Ashbee wrote of a copy of the book dated 1760 (although the dates were frequently false) and a copy in a bookseller's catalogue from the beginning of the nineteenth century. Dugdale reprinted this 1850–60, altering and adding to the text, with numerous engravings, eventually extending it to two volumes. Ashbee, vol. I, pp. 117–18.

65. PRO, KB 28428/22.

The Gender-Sex Debate: A Historiography

1. Lawrence Stone, *The Family, Sex and Marriage in England 1500–1800* (London, Weidenfeld & Nicolson, 1977); Paul-Gabriel Boucé (ed.), *Sexuality in Eighteenth-Century Britain* (Manchester, Manchester University Press, 1982); G. S. Rousseau and Roy Porter (eds.), *Sexual Underworlds of the Enlightenment* (Manchester, Manchester University Press, 1987); T. Laqueur and C. Gallagher (eds.), *The Making of the Modern Body. Sexuality and Society in the Nineteenth Century* (Berkeley, University of California Press, 1987); Robert Purks Maccubbin (ed.), *'Tis Nature's Fault. Unauthorised Sexuality during the Enlightenment* (Cambridge, Cambridge University Press, 1987); John C. Fout (ed.), *Forbidden History. The State, Society and the Regulation of Sexuality in Modern Europe* (Chicago, Chicago University Press, 1990); Roy Porter and Mikulás Teich (eds.), *Sexual Knowledge and Sexual Science. The History of Attitudes to Sexuality* (Cambridge, Cambridge University Press, 1994). More recently Thomas Laqueur, *Making Sex. Body and Gender from the Greeks to Freud* (Cambridge, MA, Harvard University Press, 1992); Michael Mason, *The Making of Victorian Sexuality* (Oxford, Oxford University Press, 1994); Roy Porter and Lesley Hall, *Facts of Life: The Creation of Sexual Knowledge in Britain, 1650–1950* (New Haven, Yale University Press, 1995); Tim Hitchcock, *English Sexualities, 1700–1800* (London, Macmillan, 1997); Franz X. Eder, Lesley A. Hall and Gert Hekma (eds.), *Sexual Cultures in Europe National Histories* (Manchester, Manchester University Press, 1999); Kim M. Phillips and Barry Reay (eds.), *Sexualities in History* (London, Routledge, 2002).

2. Katherine M. Rogers, *Feminism in the Eighteenth Century* (Brighton, Harvester Press, 1982); Leonore Davidoff and Catherine Hall, *Family Fortunes: Men and Women of the English Middle-Class, 1780–1850* (London, Routledge, 2002); Amanda Vickery, 'Golden Age to Separate Spheres? A Review of the Categories and Chronology of English Women's History', *Historical Journal*, vol. 32, no. 2 (1993), pp. 383–414; Anne Laurence, *Women in England 1500–1760. A Social History* (London, Weidenfeld & Nicolson, 1994).

3. Bridget Hill, 'A Study of Change, Continuity or Standing Still', *Women's History Review*, vol. 2, no. 1 (1993), pp. 5–22; Judith Bennett, 'Women's History. A Study

in Continuity and Change', *Women's History Review*, vol. 2, no. 2 (1993).

4. Mary Poovey, 'Feminism and Deconstruction', *Feminist Studies*, vol. 14, no. 1 (1988), pp. 51–63; Joan W. Scott, 'Deconstructing Equality-versus-Difference: Or, the Uses of Poststructuralist Theory for Feminism', *Feminist Studies*, vol. 14, no. 1 (1988), pp. 33–49; Judith Butler, *Gender Trouble, Feminism and the Subversion of Identity* (London, Routledge, 1990); Anna Clark, *The Struggle for the Breeches. Gender and the Making of the British Working Class* (London, Rivers Oram Press, 1995); Anthony Fletcher, *Gender, Sex and Subordination in England, 1500–1800* (New Haven, Yale University Press, 1995); Sommerville, Margaret, *Sex and Subjugation. Attitudes in Early-Modern Society* (London, Edward Arnold, 1995); Robert Shoemaker, *Gender in English Society, 1650–1850. The Emergence of Separate Spheres?* (London, Longman, 1998).

5. See the following for some of the arguments around the history of masculinities: Michael Roper and John Tosh, *Manful Assertions. Masculinities in Britain since 1800* (London, Routledge, 1991); R. W. Connell, *Masculinities* (Cambridge, Polity Press, 1995); John Tosh, *History Workshop Journal*, 40 (1995); Tosh, *Gender and History*, no. 8 (1996); Tosh, 'The Old Adam and the New Man. Emerging Themes in the History of English Masculinities 1750–1850', in Tim Hitchcock and Michèle Cohen (eds.), *English Masculinities, 1660–1800* (London, Longman, 1999); Phillip John Carter, 'Mollies, Fops and Men of Feeling. Aspects of Male Effeminacy and Masculinity in Britain *c.*1700–1780', PhD thesis, Magdalen College, Oxford, 1995; Randolph Trumbach, 'Erotic Fantasy and Male Libertinism in Enlightenment England' in Lynn Hunt, *The Invention of Pornography: Obscenity and the Origins of Modernity* (New York, Zone Books, 1993), pp. 253–82; and Trumbach's chapter on 'Male Libertinism' in his *Sex and the Gender Revolution: Heterosexuality and the Third Gender in Enlightenment London* (Chicago and London, University of Chicago Press, 1998), pp. 69–111; Elizabeth A. Foyster, *Manhood in Early Modern England. Honour, Sex and Marriage* (London, Longman, 1999).

6. For a good introduction to the various debates: D. Altman et al., *Which Homosexuality?* (London, GMP Publishers, 1989) and Edward Stein (ed.), *Forms of Desire. Sexual Orientation and the Social Constructionist Controversy* (London, Routledge, 1992). See also Michel Foucault, *The History of Sexuality*, vol. 1, 1976 (London, Penguin, repr. 1990); Jeffrey Weeks, *Sex, Politics and Society in the Regulation of Sexuality since 1800* (London, Longman, 1989), pp. 96–121.

7. Alan Bray, *Homosexuality in Renaissance England* (New York, Columbia University Press, 1995); Randolph Trumbach, 'Sex, Gender, and Sexual Identity in Modern Culture: Male Sodomy and Female Prostitution in Enlightenment London', *Journal of the History of Sexuality*, vol. 2, no. 2 (1991), pp. 186–203; Trumbach, 'London Sodomites: Homosexual Behaviour and Western Culture in the Eighteenth Century, *Journal of the History of Sexuality* (Spring 1978), pp. 1–33; Trumbach, 'Sodomy Transformed: Aristocratic Libertinage, Public Reputation and the Gender Revolution of the Eighteenth Century', *Journal of*

Homosexuality, vol. 19, no. 3 (1990); Trumbach 'The Birth of the Queen: Sodomy and the Emergence of Gender Equality in Modern Culture 1660–1750', in M. Duberman, M. Vicinus, and G. Chauncey Jnr (eds.), *Hidden from History. Reclaiming the Gay and Lesbian Past* (Penguin, 1991), pp. 129–40; Alan Bray, 'Homosexuality and the Signs of Male Friendship in Elizabethan England', *History Workshop Journal*, 29 (1990), pp. 1–19; Rictor Norton, *Mother Clap's Molly House: The Gay Subculture in England, 1700–1830* (London, GMP, 1992); George E. Haggerty, *Men in Love. Masculinity and Sexuality in the Eighteenth Century* (New York, Columbia University Press, 1999); Katherine O'Donnell and Michael O'Rourke, *Love, Sex, Intimacy and Friendship Between Men, 1550–1800* (Basingstoke, Palgrave, 2003).

8. Adrienne Rich, 'Compulsory Heterosexuality and Lesbian Existence', *Signs: Journal of Women in Culture and Society*, vol. 5, no. 4 (Summer 1980), pp. 631–60; Ann Ferguson, 'Patriarchy, Sexual Identity, and the Sexual Revolution', *Signs*, vol. 7, no. 1 (Autumn 1981), pp. 158–66; Lillian Faderman, *Surpassing the Love of Men. Romantic Friendship and Love Between Women from the Renaissance to the Present* (London, Junction Books, 1981); Judith C. Brown, *Immodest Acts: the Life of a Lesbian Nun in Renaissance Italy* (New York, OUP, 1986). Lynne Friedli, '"Passing Women" – A Study of Gender Boundaries in the Eighteenth Century', in Rousseau and Porter, *Sexual Underworlds*, pp. 234–60.

9. Randolph Trumbach, 'London Sapphists: from Three Sexes to Four Genders in the Making of Modern Culture', in Julia Epstein and Kristina Straub (eds.), *Body Guards: the Cultural Politics of Gender Ambiguity* (London, Routledge, 1991), pp. 112–41; Emma Donoghue, *Passions Between Women: British Lesbian Culture 1668–1801* (London, Scarlet Press, 1993); Valerie Traub, 'The Perversion of Lesbian Desire', *History Workshop*, no. 41 (1996), pp. 23–49; Alison Oram and Ann Marie Turnbull (eds.), *The Lesbian History Sourcebook. Love and Sex between Women in Britain from 1780–1970* (London, Routledge, 2001), pp. 1–2.

10. Sally Newman has identified this problem in her study of lesbianism: 'We face the danger of limiting lesbian identity solely to sexual practices, when we want to insist that it is also about cultural identity'; Sally Newman, 'Silent Witness? Aileen Palmer and the Problem of Evidence in Lesbian History', *Women's History Review*, vol. II, no. 2 (2002).

Bibliography

Primary Sources

'A Faithful Narrative Of The Proceedings In a late Affair between The Rev. Mr John Swinton, and Mr George Baker, Both of *Wadham* College, *OXFORD*' (London, n.p., 1739).

Annals of Newgate (London, 1776).

Anon., *A Commentary on the Licentious Liberty of the Press in which the recent publication, entitled 'Memoirs of Harriette W.' is severely censured* (London, 1825).

Anon., *A Flaming Whip for Lechery: or the Whoremaster's Speculum* (London, Elizabeth Harris, 1700).

Anon., *A General History of the Pyrates* (London, 1724).

Anon., *The Midnight Ramble, Or, The Adventures of Two Noble Females; Being A true and impartial Account of their late excursion through the Streets of London and Westminster* (London, B. Dickson, 1754).

Anon., *A Genuine Narrative of All the Street Robberies Committees since October last, by James Dalton and his Accomplices* (London, 1728).

Anon., *A History of Lives of the following Notorious Pirates* (London, T. Hughes, 1806).

Anon., *An Appeal to Humanity in an Account of the Life and Cruel Actions of Elizabeth Brownrigg* (London, Harrison or Ward, 1767).

Anon., *A New Atlantis for The Year 1758* (2nd edn., London, M. Thrush, 1758).

Anon., *A Spy On Mother Midnight, Or The Templar Metamorphos'd, Being A Lying-In Conversation with a Curious Adventure* (London, E. Penn, 1748).

Anon., 'Bumper Allright, Esq.', *The Honest Fellow, Or Reveller's Memorandum-Book* (London, 1790).

Anon., *Character of a Town-Miss* (London, Rowland Reynolds, 1680).

Anon., *College Sharpen'd: Or, the Head of a House with, A Sting in the Tail* (London, 1739).

Anon., *Harris's List Of Covent Garden Ladies, Or Man Of Pleasure's Kalander For The Year 1788* (London, H. Ranger, 1788).

Anon., *Hic Mulier, The Man–Woman Being a Medicine to cure the Coltish Disease of the Staggers in the Masculine-Feminines of our Times* (London, 1620?).

Anon., *History of Intriguing, From its Original* (London, T. Boreman, 1735).

Anon., *Kick Him Jenny* (London, W. France, 1737).

Anon., *Kitty's Atlantis for the Year 1766* (London, J. Harrison, 1766).

Anon., *Memoirs of the Celebrated Miss Fanny Murray* (London, J. Scott, 1759).

Anon., *The Modern Propensities; Or An Essay On The Art Of Strangling, &C. Illustrated With Several Anecdotes. With Memoirs Of Susannah Hill* (London, J. Dawson, 1791).

Anon., *Nunnery for Coquettes* (London, T. Lowndes, 1771).

Anon., *Nunnery Tales* (London, *c.*1888).

Anon., *Plain Reasons for the Growth of Sodomy* (London, A. Dodd and E. Nutt, 1728).

Anon., *Poems on Several Occasions* (Glasgow, R. & A. Foulis, 1770).

Anon., *The Court Jester, or Lady's and Gentleman's Treasure of Wit, Humour, and Amusement* (London, Britannia Printing Office, J. Roach, n.d.).

Anon., *Proposal For The Erecting A Protestant Nunnery In The City Of Dublin Utterly Rejecting and Renouncing The New Game of Quadrille*, 'By the Ladies' (Dublin, E. Waters, 1726).

Anon., *Prostitutes of Quality; or Adultery à-la-mode. Being Authentic Memoirs of several person of the Highest Quality* (J. Cook & J. Coote, London, 1757).

Anon., *Rare Verities. The Cabinet of Venus Unlocked and Her Secrets laid open* (London, P. Brigg, 1657).

Anon., *Records Of The Most Ancient And Puissant Order Of The Beggar's Benison And Merryland, Anstruther and Supplement To The Historical Portion Of The 'Records Of The Most Ancient And Puissant Order Of The Beggar's Benison And Merryland, Anstruther', Being An Account Of The Proceedings At The Meeting Of The Society, Together With Excerpts, Stories, Bon-Mots, Speeches, And Songs Delivered Thereat* (Anstruther, Leonard Smithers, Printed for Private Distribution, 1892).

Anon., *The Benefit of School Discipline* (London, R. Minors, 1741).

Anon., *The Birchen Bouquet* (London, G. Canon, 1826, 1860, 1881).

Anon., *The Case and Memoirs of the late Rev. Mr James Hackman* (London, G. Kearsly, 1779).

Anon., *The Case Between the Proprietors of Newspapers, and the Coffee-Men of London and Westminster* (London, R. Walker, n.d., c.1750).

Anon., *The, Case of John Atherton, Bishop of Waterford in Ireland, who was convicted of the sin of uncleanliness with a cow and other creatures, for which he was Hang'd at Dublin* (London, Curll, 1710).

Anon., *The Fruitshop* (London, C. Moran, 1765).

Anon., *The History of the Following Notorious Pirates* (London, 1806).

Anon., *The Life, Adventures, Intrigues, and Amours of the Celebrated Jemmy Twitcher* (London, Jonathan Brough, 1770).

Anon., *The Life and Adventures of Hannah Snell* (London, R. Walker, 1755).

Anon., *The Life and Extraordinary Adventures of Susanna Cope. The Female British Soldier* (Banbury, 1810).

Anon., *The Lives and Adventures of a German Princess, Mary Read, Anne Bonny, Joan Philips . . . etc* (London, M. Cooper, W. Reeve and C. Sympson, 1755)

Anon., *The Nun in the Cloister or, the Amours, Intrigues and Adventures of the Marchioness of Beauville* (London, W. Dugdale, 1828).

Anon., *The Phoenix of Sodom, or the Vere Street Coterie* (London, Holloway Printers, 1813).

Anon., *The Priest Gelded: Or, Popery At The Last Gasp Shewing* (London, 1747).

Anon., *Romance of a Night. Or, A Covent-Garden Adventure, The Reverie: Or, A Flight to the Paradise of Fools, Nocturnal Revels; or, A Universal Dream-Book* (London, 1744).

Anon., 'Theresa Berkeley', *Venus School-Mistress, Or Birchen Sports* (London, *c.*1808), repr. *c.*1917.

Anon., *The Tryals of John Rackham and Other Pirates* (London, 1721).

Anon., [Charles Ancillon], *Eunuchism Display'd* (London, Curll, 1718).

Archenholz, M. D., *A Picture of England; Containing a Description of the Laws, Customs and Manners of England* (Dublin, P. Byre, 1790).

Bianchi, G. P. S., *An Historical and Physical Dissertation on the Case of Catherine Vizzani, containing the adventures of a young woman who for eight years poised in the habit of a man . . . with some curious and anatomical remarks on the nature and existence of the hymen . . . On which are added certain needful remarks by the English editor.* (London, 1751); *The True History and Adventures of Catherine Vizzani* (London, W. Reeve and C. Sympson, 1755).

Blackstone, Sir William, *Commentaries on the Laws of England*, 12th edn, 4 vols. (London, 1793–5).

Bladdon, S., *The Adulteress* (London, 1773).

Boswell, James *London Journal*, 1762–1763 (repr., Harmondsworth, Penguin, 1966).

Brownrigg, Elizabeth, *Genuine and Authentic Account of the Life, Trial and Execution of Elizabeth Brownrigg who was executed for the Barbarous Murder of Mary Clifford. Together with the Sufferings of Mary Mitchell and Mary Jones* (London, R. Richards, 1767).

'By A Monk Of The Order Of St. Frances', *Nocturnal Revels, Or, The History Of*

King's-Palace and Other Modern Nunneries (London, M. Goadby, 1779).

'Captain Charles Johnson' [Daniel Defoe?], *A General History of the Pyrates* (London, 1724).

Charke, Charlotte, *A Narrative of the Life of Mrs Charlotte Charke* (London, W. Reeve, 1755).

Chesterfield, Lord, *Letters to His Sons and Others* (1774, repr., London, Everyman, 1984).

Cleland, John, *Memoirs of a Woman of Pleasure* (London, G. Fenton, 1749).

Coffey, Charles, *The Boarding-School: or, the Sham Captain. An Opera. As it is Perform'd at the Theatre-Royal in Drury-Lane, By His Majesty's Servant* (London, J. Watts, 1733).

Curll, Edmund, *Curlicism Display'd: or, an Appeal to the Church. Being just observations upon the books publish'd by Mr Curll.* (London, Curll, 1718).

D.'Archenholz, M., *A Picture of England; Containing a Description of the Laws, Customs and Manners of England* (Dublin, P. Byre, 1790).

Defoe, Daniel, *Augusta Triumphans* (1728).

Franklin, Benjamin, *Old Mistresses Apologue, or Advice to a Young Man on the Choice of a Mistress.*

Fuller, William, *Mr. William Fuller's Trip to Bridewell* (London, n.p., 1703).

Halifax, Lord, *The Lady's New Year Gift: or advice to a Daughter 1688* (London, 1688).

Hickes, G., *Rabillac Redivivus* (London, Henry Hills, 1678).

Johnston, Charles, *Chrysal; or the Adventures of a Guinea* (London 1760).

Johnstone, Julia, *Confessions of Julia Johnstone . . . in contradiction of the fables of Harriette Wilson* (London, Benbow, 1825).

Lyons, Mary (ed.), *The Memoirs of Mrs Leeson, Madam 1727–1797* (Dublin, Lilliput Press, 1995).

'M. Ludovicus' [John Campbell], *A Particular but Melancholy Account of the Great Hardships, Difficulties and Miseries, That Those Unhappy and Much-To-Be Pitied Creatures, The Common Women of the Town, Are Plung'd into at this Juncture* (London, 1752).

Marten, John, *A Treatise of all the degrees and symptoms of the venereal disease* (London, 1704).

More, Hannah, *Works of* (London, 1801).

Pope, Alexander, *The Second Satire of Dr John Donne, Versifyed* (1733).

Scott, Walter, *Journal*, 9 December 1825.

Smollett, Tobias, *The Expedition of Humphry Clinker* (repr., London, Everyman, 1966).

Society for the Suppression of Vice Report, 1825.

Stevenson, John Hall, *Confessions of Sir Francis and Lady Mary his wife* in *Crazy Tales and Fables for Grown Gentlemen* (London, J. Dodsley, 1780).

Stevenson, John Hall, *New Crazy Tales Or Ludicrous Strokes* (Mulberry Hill, Printed at Crazy Castle, 1783).

The Trial of Richard Branson for An Attempt to Commit Sodomy on the Body of James Fassett (London, H. Serjeant and T. Drake, 1760).

Walpole, Horace, *Memoirs of King George III* (London, Colburn, 1847, 4 vols.).

Ward, Ned, *The History of the London Clubs* (London, n.p., 1709).

Ward, Ned, *The London Spy ed. Paul Hyland* (repr. of 4th edn of 1709; East Lansing, Colleagues Press, 1993).

Welch, Saunders, *A Proposal To Render Effectual A Plan To Remove The Nuisance Of Common Prostitutes From The Streets Of This Metropolis* (London, 1758).

Wilkes, John, *An Essay on Woman* (Aberdeen, James Hry, 1788).

Wilson, Harriette, *The Interesting Memoirs and Amorous Adventures of Harriette Wilson* (London, W. Chubb, T. Blacketer, and T. Reed, 1825).

Wilson, Harriette, *The Interesting Memoirs and Amorous Adventures of Harriette Wilson* (London, William Stockdale, 1925, reprinted in Lesley Blanch (ed.), *The Game of Hearts, Harriette Wilson and Her Memoirs* (London, Grypton Books, 1957).

Secondary Sources

Altman, D. et al., *Which Homosexuality?* (London, GMP, 1989).

Ash, Geoffrey, *The Hell-Fire Club. A History of Anti-Morality* (1974; repr., Stroud, Sutton, 2000).

Aston, John, *Chapbooks of the Eighteenth Century* (1882; repr., London, Skoob Books, n.d.).

Aubrey, John, *Brief Lives* (repr., Bury St Edmunds, Boydell Press, 1998).

Balderston (ed.), *Katharine C., Thraliana. The Diary of Mrs Hester Lynch Thrale,* 1776–1809 (Oxford, Clarondon Press, 1951).

Baldrick, Robert (ed.), Fredéric Gaillardet, *The Memoirs of the Chevalier D'Eon* (London, Anthony Blond, 1970).

Barbier, Patrick, *The World of the Castrati. The History of an Extraordinary Operatic Phenomenon* (London, Souvenir Press, 1996).

Bence-Jones, Mark, *The Catholic Families* (London, Constable, 1992).

Bennett, Judith, 'Women's History. A Study in Continuity and Change', *Women's History Review*, vol. 2, no. 2 (1993).

Berry, Helen, 'Rethinking Politeness in Eighteenth-Century England: Moll King's Coffee House and the Significance of Flash Talk', in *Royal Historical Society Transactions*, 2001, pp. 65–81.

Black, Jeremy, *The British Abroad The Grand Tour in the Eighteenth Century* (Stroud, Alan Sutton, 1992).

Black, Jeremy, *Illustrated History of Britain, 1688–1793* (Manchester, Manchester University Press, 1996).

Blackwell, Bonnie, '"An Infallible Nostrum": Female Husbands and Greensick Girls in Eighteenth-Century England', in *Literature and Medicine*, vol. 21, no. 1 (Spring 2002), pp. 56–77.

Blanch, Lesley (ed.), *The Game of Hearts. Harriette Wilson and Her Memoirs* (London, Gryphon Books, 1957).

Bleackley, H., *Life of John Wilkes* (London, John Lane 1917).

Bold, Alan (ed.), *Records of the Most Ancient and Puissant Order of the Beggar's Benison and Merryland, Anstruther* (London, Paul Harris, 1982).

Boswell, James, *Life of Samuel Johnson* (Calcutta, British India Publishing Company, n.d.).

Boucé, Paul-Gabriel (ed.), *Sexuality in Eighteenth-Century Britain* (Manchester: Manchester University Press, 1982), pp. 1–27.

Brady, Frank, and Frederick A. Pottle (eds.), *Boswell on the Grand Tour* (London, Heinemann, 1955).

Bray, Alan, *Homosexuality in Renaissance England* (New York, Columbia University Press, 1995).

Bray, Alan, 'Homosexuality and the Signs of Male Friendship in Elizabethan England', *History Workshop Journal*, 29 (1990), pp. 1–19.

Brewer, John, *The Pleasures of the Imagination. English Culture in the Eighteenth Century* (London, HarperCollins, 1997).

Brewer's Dictionary of Phrase and Fable (London, Cassell, 1957).

Brown, Judith, 'Lesbian Sexuality in Renaissance Italy: The Case of Sister Benedetta Carlini, *Signs* (Summer 1984), pp. 751–8.

Brown, Judith C., *Immodest Acts: the Life of a Lesbian Nun in Renaissance Italy* (New York, Oxford University Press, 1986).

Browne, Alice, *The Eighteenth Century Feminist Mind* (Brighton, Harvester Press, 1987).

Bullough, Vern L., *Cross Dressing, Sex and Gender* (Philadelphia, University of Pennsylvania Press, 1993).

Bullough, Vern L., and Bonnie Bullough, *Sin, Sickness and Sanity* (New York, New American Library, 1977).

Burford, E. J., *Wits, Wenches and Wantons. London's Low Life: Covent Garden in the Eighteenth Century* (London, Robert Hale, 1986).

Carter, Phillip John, 'Mollies, Fops and Men of Feeling. Aspects of Male Effeminacy and Masculinity in Britain *c.*1700–1780', PhD thesis, Magdalen College, Oxford, 1995.

Childs, J. Rives, *Casanova. A New Perspective* (London, Constable, 1989).

Clark, Anna, *Women's Silence, Men's Violence. Sexual Assault in England 1770–1845* (London, Pandora Press, 1987).

Clark, Anna, 'Humanity or Justice? Wife-beating and the Law in the Eighteenth and Nineteenth Centuries', in Carol Smart (ed.), *Regulating Womanhood. Historical Essays on Marriage, Motherhood and Sexuality* (London, Routledge, 1992), pp. 187–206.

Cockburn, H. A, 'An Account of the Friday Club' in *Book of the Old Edinburgh Club* (1910).

H. G. Cocks, *Nameless Offences. Homosexual Desire in the Nineteenth Century* (London, I. B. Tauris, 2003).

Connell, R. W., *Masculinities* (Cambridge, Polity Press, 1995).

Cooper, Rev. William. M., *Flagellation and the Flagellants. A History of the Rod* (London, William Reeves, 1870).

Crawford, Patricia, 'Sexual Knowledge in England, 1500–1750', in Roy Porter and Mikulás Teich (eds.), *Sexual Knowledge and Sexual Science. The History of Attitudes to Sexuality* (Cambridge, Cambridge University Press, 1994).

Creighton, Margaret S., and Lisa Norling, *Iron Men, Wooden Women. Gender and Seafaring in the Atlantic World, 1700–1920* (Baltimore, John Hopkins Press, 1996).

Cunnington, C. Willett and Phillis Cunnington, *Handbook of English Costume in the Eighteenth Century* (London, Faber & Faber, 1957).

Dashwood, Sir Francis, *The Dashwoods of West Wycombe* (London, Aurum Press, 1987).

Dekker, Rudolph M., and Lotte C. van de Pol, *The Tradition of Female Transvestism in Early Modern Europe* (Basingstoke, Macmillan, 1989).

Doherty, Francis, *A Study in Eighteenth-Century Advertising Methods: the Anodyne Necklace* (New York, Edwin Mellen Press, 1992).

Dollimore, John, *Sexual Dissidence. Augustine to Wilde, Freud to Foucault* (Oxford, Clarendon Press, 1991).

Donoghue, Emma, *Passions Between Women: British Lesbian Culture, 1668–1801* (London, Scarlet Press, 1993).

Dowie, Ménie Muriel (ed.), *Women Adventurers* (London, 1893), pp. 97–8.

Dreger, Alice Domurat, *Hermaphrodites and the Medical Invention of Sex* (Cambridge, MA., Harvard University Press, 1998).

Durova, Nadezhda, *The Cavalry Maiden. Journals of a Female Russian Officer in the Napoleonic Wars* (London, Angel Books, 1988).

Epstein, Julia and Kristina Straub (eds.), *Body Guards: the Cultural Politics of Gender Ambiguity* (London, Routledge, 1991).

Eriksson, Brigette, 'A Lesbian Execution in Germany, 1721. The Trial Records', *Journal of Homosexuality*, vol. 6, no. 1–2 (1980/81), pp. 27–40.

Evans, E. P., *The Criminal Prosecution and Capital Punishment of Animals. The Lost History of Europe's Animal Trials* (1906; repr., London, Faber & Faber, 1987).

Faderman, Lillian, *Surpassing the Love of Men. Romantic Friendship and Love Between Women from the Renaissance to the Present* (London, Junction Books, 1981).

Ferguson, Ann, 'Patriarchy, Sexual Identity, and the Sexual Revolution', *Signs*, vol. 7, no. 1 (Autumn 1981), pp. 158–66.

Fielding, Henry, *The Female Husband: or the Surprising History of Mrs Mary, alias Mr George Hamilton* (London, M. Cooper, 1746).

Fletcher, Anthony, *Gender, Sex and Subordination in England, 1500–1800* (New Haven, Yale University Press, 1995).

Ford, Boris (ed.), *Cambridge Cultural History of Britain: Eighteenth Century* (Cambridge, Cambridge University Press, 1992), p. 32.

Foucault, Michel, *The History of Sexuality*, vol. I, 1976 (London, Penguin, repr. 1990).

Fout, John C. (ed.), *Forbidden History. The State, Society and the Regulation of Sexuality in Modern Europe* (Chicago, Chicago University Press, 1993).

Foxon, David, *Libertine Literature in England 1660–1745* (New York, University Books, 1965).

Foyster, Elizabeth A., *Manhood in Early Modern England. Honour, Sex and Marriage* (London, Longman, 1999).

Fryer, Peter, *The Birth Controllers* (London, Secker & Warburg, 1965).

Fuller, Ronald, *Hell-Fire Francis* (London, Chatto & Windus, 1939).

Fyvie, John, *Wits, Beaux, and Beauties of the Georgian* Era (London, John Lane, 1909).

Garber, Marjorie B., *Vested Interests. Cross-dressing and Cultural Anxiety* (London, Routledge, 1992).

Kates, Gary, *Monsieur D'Eon Is a Woman. A Tale of Political Intrigue and Sexual* Masquerade (London, HarperCollins, 1995).

George, M. Dorothy, *London Life in the Eighteenth-Century* (1925; repr. Harmondsworth, Penguin, 1976).

Gilbert, A. N., 'Buggery and the British Navy, 1700–1861', *Journal of Social*

History, vol. X, no. 1 (1978), pp. 71–98.

Gilbert, A. N., 'Conceptions of Homosexuality and Sodomy in Western History', *Journal of Homosexuality*, vol. VI (1980/81), pp. 57–68.

Gillis, John, *For Better For Worse: British Marriages, 1600 to the Present* (New York, OUP, 1985).

Goldsmith, Netta Murray, *The Worst of Crimes: Homosexuality and the Law in Eighteenth-Century London* (Aldershot, Ashgate, 1998).

Gowing, Laura, 'Gender and the Language of Insult in Early Modern London', *History Workshop Journal*, 35 (1993).

Gowing, Laura 'Language, Power and the Law: Women's Slander Litigation in Early Modern London, in Kermode, J. and G. Walker (eds.), *Women, Crime and the Courts in Early Modern England* (London, UCL Press, 1994).

Green, Martin (ed.), *The Further Memoirs of Casanova. Casanova in London* (London, Mayflower, 1969).

Green, Vivian, *The Madness of Kings. Personal Trauma and the Fate of Nations* (Stroud, Alan Sutton, 1993).

Grosley, P. J., *A Tour to London* (London, 1772).

Gross, F., *Guide to Health and Beauty* (London, 1783).

Grundy, Isobel, *Lady Mary Wortley Montagu. Comet of the Enlightenment* (Oxford, OUP, 1999).

Haggerty, George E., *Men in Love. Masculinity in the Eighteenth Century* (New York, Columbia University Press, 1999).

Halsband, Robert (ed.), *The Complete Letters of Lady Wortley Montagu* (Oxford, Clarendon Press, 1965).

Hamilton, Adrian, *The Infamous Essay on Woman, or, John Wilkes seated between Vice and Virtue* (London, André Deutsch, 1972).

Harvey, A. D., 'Prosecutions for Sodomy in England at the Beginning of the Nineteenth Century', *Historical Journal*, 21 (1978), pp. 939–48.

Haswell, Jock, *The British Army. A Concise History* (London, Thames & Hudson, 1975), pp. 28–29.

Henderson, A. R., *Female Prostitution, 1730–1830*, RHBNC, PhD thesis, 1982.

Henderson, Tony, *Disorderly Women in Eighteenth-Century London. Prostitution and Control in the Metropolis, 1730–1830* (London, Longman, 1999), p. 45.

Hickman, Katie, *Courtesans* (London, HarperCollins, 2003).

Hill, Bridget, 'A Study of Change, Continuity or Standing Still', *Women's History Review*, vol. 2, no. 1 (1993), pp. 5–22.

Hitchcock, Tim, *English Sexualities, 1700–1800* (Basingstoke, Macmillan, 1997).

Hitchcock, Tim and Michèle Cohen (eds.), *English Masculinities, 1660–1800* (London, Longman, 1999).

Holcombe, Lee, *Wives and Property: Reform of the Married Woman's Property Law in Nineteenth-Century England* (Oxford, Martin Robertson, 1983).

Innes, Joanna, 'Politics and Morals: the Reformation of Manners Movement in Later Eighteenth-Century England', in Eckhart Hellmuth, ed., *The Transformation of Political Culture: England and Germany in the Late Eighteenth Century* (Oxford, OUP, 1990).

Jenkins, Roy, *Gladstone* (London, Macmillan, 1995), pp. 100–15.

Jones, Vivien (ed.), *Women in the Eighteenth Century* (London, Routledge, 1990).

Kaplan, Louise, *Female Perversions: The Temptations of Madame Bovary* (London, Penguin, 1991).

Kearney, Patrick, *The History of Erotic Literature* (London, Macmillan, 1982), p. 22.

Kelly, H. A., 'English Kings and the Fear of Sorcery', in *Mediaeval Studies*, vol. 39 (1977), pp. 206–38.

Kemp, Betty, *Sir Francis Dashwood: An Eighteenth-Century Independent* (London, Macmillan, 1967).

Kraakman, Dorelies, 'A Critical History of Sexual Knowledge for Girls in French Erotic Fiction, 1750–1840', *Journal of the History of Sexuality*, vol. 4, no. 4, 1994, pp. 517–48.

Laqueur, Thomas W., *Solitary Sex. A Cultural History of Masturbation* (New York, Zone Books, 2003).

Latham, Robert, and William Matthews (ed.), *The Diary of Samuel Pepys* (London, George Bell, 1971).

Laurence, Anne, *Women in England 1500–1760. A Social History* (London, Weidenfeld & Nicolson, 1994).

Legman, G., *The Horn Book: Studies in Erotic Folklore and Bibliography* (London, Jonathan Cape, 1970).

Lindsay, Lord, *Lives of the Lindsays: or a Memoir of the Houses of Crawford and Blacarres* (London, John Murray, 1849).

Lough, John, *French Travellers in the Seventeenth Century by British Travellers* (London, Oriel Press, 1985).

Lucas C. B. (ed.), *Letters of Horace Walpole*, (London, George Newnes, 1904).

Lucey, Janet Camden, *Lovely Peggy. The Life and Times of Margaret Woffington* (London, Hurst & Blackett, 1952).

Lyon, Mary (ed.), *The Memoirs of Mrs Leeson, Madam, 1727–1797* (Dublin, Lilliput Press, 1995).

Maccubbin, R. P. (ed.), *'Tis Nature's Fault. Unauthorized Sexuality During the Enlightenment* (Cambridge, Cambridge University Press, 1987).

McLaren, Angus *Reproductive Rituals. The Perception of Fertility in England from the Sixteenth to the Nineteenth Century* (London, Methuen, 1984).

Mannix, Daniel P., *The Hell-Fire Club* (London, New English Library, 1964).

Martin, Peter, *A Life of James Boswell* (London, Weidenfeld & Nicolson, 1999).

Masters, John, *Casanova* (London, Michael Joseph, 1969).

Mavor, Elizabeth, *The Ladies of Llangollen* (London, Penguin, 1973).

McCormack, Donald, *The Hellfire Club* (Jarrolds, 1958).

McLynn, Frank, *Crime and Punishment in Eighteenth-Century England* (Oxford, OUP, 1991).

Merians, Linda E. (ed.), *The Secret Malady: Venereal Disease in Eighteenth Century Britain and France* (Lexington, University Press of Kentucky, 1996).

Moore, Lisa A., *Dangerous Intimacies. Towards a Sapphic History of the British Novel* (London, Duke University Press, 1997).

Morgan, Fidelis, *The Well-Known Trouble-maker: A Life of Charlotte Charke* (London, Faber or Faber, 1988).

Myer, Valerie Grosvenor, *Harriette Wilson, Lady of Pleasure* (Ely, Fern House, 1999).

Naphy, William, *Sex Crimes. From Renaissance to Enlightenment* (Stroud, Tempus, 2002).

Nash, S., 'Prostitution and Charity: the Magdalene Hospital, a case study', *Journal of Social* History, 17 (1984), p. 624.

Newman, Sally, 'Silent Witness? Aileen Palmer and the Problem of Evidence in Lesbian History', *Women's History Review*, vol. II, no 2 (2002).

Nixon, Edna, *Royal Spy* (London, Heinemann, 1966).

Norton, Rictor, *Mother Clap's Molly House: The Gay Subculture in England, 1700–1830* (London, GMP, 1992).

Ober, William B., *Bottoms Up! A Pathologist's Essays on Medicine and Humanities* (London, Alison or Busby, 1987).

O'Donnell, Katherine, and Michael O'Rourke, *Love, Sex, Intimacy and Friendship Between Men, 1550–1800* (Basingstoke, Palgrave, 2003).

Oram Alison, and Ann Marie Turnbull (eds.), *The Lesbian History Sourcebook. Love and Sex between Women in Britain from 1780–1970* (London, Routledge, 2001).

Ousby, Ian, *The Cambridge Guide to English Literature* (Cambridge, Cambridge University Press, 1998).

Parsons, James, *A Mechanical and Critical Enquiry into the Nature of Hermaphrodites* (London, J. Watthoe, 1741).

Peakman, Julie, *Mighty Lewd Books. The Development of Pornography in Eighteenth-Century England* (London, Palgrave, 2003).

Peakman, Julie, 'Initiation, Defloration and Flagellation: Sexual Propensities in *Memoirs of a Woman of Pleasure*', in Patsy Fowler and Alan Jackson (eds.), *This Launch into the Wide World: Essays on Fanny Hill*, (New York, AMS Press, 2003).

Picard, Lisa, *Dr Johnson's London: Life in London, 1710–1770* (London, Weidenfeld & Nicolson, 2000), p. 200.

Porter, Roy, *English Society in the Eighteenth Century* (Harmondsworth, Penguin, 1982).

Porter, Roy, *English Society in the Eighteenth Century* (London, Penguin, 1990).

Porter, Roy (ed.), *Cambridge Illustrated History of Medicine* (Cambridge, Cambridge University Press, 1996).

Porter, Roy, *A Social History* (London, Penguin, 1996).

Porter, Roy, *Bodies Politic. Disease, Death and Doctors in Britain, 1650–1900* (London, Reaktion, 2001).

Porter, Roy, and Lesley Hall, *Facts of Life: The Creation of Sexual Knowledge in Britain, 1650–1950* (New Haven, Yale University Press, 1995).

Porter, Roy and Dorothy Porter, *In Sickness and in Health: the British Experience, 1650–1850* (London, Fourth Estate, 1988).

Porter, Roy, and Marie-Mulvey Roberts, *Pleasure in the Eighteenth Century* (Basingstoke, Macmillan, 1996).

Postgate, Raymond, *That Devil Wilkes* (1930; rep., London, Dobson, 1956).

Quennell, Peter, *The Profane Virtues. Four Studies of the Eighteenth Century* (1905; repr., CT, Greenwood Press, 1945).

Quennell, Peter (ed.), *Memoirs of William Hickey* (London, Routledge & Kegan Paul 1975).

Rich, Adrienne, 'Compulsory Heterosexuality and Lesbian Existence', *Signs: Journal of Women in Culture and Society*, vol. 5, no. 4 (Summer 1980), pp. 631–60.

Richardson, Maj. Gen. Frank M., *Mars Without Venus: a Study of Some Homosexual Generals* (London, Blackwood, 1981).

Richardson, Joanna, *The Courtesans: The Demi-Monde in Nineteenth-Century France* (London, Weidenfeld & Nicolson, 1967).

Roberts, M. J. D., 'The Society for the Suppression of Vice and its Early Critics, 1802–1812', *Historical Journal*, vol. 26, pp. 159–76.

Rogers, Katherine M., *Feminism in the Eighteenth-Century* (Brighton, Harvester Press, 1982).

Rogers, N. A. M., *The Insatiable Earl. A Life of John Montagu, 4th Earl of Sandwich* (London, W. W. Norton, 1994), pp. 122–3.

Rogers, Pat, 'The Breeches Part', in Paul-Gabriel Boucé, *Sexuality in Eighteenth-century Britain*, (Manchester, Manchester University Press, 1982), pp. 244–58.

Roper, Michael, and John Tosh, *Manful Assertions. Masculinities in Britain since 1800* (London, Routledge, 1991).

Rosario, Vernon A., *The Erotic Imagination. French Histories of Perversity* (Oxford, OUP, 1997).

Rousseau, G. S., and Roy Porter (eds.), *Sexual Underworlds of the Enlightenment* (Mancester, Manchester University Press, 1987).

Rousseau, Jean-Jacques, *Confessions* (repr., London, Everyman, 1931).

Rousseau, Jean-Jacques, *Emile* (1762).

Scott, George Ryley, *The History of Corporal Punishment* (London, Tallis Press, 1968).

Scott, R. H. F. (ed.), *The Transvestite Memoirs of the Abbé De Choisy* (London, Peter Owen, 1973).

Sharpe, J. A., *Judicial Punishment in England* (London, Faber & Faber, 1990).

Simpson, A., *Biographical Dictionary of Common Law* (London, Butterworth, 1984).

Sissman, Adam, *Boswell's Presumptuous Task. Writing the Life of Mr Johnson* (London, Penguin, 2000).

Speck, W., 'The Harlot's Progress in Eighteenth-Century England', *British Eighteenth-Century Studies*, vol. 3 (1980), pp. 127–39.

Spencer, Colin, *Homosexuality, A History* (London, Fourth Estate, 1995).

Stanhope, Philip Henry, *History of England* (London, 1836–54, 7 vols.).

Stark, Suzanne J., *Female Tars. Women Aboard Ship in the Age of Sail* (London, Constable 1996).

Stein, Edward (ed.), *Forms of Desire, Sexual Orientation and the Social Constructionist Controversy* (London, Routledge, 1990).

Stevenson, David, *The Beggar's Benison. Sex Clubs of Enlightenment. Scotland and their Rituals* (East Linton, Tuckwell Press, 2001).

Stone, Lawrence, *The Family, Sex and Marriage in England 1500–1800* (London, Weidenfeld & Nicolson, 1977).

Stone, Lawrence, *Road to Divorce, England 1530–1987* (Oxford, Clarendon Press, 1990).

Stone Lawrence, 'Libertine Sexuality in Post-Restoration England: Group Sex and Flagellation among the Middling Sort in Norwich in 1706–7', *Journal of the History of Sexuality*, vol. 2, no. 4 (1992), pp. 511–25.

Straub, Kristina, 'The Guilty Pleasures of Female Theatrical Cross-Dressing and the Autobiography of Charlotte Charke', in Epstein and Straub (eds), *Body Guards*, 1991).

Straus, Ralph, *The Unspeakable Curll* (London, Chapman & Hall, 1927).

Strohm, Paul, *Hochon's Arrow. The Social Imagination of Fourteenth-Century*

Texts (Princeton, NJ., Princeton University Press, 1992).

Suster, Gerald, *The Hell-fire Friars. Sex, Politics and Religion* (London, Robson, 2000).

Thomas, Keith, 'The Double Standard', *Journal of the History of Ideas*, 20 (1959).

Thomas, Peter D. G., *John Wilkes. A Friend to Liberty* (Oxford, Clarendon Press, 1996), p. 4.

Thompson, E. P., *Customs in Common* (London, Penguin, 1993).

Thompson Grace E., *The Cyprian. The Life of a Covent Garden Lady* (London, Hutchinson, 1932), p. 122.

Thomson, Roger, *Samuel Pepys Penny Merriments* (London, Constable, 1976).

Tillyard, Stella, *Aristocrats* (London, Vintage, 1995).

Tosh, John, *History Workshop Journal, 40 (1995); Tosh, John,* Gender and History, no. 8 (1996).

Towers, Eric, *Dashwood, The Man and the Myth* (Wellingborough, Crucible, 1986).

Traub, Valerie, 'The Perversion of Lesbian Desire', *History Workshop*, no. 41 (1996), pp. 23–49.

Trudgill, Eric, *Madonnas and Magdalens: the Origins and Development of Victorian Sexual Attitudes* (London, Heinemann, 1976).

Trumbach, Randolph, 'London Sodomites: Homosexual Behaviour and Western Culture in the Eighteenth Century', *Journal of the History of Sexuality* (Spring 1978), pp. 1–33.

Trumbach, Rudolph (ed.), Anon., *the Wandering Whore* (London, 1660–3; repr., New York, Garland, 1986).

Trumbach, Randolph, 'Sodomy Transformed: Aristocratic Libertinage, Public Reputation and the Gender Revolution of the Eighteenth Century', *Journal of Homosexuality*, vol. 19, no. 3 (1990), pp. 105–24.

Trumbach, 'Sodomy Transformed: Aristocratic Libertinage, Public Reputation and the Gender Revolution of the Eighteenth Century', *Journal of Homosexuality* vol. 19, no. 3 (1990).

Trumbach, Randolph, 'London Sapphists: from Three Sexes to Four Genders in the Making of Modern Culture,' in Epstein and Straub (eds.), *Body Guards*, pp. 112–41.

Trumbach, Randolph, 'Sex, Gender, and Sexual Identity in Modern Culture: Male Sodomy and Female Prostitution in Enlightenment London', *Journal of the History of Sexuality* vol. 2, no. 2 (1991), pp. 186–203.

Trumbach, Randolph, *Sex and the Gender Revolution. Heterosexuality and the Third Gender in Enlightenment London* (Chicago and London, University of Chicago Press, 1998).

Trumbach, Randolph, 'Erotic Fantasy and Male Libertinism in Enlightenment England', in Hunt, Lynn, *The Invention of Pornography: Obscenity and the Origins of Modernity, 1500–1800* (New York, Zone Books, 1993), pp. 253–82.

Turner, James G., 'The Properties of Libertinism', *Eighteenth-Century Life*, vol. IX (1989).

Van der Meer, Theo, 'Tribades on Trial: Female Same-Sex Offenders in Late Eighteenth-Century Amsterdam', in *Forbidden History*, ed. John C. Fout, pp. 189–210.

Vicinus, Martha, '"They Wonder to Which Sex I Belong": The Historical Roots of the Modern Lesbian Identity', in Dennis Altman et al., *Which Homosexuality?* (London, GMP, 1989), pp. 171–98.

Vickery, Amanda, 'Golden Age to Separate Spheres? A Review of the Categories and Chronology of English Women's History', *Historical Journal*, vol. 32, no. 2 (1993), pp. 383–414.

Wagner, Peter, 'The Hang-up of Franz Kotzwara and its Relationship to Sexual Quackery in Late Eighteenth Century London', in H. T. Mason (ed.), *Sex and Eighteenth-Century English Culture, Studies on Voltaire and the Eighteenth Century*, vol. CCXXVIII, 1984, pp. 47–67.

Wagner, Peter, 'The Discourse on Sex – or Sex as Discourse: Eighteenth-Century Medical Paramedical Erotica', in Rousseau and Porter (eds.), *Sexual Underworlds* pp. 46–68; see pp. 52–3.

Wagner, Peter, *Eros Revived: Erotica of the Enlightenment in England and America* (Secker & Warburg, 1988).

Warner, Jessica, *Craze. Gin and Debauchery in an Age of Reason* (New York, Four Walls, Eight Windows, 2002).

Weeks, Jeffrey, *Sex, Politics and Society in the Regulation of Sexuality since 1800* (London, Longman, 1989).

Wheelwright, Julie, *Amazons and Military Maids* (London, Pandora Press, 1989).

Whitbread, Helena (ed.), '"*I Know My Own Heart*"': *The Diaries of Anne Lister 1791–1840* (New York, New York University Press, 1992).

Wilson, Frances, *The Courtesan's Revenge* (London, Faber or Faber, 2003).

Wrigley, E. A. and R. S. Schofield, *The Population History of England, 1541–1871* (London, Edward Arnold, 1981).

Yoseloff, Thomas, *Laurence Sterne, A Fellow of Infinite Jest* (London, Francis Aldor, 1948).

Bibliographies, Directories and Encyclopaedias

Bibliography of Forbidden Books (New York, Jack Brussel, 1962).

Britain in the Hanoverian Age, 1714–1837. An Encyclopaedia (New York and London, Garland Publishing, 1997).

Fraxi, Pisanus [Henry Spencer Ashbee], *Index Librorum Prohibitorum–Centuria Librorum Absconditorum–Catena Librorum Tacendorum* (London, privately printed, 1877)

Newspapers and Magazines

Bon Ton March 1793.

Bon Ton, April 1793.

Bon Ton, November 1793.

British Magazine, September 1748, vol. 3.

Female Tatler, no. 37, 28–30 September 1709.

General Evening Post, 24 July 1790.

Gentleman's Magazine, January 1735, Vol. I.

Gentleman's Magazine, July 1732.

Gentleman's Magazine 1762.

Gentleman's Magazine 1763 (all).

London Chronicle, 7–9 June 1764.

London Journal, 8 February 1724.

London Journal 7 May 1726.

London Journal, 14 May 1726.

North Briton, no. 1, Saturday 5 June, 1762.

Notes and Queries, 226 (1981)

Rambler's Magazine January 1783, Vol. 1.

Stockdale's Budget, no. III, 27 December 1826.

Times, The, 1 January 1785.

Times, The, 18 September 1788.

Times, The, 2–4 July 1788.

Manuscripts

Dashwood, Sir Francis, Private Papers held at Dashwood Estate, West Wycombe.

MSS 30872, fo. 92–3, BL.

MSS 30891 ff. 2, 9–10, BL.

MSS 38351, St Andrews University Muniments, Robert Maxwell Canach Kanavegh.

MSS 38351, St Andrews University Muniments, *Nos. 2, 3, 4 and 7 minutes of the Wig Club for 13 April 1801, 18 July 1801, 9 January 1802 and 8 April 1805.*

MSS Minutes of the Wig Club 1775–7.

MSS notes of M. R. C. Kavaugh's *Army Book 135 – The Untied Service Club Edinburgh.*

Notes on The Records of the Beggar's Benison Society and Merryland of Anstruther, Fife, 1739–1836' (Anstruther, Printed for Private Circulation, 1892).

Other Printed Material

Collection of Tracts: BL (1690 816 m 19 (44)).

Collection of Tracts: BL (816m19).

Historical Collections Relating to Ranelagh: BL (CUP 401 k8).

Trial Records

Annual Register, 19 June 1773, 5 July 1777, 1 September 1815.

KB 28/347/4 Michaelmas Term 1788.

KB/28/445/10, 1813.

Middlesex Sessions, February 1792.

New Newgate Calendar, London, 1818.

Old Bailey February Session, 1792.

PRO, Criminal Register for Middlesex, 1791, HO26/2.

PRO, KB 28428/22.

PRO, Register of all the Prisoners of the Gaol of Newgate from 28 September 1793, HO26/3.

Proceedings from the Old Bailey, 11 July 1726.

Proceedings on the King's Commissions of the Peace, Oyer and Terminer, and Gaol Delivery for the City of London; And also the Gaol Delivery for the County of Middlesex, held at Justice-Hall in the Old-Bailey, on Wednesday the 10th, and

Thursday the 11th of July [1745], London, M. Cooper, 1745).

Select Trials for Murders, Robberies, Rapes, Sodomy, Coining, Frauds and other offences at the Sessions-House in the Old Bailey from 1724–1732 (London, J. Wilford, 1735)

Trials for Adultery, or the History of Divorces . . . From 1760 to the Present Time (London, S. Bladon, 1779–1780).

Whole Proceeding on the King's Commission of the Peace, Oyer and Terminer, and Gaol Delivery for the City of London; Old Bailey No VII, Part I (London, J. Wilkins, 1767).

Index